The Herbal Remedies & Natural Medicine Bible

15 books in 1

The Bible of Herbal Remedies and Natural Medicine: Unlock nature's healing power with this definitive collection of potions and herbal remedies for optimal vitality and health!

LUNA STEVENSON

Dear reader, thank you so much for delving into 'The Herb Bible.' Your support means the world to me! I hope this book has sparked your interest in the fascinating world of herbs and natural wellness.

Your feedback is valuable, so I invite you to share your experience through a review. As a token of gratitude, you can download the 'Guide to Anti-Inflammatory Herbs' for free.

It's a special gift for you, a way to further explore the benefits of herbs. Thank you again for choosing this book and being a part of this incredible journey into the world of herbs!

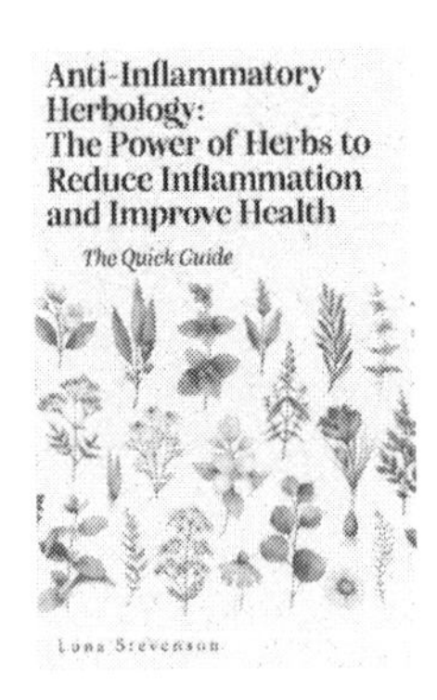

Table of Contents

INTRODUCTION

The natural medicine bible, "Herbal Remedies," welcomes you. In this detailed manual, we'll investigate the alluring field of herbal medicine and learn about the restorative powers of plant life. Humans have used herbal remedies for centuries to improve health, combat disease, and restore emotional and mental equilibrium.

The incredible diversity of plants offered by Mother Nature can aid in many ways, including physical and mental wellness. Teas, tinctures, extracts, essential oils, and poultices are all forms of herbal medicine that can be used to reap the medicinal advantages of plants.

This Natural Medicine Bible is meant to be a reliable resource packed with information about the healing powers of common plants. This book will give you a firm footing from which to explore the world of herbal treatments, whether you are a seasoned herbalist or a curious beginner.

BOOK 1: INTRODUCTION TO HERBAL APOTHECARY

An herbal apothecary is a store that sells and prepares medical herbs, plants, and natural medicines for various health conditions. It is a traditional style of medicine that promotes well-being and addresses various conditions by utilizing the medicinal powers of plants.

Herbal medicine has been practiced for thousands of years and is found in cultures worldwide. It entails extracting active compounds from plants, such as leaves, flowers, stems, roots, and seeds, which are thought to have medicinal benefits on the body.

The herbal apothecary concept is based on the belief that nature offers us a diverse range of plants and herbs that can be used to support and enhance our health. Herbalists and traditional medicine practitioners research and comprehend the qualities of various herbs and their effects on the human body.

An herbal apothecary will have many dried herbs, concoctions, tinctures, teas, salves, and oils. These are frequently created by carefully choosing, harvesting, and processing herbs to maintain their medicinal properties.

An apothecary's herbalists and skilled practitioners work closely with those looking for natural cures. Based on their knowledge and expertise, they examine each person's individual health needs and problems and prescribe or produce custom herbal medicines. The purpose is to promote overall well-being by providing natural alternatives to traditional medicine.

A herbal apothecary often uses Chamomile, lavender, echinacea, ginger, turmeric, ginseng, peppermint, and many other herbs. Each herb has distinct qualities used to treat various health issues such as digestive troubles, sleep disorders, immune system support, stress alleviation, and skin ailments.

While herbal medicine can be beneficial, it is critical to contact experienced specialists and practitioners before utilizing any herbal remedies, particularly if you have pre-existing medical conditions or are taking drugs. They can advise you on the appropriate dosage, potential interactions, and any potential side effects.

An herbal pharmacy, in general, is a site where the ancient expertise of herbal medicine is preserved and shared, offering natural options for maintaining health and well-being.

Chapter 1: Importance Of Having A Herbal Apothecary In The Home

A home herbal apothecary can be useful for enhancing health and well-being and providing many advantages. Here are a few factors emphasizing the value of having a herbal pharmacy:

1. Natural Medicines: For millennia, herbal remedies have been utilized to treat various health issues. You can access a variety of herbal medicines for common conditions, including colds, digestive difficulties, headaches, stress, sleep troubles, and more, by keeping a herbal apothecary at home. Unlike pharmaceutical pharmaceuticals, herbal medicines can offer effective relief with fewer adverse effects.
2. Self-Sufficiency: A well-stocked herbal apothecary gives people and families the power to take charge of their health. You can research natural solutions and self-treat as necessary rather than relying only on over-the-counter drugs or seeing a doctor for minor ailments. Your general well-being can be improved, and your reliance on outside resources can be decreased with this self-sufficiency.
3. Herbal training: Learning about the characteristics, applications, and preparations of various herbs is encouraged by creating a herbal apothecary. Ayurveda, Traditional Chinese Medicine, and Native American medicine are just a few examples of traditional herbal medicine systems that are encouraged to be studied in schools. Due to this information, you are more equipped to investigate holistic wellness methods and make wise decisions about your health.
4. Emergency Preparedness: Having a herbal apothecary can be especially helpful in times of crisis or when there may be restricted access to medical care due to a natural disaster. While you wait for medical attention, you can treat minor injuries or illnesses. In times of emergency, common first-aid herbs and mixtures can help relieve pain, encourage healing, and boost general wellbeing.
5. Cost-Effectiveness: A herbal pharmacy is a cost-effective way to handle minor health issues because herbal medicines are frequently less expensive than pharmaceutical pharmaceuticals. You can save costs over time while still keeping a full and potent natural medicine cabinet by growing your herbs or buying them from dependable vendors.
6. Sustainability: Growing and using herbs at home can help you live more sustainably and leave a smaller environmental footprint. You can choose natural, plant-based substitutes that are less harmful to the environment rather than relying on goods that come in single-use plastic or adding to the

demand for commercially manufactured pharmaceuticals.

7. Mind-Body Connection: By highlighting the holistic aspect of health and emphasizing the interdependence of the mind, body, and spirit, herbal medicine stresses the mind-body connection. Herbs can help cultivate awareness, strengthen your relationship with nature, and improve your general wellbeing. Maintaining your herbal pharmacy can be therapeutic in and of itself.

While there are many health issues for which herbal medicines might be helpful, it's vital to remember that there are times when seeking expert medical guidance is necessary. Speaking with a healthcare professional about any potential interactions between herbal medicines and prescription pharmaceuticals is critical, especially for serious or chronic diseases.

The benefits and possibilities of creating your herbal remedy pantry.

Chapter 2:
List Of The Most Popular And Widely Used Natural Remedies.

Essential Herbs:

- Chamomile
- Calendula
- Lavender
- Echinacea
- Turmeric
- Ginger
- Sage

Chamomile:

The daisy-like flowering plant known as chamomile is prized for its meditative and soothing qualities. It is frequently employed to encourage relaxation, reduce stress, and support sleep. Because of its pleasant, apple-like flavor, chamomile tea is popular and frequently used to ease stomach discomfort and enhance general wellbeing.

Calendula:

Calendula, sometimes called marigold, is a colorful and upbeat herb with many therapeutic benefits. It is frequently applied topically as a cream or ointment to relieve rashes, skin irritations, and minor wounds. Calendula is a great natural cure for skin health because it is said to have anti-inflammatory and antibacterial properties.

Lavender:

An aromatic herb known for its relaxing aroma and relaxation-inducing qualities is lavender. It is frequently applied in aromatherapy to help with stress alleviation and better sleep. The lavender essential oil has been linked to possible advantages for anxiety and mood problems and can be administered topically to ease mild skin irritations.

Echinacea:

A flowering plant, echinacea, is frequently used as an herbal immune system booster. It is frequently used to prevent or shorten the duration of colds and upper respiratory infections since it is thought to have immune-stimulating qualities. There are several ways to get echinacea, including capsules, extracts, and teas.

Turmeric:

The bright yellow spice known as turmeric is frequently used in cooking, especially in Asian and Indian dishes. It contains a substance called curcumin, which is highly effective, anti-inflammatory, and antioxidant. Turmeric has been linked to several health advantages, including lowering inflammation, promoting joint health, and even helping treat long-term illnesses like arthritis.

Ginger:

Ginger is a versatile herb frequently used in cooking and medicine. It is well renowned for its capacity to treat nausea, including motion sickness and morning sickness during pregnancy, and has a distinctive, spicy flavor. Additionally used to treat bloating, gas, and menstruation discomfort, ginger is a natural anti-inflammatory and digestive aid.

Sage:

Sage has a warm, earthy flavor and is a fragrant herb. It has been utilized for ages for both culinary and medicinal purposes. Sage is frequently used as an all-natural treatment for cold, cough, and sore throat symptoms because of its antibacterial and antioxidant characteristics. Additionally, it is used in cooking to flavor a variety of meals.

These vital herbs have historically been utilized for their healing powers and provide a variety of health advantages. A healthcare practitioner should always be consulted before using herbs for any specific medical ailments or if you have any concerns because individual experiences and responses to herbs might vary.

Essential oils:

- Tea tree oil
- Lavender oil
- Peppermint oil
- Eucalyptus oil
- Rosemary oil
- Lemon oil
- Sweet orange oil

Tea Tree Oil:

Australia-native Melaleuca alternifolia tree leaves are used to make tea tree oil. It is frequently found in cosmetics products, shampoos, and household cleansers due to its potent antibacterial qualities. According to some theories, tea tree oil has antibacterial, anti-inflammatory, and antifungal characteristics that effectively treat skin disorders like dandruff, athlete's foot, and acne.

Lavender Oil:

The lavender plant's blooms are used to make lavender oil. One of the most adaptable essential oils, it's known for its calming and soothing properties. Aromatherapy frequently employs lavender oil to encourage relaxation, lessen anxiety and stress, and enhance sleep quality. Additionally, it can be applied topically to accelerate wound healing and calm mild skin irritations.

Peppermint Oil:

The leaves of the peppermint plant, a cross between spearmint and water mint, are used to make peppermint oil. When applied to the skin, it feels cold and refreshing. Because of its energizing scent, peppermint oil is frequently used in aromatherapy to improve attention, increase energy, and treat headaches and migraines. It can also be applied topically to relieve stomach problems and muscle aches.

Eucalyptus Oil:

The eucalyptus tree's leaves are used to make eucalyptus oil. It is frequently used to help the respiratory system and has a powerful, fresh aroma. Eucalyptus oil inhalation might assist in opening up the sinuses and reduce congestion. It is frequently used for colds and respiratory illnesses, such as cough drops, chest rubs, and steam inhalations. Additionally, eucalyptus oil has anti-inflammatory and antibacterial effects.

Rosemary Oil:

The leaves of the rosemary plant are used to make rosemary oil. It is renowned for its energizing and stimulating qualities and has a woodsy, herbal aroma. In aromatherapy, rosemary oil is frequently used to enhance focus, memory, and mental clarity. Additionally, it can be applied topically to improve healthy circulation, encourage hair development, and relieve muscle pain.

Lemon Oil:

Lemon peels are used to make lemon oil. It has a fresh, lemony perfume and is renowned for energizing and reviving. In aromatherapy, lemon oil is frequently used to uplift mood, enhance mental clarity, and lessen stress. As a result of its antibacterial qualities, it can also be used as a natural cleanser.

Sweet Orange Oil:

Orange peel is used to make sweet orange oil. Because of its uplifting and stimulating properties, it is frequently used in aromatherapy. It has a sweet, fruity perfume. It's thought that sweet orange oil has antidepressant and anxiety-reducing qualities. Additionally, it can be applied topically to lessen minor inflammation and enhance skin brightness.

Although essential oils provide some advantages, it's crucial to use them carefully, adhere to the recommended dilution levels, and consider each person's sensitivity. Before using essential oils, it's also a good idea to speak with a healthcare provider, especially if you have any underlying medical issues or are pregnant or nursing.

Tinctures:

- Echinacea tincture
- Valerian tincture
- Tincture of passion flower
- Tincture of hawthorn
- Tincture of dandelion
- Tincture of echinacea and propolis

Tinctures are herbal extracts created by steeping plant material in a solvent, usually alcohol, to draw out the plant's therapeutic components. They are a popular method of ingesting medicinal plants in conventional and alternative medicine.

Echinacea Tincture:

The popular herb echinacea is well known for enhancing the immune system. Alcohol is used to extract the active elements of the Echinacea plant, including echinoids and alkamides, to create tinctures. It is frequently used to boost immunity, improve general health, and lessen cold and flu symptoms.

Valerian Tincture:

Since ancient times, the plant valerian has naturally treated anxiety and sleep disturbances. The valerian root is steeped in alcohol to create valerian tinctures. It is frequently employed as a sedative and sleep aid, promoting relaxation and raising the caliber of sleep.

Tincture of Passionflower:

A blossoming plant called passionflower is renowned for its relaxing and anxiety-reducing properties. Alcohol is used to extract the plant's active ingredients, such as flavonoids and alkaloids, to create the tincture of passionflower. It is frequently used to treat uneasiness, sleeplessness, and anxiety.

Tincture of Hawthorn:

A hawthorn tree or shrub produces tiny berries that have long been used to support cardiovascular health since they are highly antioxidants. Alcohol extracts the therapeutic elements from hawthorn berries, leaves, or blossoms to create the tincture. It is frequently employed to maintain cardiovascular health, enhance circulation, and control blood pressure.

Tincture of Dandelion:

Common weeds like dandelions provide some health advantages. The beneficial elements, including vitamins, minerals, and bitter chemicals, are extracted with alcohol from the dandelion root or leaves to create the tincture. It is frequently used as a digestive tonic, liver detoxifier, and diuretic to promote general liver and kidney function.

Tincture of Echinacea and Propolis:

Echinacea and propolis, two herbal treatments, are combined in this tincture. As was previously noted, the immune system is supported by echinacea, and the bees' resinous product propolis contains antibacterial and anti-inflammatory effects. Alcohol is used to extract the medicinal properties of both herbs to create the tincture. It is frequently used to boost immune response, accelerate wound healing, and ease respiratory infection symptoms.

While tinctures may offer some possible health advantages, it's always wise to speak with a doctor or herbalist before beginning any herbal supplement to ensure it's suitable for your needs and to establish the right dosage. Echinacea and propolis, two herbal treatments, are combined in this tincture. As was previously noted, the immune system is supported by echinacea, and the bees' resinous product propolis contains antibacterial and anti-inflammatory effects. Alcohol is used to extract the medicinal properties of both herbs to create the tincture. It is frequently used to boost immune response, accelerate wound healing, and ease respiratory infection symptoms.

While tinctures may offer some possible health advantages, it's always wise to speak with a doctor or herbalist before beginning any herbal supplement to ensure it's suitable for your needs and to establish the right dosage. Echinacea and propolis, two herbal treatments, are combined in this tincture. As was previously noted, the immune system is supported by echinacea, and the bees' resinous product propolis contains antibacterial and anti-inflammatory effects. Alcohol is used to extract the medicinal properties of both herbs to create the tincture. It is frequently used to boost immune response, accelerate wound healing, and ease respiratory infection symptoms.

While tinctures may offer some possible health advantages, it's always wise to speak with a doctor or herbalist before beginning any herbal supplement to ensure it's suitable for your needs and to establish the right dosage.

Infusions and herbal teas:

- Chamomile
- Peppermint
- Lemon balm
- Fennel
- Mallow
- Elderberry

Because of their calming flavors and potential health advantages, infusions and herbal teas are popular options. Regarding the infusions and herbal teas you suggested, here is some information:

Chamomile:

The well-known herbal tea chamomile is frequently drunk for its relaxing effects. It has a mildly flowery flavor and is created from dried chamomile flowers. Before bed, many people drink chamomile tea to aid in relaxation and sleep.

Peppermint:

The peppermint plant's leaves make peppermint tea with a cooling, minty flavor. It is renowned for its capacity to relieve digestive problems like bloating and indigestion. Additionally calming and effective for reducing headaches and nasal congestion is peppermint tea.

Lemon balm:

The leaves of the lemon balm plant, which have a lemony flavor and aroma, are used to make lemon balm tea. Consuming it frequently can help you unwind, reduce tension, and feel better. Tea made from lemon balm can be consumed before night because it has soothing qualities.

Fennel:

The fennel plant's seeds make fennel tea with a sweet, licorice-like flavor. It is frequently employed to promote healthy digestion, reduce bloating, and ease stomach discomfort. After meals, fennel tea can be consumed to promote a healthy digestive system.

Mallow:

The blooms and leaves of the mallow plant are used to make mallow tea, often called marshmallow tea. It tastes moderate and a little bit sweet. Mallow tea is frequently drunk because of its calming qualities, which may help soothe the throat and digestive system irritability. Additionally, it is thought to have weak anti-inflammatory properties.

Elderberry:

The dried berries of the elderberry plant are used to make elderberry tea. It has a rich, fruity flavor and is frequently consumed in winter. The immune system is thought to be supported by elderberry tea, which may also lessen the intensity and duration of cold and flu symptoms. Additionally, it has plenty of antioxidants.

Stepping herbal teas in hot water for a few minutes is normally advised before filtering and consuming. Although most people find these herbal teas safe, it's always a good idea to talk to a doctor, especially if you have any underlying medical issues or are on any drugs that might interact with the herbs.

Ointments and balms:

- Tiger balm
- Calendula ointment
- Aloe vera lip balm
- Arnica ointment
- Muscle and joint pain balm

Topical preparations like ointments and balms are frequently used for various functions, including pain treatment, calming inflammation, and accelerating healing.

Tiger Balm:

A popular ointment called Tiger Balm has its roots in conventional Chinese medicine. Camphor, menthol, cajuput oil, and clove oil are among the mixture of botanical compounds that it contains. Tiger balm is frequently used to soothe insect bites, treat migraines, ease stress and muscle aches and pains, and provide a cooling effect.

Calendula Ointment:

The calendula flower, often known as marigold, makes calendula ointment. Calendula is frequently used to promote healing of small wounds, burns, and skin irritations because of its anti-inflammatory and calming characteristics. It can also be applied to skin that is dry or chapped.

Aloe Vera Lip Balm:

A moisturizing balm made especially for the lips is aloe vera lip balm. Aloe vera is a popular component for lip care because of its well-known moisturizing and calming qualities. It provides hydration and eases discomfort, preventing dryness, chapping, and cracking of the lips.

Arnica Ointment:

Arnica ointment, which is made from the arnica herb, is frequently used for its capacity to reduce inflammation and relieve pain. It is frequently given topically to muscle discomfort, bruises, sprains, and strains. Arnica ointment is thought to lessen swelling and speed up recovery.

Muscle and Joint Pain Balm:

To treat the pain and discomfort brought on by muscle pains, strains, and joint issues, topical formulations known as "muscle and joint pain balms" were developed. These balms frequently contain menthol, camphor, or capsaicin, which produce a cooling or warming sensation and reduce pain. To deliver specialized alleviation, they are often massaged onto the afflicted area.

These ointments and balms may not be appropriate for everyone, even though they can temporarily alleviate some ailments. It is advised to read the directions, abide by them, and get medical advice if you have any particular medical issues or worries.

Herbal blends:

- Blends for sleep and relaxation
- Blends for digestion and intestinal well-being
- Blends for the immune system
- Blends for respiratory health
- Blends for energy support and vitality

Blends for Sleep and Relaxation:

- The blend of chamomile, lavender, and lemon balm encourages rest and aids with sleep.
- Hops, passionflower, and valerian root are relaxing herbs that improve sleep quality.
- Skullcap, catnip, and chamomile: This combination eases tension and encourages calm.
- Blends for Healthy Digestive and Intestinal Function:
- Combining peppermint, ginger, and fennel promotes digestion and relieves gastrointestinal discomfort and bloating.

- Burdock root, licorice, and dandelion root are all herbs that help the liver function, aid in detoxification, and maintain a healthy digestive system.
- This combination of chamomile, marshmallow root, and slippery elm aids in calming and healing the digestive tract, especially for people with gastritis or irritable bowel syndrome.

Blends for the Immune System:

- Elderberry, astragalus, and echinacea all work to strengthen the immune system and ward off diseases.
- Combining ginseng, reishi, and ashwagandha boosts general immunity and helps the body deal with stress.
- Garlic, oregano, and olive leaf: These herbs maintain a strong immune system and have antimicrobial characteristics.

Blends for Respiratory Health:

- Thyme, eucalyptus, and peppermint: This combination promotes respiratory health and relieves coughs and congestion.
- Mullein, marshmallow root, and licorice are three herbs that help the respiratory system, especially in bronchitis or asthma.
- Black pepper, ginger, and turmeric are anti-inflammatory and can help with respiratory issues.

Blends for Energy Support and Vitality:

- Ginseng, green tea, and gotu kola are three herbs that improve mental clarity, increase vigor, and raise energy.
- This combination of rhodiola rosea, maca root, and ashwagandha promotes adrenal health, increases stamina, and lessens fatigue.
- Guarana, yerba mate, and cacao are all natural energy and focus boosters without the caffeine crash.
- Before introducing any new herbal blends into your routine, remember to speak with a healthcare provider or herbalist, especially if you have existing medical concerns or are using prescription drugs.

Chapter 3:
How Medicinal Plant And Herbs Work

Different chemical compounds found in medicinal plants and herbs can have therapeutic effects on the human body. These substances have the potential to interact with biological systems and processes to encourage recovery, reduce symptoms, and support general health. Here is a broad explanation of how herbs and medicinal plants work:

1. Bioactive substances: Alkaloids, flavonoids, terpenoids, phenolics, and essential oils are only a few examples of the bioactive substances found in medicinal plants and herbs. The therapeutic qualities of the plants are caused by these substances.
2. The active components in medicinal plants have a variety of ways by which they can exert their effects. Typical forms of action include:

- Specific chemicals have the ability to bind to certain receptors in the body, activating or inhibiting particular biological processes. For instance, alkaloids from the opium poppy, such as morphine, link to opioid receptors in the brain to relieve pain.
- Enzymes that regulate numerous biochemical processes in the body can either be inhibited or activated by certain plant chemicals. These substances can have an impact on signaling pathways or metabolic processes by altering enzyme activity.
- Medicinal plants and herbs are abundant sources of antioxidants, which work to combat dangerous free radicals and lessen oxidative stress and inflammation in the body. This antioxidant activity may help promote overall health and prevent disease.
- Effects on inflammation: A number of plants have anti-inflammatory qualities that can help lower inflammation in the body. Flavonoids and polyphenols, which are present in plants, can block inflammatory mediators and enzymes, reducing inflammation-related symptoms.
- Immune system control: Certain plants have the ability to control the immunological system, either by enhancing immune function or by controlling an overzealous immune response. For instance, it is thought that herbs like echinacea can boost immunological function.

3. Pharmacokinetics: After ingestion, the active ingredients in medicinal plants and herbs are transported throughout the body by the bloodstream. Similar to medicinal medications, they might go through several processes like metabolism and excretion. The strength and length of exposure to various substances can affect how effective they are.
4. Effects of synergism: Medicinal plants frequently contain a number of active

ingredients that combine to improve their overall medicinal effects. When compared to single drugs, this synergy can produce a reaction that is more evenly distributed and moderate.

5. Individual variations: It's significant to note that each person will respond differently to therapeutic plants and herbs. The way the body reacts to these substances can be affected by a number of variables, including heredity, general health, and any drugs being taken.

Before utilizing medicinal plants and herbs, it is essential to seek advice from medical professionals or herbal medicine specialists, especially if you have a particular health problem or are taking medication. They can offer you specialized counsel and advise based on your situation.

Chapter 4:
What Not To Miss

Purchasing top-notch ingredients is essential when putting up a herbal apothecary. To make sure you don't overlook the crucial details, consider the following factors:

- Find trustworthy vendors: Look for vendors who are known for offering high-quality herbs and botanicals. Find more about their sourcing processes, such as organic certification, environmentally friendly harvesting methods, and adherence to quality standards.
- Herb potency and freshness: Prioritize using fresh ingredients because dried herbs lose their strength over time. To make sure the herbs are as fresh as possible, check the packaging date or ask about the harvesting and processing procedures.
- Options that are organic and sustainable: To avoid potential pesticide residues, select organic herbs whenever possible. Prioritize vendors who practice sustainable harvesting as well to promote biodiversity and safeguard the environment.
- Ethical sourcing: Look for vendors who value fair trade principles and collaborate with farmers and producers directly. As a result, the farmers are paid fairly, and the ingredients are sourced morally.
- Assurance of quality: It is advantageous to work with suppliers who carry out quality inspections and offer certificates of analysis (COA) for their goods. These records attest to the herb's veracity, purity, and lack of impurities or adulteration.
- Look for well-known herbal brands or companies that have a good reputation in the herbal world while conducting research on trustworthy herbal businesses. They are more likely to produce goods that are of a high caliber.
- Herbs that are in season and locally sourced: Look into growing your own herbs in your garden or finding local sources for them. This gives you complete control over the herbs' quality and freshness while also promoting regional growers.

Proper handling and storage are essential for maintaining the effectiveness of high-quality substances after purchase. To keep track of their freshness, store them in airtight containers, shield them from moisture, light, and heat, and label them with the date of purchase.

Tools and equipment needed for preparing and storing herbal remedies-

To liberate the active compounds contained in herbs, roots, and other plant materials, a mortar and pestle is used. Choose a glass or porcelain mortar and pestle if you want to avoid reactions.

- Herb Grinder: An herb grinder can be used to ground dried herbs rapidly and effectively as an alternative to a mortar and pestle.

- Using a kitchen scale, you may precisely weigh the herbs and other components you use in herbal medicines.
- To measure liquid and powdered substances in precise amounts, measuring spoons and cups are required.
- Glass Jars or Bottles: To shield the herbs from light and air, choose dark-colored glass jars or bottles with airtight covers. Glass in shades of amber or cobalt blue is frequently used for this.
- Identify the plants and medicines on the labels, and be sure to indicate the date of preparation. This makes it easier for you to monitor the potency and freshness of your herbal medicines.
- Cheesecloth or a strainer are used to separate the liquid from the solid plant material in herbal tinctures, decoctions, and infusions.
- The use of a funnel facilitates the spill-free transfer of liquid preparations into bottles or jars.
- Making herbal oils or salves? Use a double boiler or mason jars that can withstand heat for the gentle heat infusion operations.
- Dehydrator or Drying Rack: When drying fresh herbs, a dehydrator or a drying rack with adequate ventilation can aid in removing moisture and halt the development of mold.
- Herb Shears or Scissors: These specialist shears or scissors are useful for swiftly and accurately chopping herbs into tiny bits.
- Gloves and face mask: To prevent allergies or respiratory problems when handling some strong or irritating plants, gloves and a face mask are recommended.
- Storage Jars: In addition to glass jars, you may need other jars to store dried herbs or herbal powders, such as resealable plastic bags or airtight jars.
- Find a cool, dark place to store your herbal treatments because heat, light, and humidity can reduce their effectiveness.

Identifying and selecting essential herbs for your herbal apothecary

- Establish your objectives: Clarify the goal of your herbal apothecary to start. Do you have a preference between culinary and medicinal plants, or both? Decide which particular areas you want to concentrate on, such as increasing culinary creations, curing particular illnesses, or encouraging overall wellness.
- If you're interested in using herbs as medicines, learn about their therapeutic benefits and historical applications. Look for herbs that can help you achieve your objectives, such as those that are known to promote skin health, digestion, stress reduction, or the immune system. Books, trustworthy websites, herbalists, and conventional medical systems like Ayurveda or

Traditional Chinese Medicine are examples of reliable information sources.

- Examine native plants and herbs that thrive in your area by considering the surroundings. Native plants frequently offer special qualities and might be more accessible and sustainable. Growing local herbs in your pharmacy can also strengthen your relationship with the soil and encourage environmental care.
- Start with adaptable herbs: To get the most out of your apothecary, pick plants that can be used in a variety of ways. For instance, herbs like lavender, chamomile, and peppermint are useful complements because they have both culinary and medical uses.
- Personal preferences: Consider your individual tastes. Think about the herbs you like to use or that have an appealing aroma, flavor, or appearance. Herbs that speak to you can help you work more effectively and be more motivated.
- Choose herbs that can help with common health issues that you or your loved ones may be experiencing. For instance, if you frequently have sleep problems, you might want to use herbs like valerian root or passionflower. Similarly, ginger or fennel may be helpful if digestion is a problem.
- Think about safety: When selecting herbs, take into account their safety characteristics. Some herbs could interact with prescription drugs or be harmful if you have a certain disease. Make sure you are informed of any possible hazards, and if you have any questions, speak with a licensed herbalist or healthcare provider.
- Start with a manageable number: Based on your study and objectives, start with a manageable selection of important herbs. Aim for a well-rounded selection that includes a variety of medicinal qualities and uses.
- Remember to grow over time: Creating a herbal apothecary is a continuous process. You can progressively add more herbs that catch your attention or address particular needs to your collection as you gain knowledge and expertise.

Chapter 5:
Preparation Of Herbal Remedies

1. Begin by doing some research on and identifying the plants you plan to utilize in your treatment. Find out about their therapeutic benefits, possible side effects, and suitable dosages. It's crucial to choose herbs that are secure and appropriate for the particular disease you're treating.
2. Collect top-notch herbs: Buy fresh or dried herbs from reliable vendors. Make sure the herbs are pesticide- and contaminant-free and organic. If you're picking your own herbs, be sure you can correctly identify them and gather them at the appropriate time.
3. Select an extraction technique: The medicinal properties of herbs can be extracted using a variety of techniques. The most popular techniques include:

- For delicate plant parts like leaves and blossoms, use infusion. The herbs should be covered with boiling water and steeped for 10 to 20 minutes. After straining, sip the drink.
- b. Decoction: This method works well with harder plant components like seeds, roots, or bark. Herbs should be infused in water for 20 to 30 minutes, strained, and then used as a drink.
- Using alcohol, such as vodka or brandy, to extract the therapeutic components, a tincture is created. Put the herbs in a glass jar, pour the alcohol over them, and let the concoction sit for a few weeks while occasionally stirring it. In a bottle made of dark glass, keep the tincture after straining.
- d. Oil infusion: Useful for plants that have components that are oil soluble. Put the herbs in a jar and pour a carrier oil, like coconut or olive oil, over them. Shake the mixture occasionally as it sits for several weeks in a warm location. The oil should be strained and kept in a bottle made of dark glass.

4. Useful dosage and usage: Find out the right dosage for the herbs you've picked and the disease you're trying to treat. To ensure safety and effectiveness, it's imperative to adhere to suggested criteria. Remember that herbal remedies and pharmaceuticals can interact, so if you have any questions or are on medication, go to a healthcare provider.

5. Storage and shelf life: To preserve the strength of your herbal treatments, store them correctly. Away from heat, moisture, and bright light, store them in airtight containers. Indicate the herb(s), extraction technique, and preparation date for each preparation. The shelf lives of various herbal treatments vary, so make sure to verify the suggested time frame for each individual remedy.

Chapter 6: Variety Of Modalities Of Use

Oral administration

The term "oral administration" describes a method of drug or substance delivery in which the substance is ingested and swallowed. One of the most popular and practical ways to take prescription drugs, dietary supplements, or herbal medicines is through this manner.

Here are some common forms of oral administration:

- ✓ Infusions: To extract the active ingredients from plant material (such as herbs), infusions entail steeping the material in hot water. After that, the resulting liquid is taken orally. Herbal teas like chamomile or mint tea are two examples.
- ✓ Decoctions: Like infusions, decoctions are made by boiling plant material—such as roots, bark, or seeds—in water to draw out the active ingredients. Orally ingesting the strained liquid. For herbal treatments, decoctions are frequently used in traditional Chinese medicine.
- ✓ Tablets and capsules: Tablets and capsules are solid dosage forms that each have a pre-measured amount of the active ingredient. They are ingested whole, and once in the digestive tract, they dissolve or break down, releasing the drug or supplement for absorption. Tablets are crushed powders, whereas capsules typically include gelatin-based shells with liquid or powdered contents.
- ✓ Tablets are comparable to pills, but pills are normally smaller and sometimes shaped differently. They are ingested whole and include a pre-measured dose of drug or supplement.
- ✓ Some prescription drugs and dietary supplements are available as powders. Before consumption, they can be blended with water or other beverages. Powders are frequently used to rehydrate medicines or nutritional supplements.
- ✓ Suspension: A liquid mixture that has insoluble particles scattered throughout it is called a suspension. To ensure that the particles are distributed evenly, they must be shaken prior to delivery. Certain medications may be administered as suspensions, particularly for kids or those who have trouble swallowing pills or capsules.
- ✓ Syrups: To make them more palatable, syrups, which are thick, viscous liquids, are sweetened with sugar or a sugar substitute. For pediatric drugs or cough syrups, they are frequently utilized.
- ✓ The effectiveness and safety of herbal teas, infusions, and decoctions—which are often used oral administration methods for herbal remedies—can vary. Before utilizing herbal preparations for therapeutic purposes, it is essential to seek advice from a medical practitioner or a certified herbalist to guarantee adequate dosage, avoid potential

interactions, and determine their suitability for a given situation.

Topical use

Topical use is when different substances are applied directly to the surface of the body, typically for therapeutic, cosmetic, or medicinal purposes. This can be applied to creams, lotions, gels, ointments, balms, oils, cataplasms (poultices), and other like goods. To deliver targeted effects, topical formulations are intended to be applied to the skin, mucous membranes, or exterior body parts.

Here are some commonly used topical products and their purposes:

- ✓ Ointments: Ointments are often manufactured with an oil or petroleum jelly base and are semi-solid treatments. They are used to provide drugs to the skin and are frequently successful in treating minor cuts, burns, dry skin, eczema, and psoriasis.
- ✓ The calming substances beeswax, shea butter, or essential oils are frequently included in balms, which are comparable to ointments in texture. Like lip balms or muscle balms for aching muscles, they are frequently used for hydrating and calming purposes.
- ✓ Oils: A variety of oils, including carrier and essential oils, can be used topically for aromatherapy, massage, and skincare. While carrier oils dilute the essential oils and assist in delivering them to the skin, essential oils are concentrated plant extracts known for their medicinal powers.
- ✓ Poultices, also referred to as cataplasms, are a sort of moist preparation created by combining herbs, clays, or other substances with water or other liquids. In order to have local therapeutic benefits on the skin, such as lowering inflammation, drawing out toxins, or calming irritations, they are applied to the skin.
- ✓ Creams and lotions are water-based or oil-in-water emulsions that can be applied to the skin more easily. They are frequently employed to hydrate, moisturize, or administer drugs to the skin. Lotions have a lighter consistency than creams, which are thicker and more emollient.
- ✓ Gels: Because of their calming or cooling effects, gels, which have a consistency similar to jelly, are frequently utilized. They may include active components for pain management, such as topical NSAIDs (nonsteroidal anti-inflammatory medications) for joint pain or aloe vera gel for sunburns.
- ✓ It's crucial to adhere to the instructions included with each product and seek medical advice if you have any particular conditions or worries. The right topical product must be chosen depending on your demands because different topical medications have varied functions.

Inhalation

Substances can be inhaled into the body and absorbed via the respiratory system. Essential oils, aromatherapy mixtures, and vapors are just a few examples of what can be inhaled for either therapeutic or recreational purposes. Methods of inhaling are discussed below.

Essential oils have potent aromatic characteristics and can be inhaled through inhalation. Essential oils can be inhaled in a variety of ways:

You can inhale the aroma of an essential oil by placing a few drops on a tissue or in your palms and sniffing. Inhale deeply while holding your hands over your nose. This is a straightforward and useful strategy.

- ✓ Essential oils can also be inhaled by diffusion into the air using a device called a diffuser. This allows the scent to permeate the entire room.
- ✓ c. Steam inhalation: add a few drops of essential oil to a bowl of hot water and inhale the vapors. Put a towel over your face, close your eyes, and inhale the steam. Congestion of the sinuses or the airways is often treated with this method.

Inhalation aromatherapy: Aromatherapy uses essential oils to support both physical and mental well-being. Since the aroma of essential oils can have a direct impact on mood and emotions, inhalation is a prominent technique in aromatherapy. It can be used to unwind, relieve stress, or improve mood. Diffusers or steam inhalation are two of the previously stated techniques for inhalation.

Inhaling smoke or fumes produced by burning materials is the process of fumigation. Herbs, resins, or incense are traditionally burned, and the smoke is inhaled for therapeutic or spiritual reasons. Examples include burning incense or participating in sage smudging rituals.

While certain compounds, such as essential oils, can have potential benefits when inhaled, it's crucial to utilize them responsibly and sparingly. Before utilizing inhalation techniques frequently, it is advised to conduct a patch test or get advice from a licensed aromatherapist or healthcare provider. Some persons may have sensitivities or allergies to particular oils or fumes.

Chapter 7:
How medicinal plants and herbs work

Active ingredients and chemical compounds found in medicinal plants and herbs

- ✓ Nitrogen-containing substances called alkaloids have strong pharmacological effects. They are frequently present in plants including belladonna, quinine-containing cinchona, and the opium poppy (atropine).
- ✓ Terpenoids are a broad class of substances generated from isoprene units. They consist of essential oils and are crucial to the flavor, smell, and healing abilities of plants. Menthol from mint, limonene from citrus fruits, and artemisinin from Artemisia annua are a few examples (sweet wormwood).
- ✓ Phenolic Compounds: Phenolic compounds include a sizable class of substances with anti-inflammatory and antioxidant effects. They consist of phenolic acids, tannins, and flavonoids like quercetin and catechins (e.g., salicylic acid). Many fruits, vegetables, and herbs, such green tea (epigallocatechin gallate) and turmeric, contain phenolic chemicals (curcumin).
- ✓ Glycosides are substances made up of a glycone, a sugar molecule, and a non-sugar molecule (aglycone). They are abundant in medicinal plants and frequently have healing benefits. Examples include saponins, anthraquinone glycosides, and cardiac glycosides (such as digoxin from Digitalis purpurea and aloe emodin from Aloe vera) (e.g., ginsenosides from Panax ginseng).
- ✓ Essential Oils: Many fragrant plants contain volatile chemicals called essential oils. They endow plants with their distinctive flavor and smell. Lavender oil, eucalyptus oil, and tea tree oil are a few of the often used essential oils in aromatherapy and herbal medicine.
- ✓ Allicin: An ingredient in garlic that contains sulfur is called allicin (Allium sativum). It has antibacterial, antioxidant, and heart health advantages.
- ✓ The substances present in turmeric that are active are known as curcuminoids (Curcuma longa). The most well-known curcuminoid, curcumin, is renowned for its antioxidant and anti-inflammatory qualities.
- ✓ Cannabinoids: Cannabinoids are substances that cannabis plants contain (Cannabis sativa). The most well-known cannabinoids are cannabidiol (CBD) and delta-9-tetrahydrocannabinol (THC) (CBD). They have a variety of therapeutic effects, such as the ability to reduce pain and reduce anxiety.
- ✓ The active elements in ginseng are known as ginsenosides (Panax ginseng). They are thought to have immune-modulating and adaptogenic qualities.

✓ Resveratrol is a polyphenol that can be found in peanuts, berries, and grapes. It has been investigated for its possible cardiovascular benefits and possesses anti-inflammatory and antioxidant effects.

Role of medicinal plants and herbs as a source of natural medicines and therapeutic alternatives

- Traditional Medicine: Ayurveda, Traditional Chinese Medicine, and indigenous medicine are just a few examples of traditional treatment systems that mainly rely on medicinal plants and herbs. These systems have a long history of treating a variety of illnesses with natural treatments derived from plants.
- Active Pharmaceutical Ingredients (APIs): The discovery and development of novel pharmaceuticals rely heavily on the use of medicinal plants. The discovery of prospective APIs can result from the isolation and purification of bioactive chemicals from plants. Many pharmacological medications used today are either derived from plant components or were inspired by the chemical makeup of plants.
- Treatment of Common Illnesses: Common illnesses including cough, cold, digestive difficulties, skin conditions, and pain alleviation are frequently treated with medicinal plants and herbs. Examples are chamomile for relaxation and sleep, aloe vera for skin issues, and ginger for nausea.
- Complementary and Alternative Medicine (CAM): Many complementary and alternative medicine procedures make use of medicinal plants and herbs. For people looking for non-pharmaceutical ways to manage their health concerns, they provide natural options.
- Nutraceuticals and dietary supplements: The creation of nutraceuticals and dietary supplements frequently involves the use of medicinal plants and herbs. These items are designed to offer particular health advantages, such enhancing immunity, enhancing digestion, or increasing general wellbeing.
- Antibacterial Characteristics: Many medicinal plants have antimicrobial properties, which makes them useful for creating all-natural antibiotic alternatives. Certain plants have demonstrated effectiveness against bacteria, viruses, fungus, and parasites, making them potential anti-infective agents.
- Several plants and herbs are abundant in antioxidants and have anti-inflammatory qualities. These characteristics make them advantageous in lowering oxidative stress, inflammation, and associated illnesses like cardiovascular diseases, rheumatoid arthritis, and some malignancies.

- Palliative Care: Patients with chronic illnesses receive symptom relief and improved quality of life thanks to the frequent use of medicinal plants and herbs in palliative care. They can support the management of various symptoms of chronic illnesses, such as fatigue, nausea, and pain.

Chemical compounds and active ingredients in medicinal plants and herbs

1. Flavonoids are a large and varied class of plant pigments that have been shown to have beneficial effects as antioxidants and inflammation fighters. Fruits, veggies, and herbs all contain them. Onions, apples, and citrus fruits all contain the flavonoid quercetin, while chamomile and parsley are good sources of apigenin and catechins (found in green tea).
2. The alkaloids are a class of nitrogen-containing chemicals with well-documented medicinal uses. They can have profound consequences on human physiology. Morphine (from opium poppies), caffeine (from coffee and tea), and nicotine are all examples of alkaloids (found in tobacco).
3. Many plant scents and fragrances can be traced back to a group of chemicals called terpenes. Essential oils include these compounds, which have a variety of medical uses including anti-inflammatory and antibacterial actions. Terpenes include, but are not limited to, menthol (from mint), limonene (from citrus fruits), and camphor (found in camphor laurel).
4. Polyphenols are a large and varied family of chemicals that have been shown to have antioxidant effects. They're common in edible plants like berries, greens, and herbs, and research has linked them to a variety of health advantages. Resveratrol, which is found in grapes and red wine, curcumin, which is found in turmeric, and epigallocatechin gallate (EGCG) are all examples of polyphenols (found in green tea).
5. Compounds called glycosides have another functional group linked to a sugar molecule. They are usually to blame for a plant's therapeutic qualities. Plants like foxglove, which contain cardiac glycosides like digoxin, are used to treat heart disorders.
6. Polyphenols like phenolic acids have antioxidant and anti-inflammatory properties. Fruits, vegetables, and whole grains aren't the only plant-based foods that contain them, though. Caffeic acid (which is found in coffee and fruits), rosmarinic acid (which is found in rosemary and sage), and ferulic acid are all examples of phenolic acids (found in wheat bran and rice bran).

The Functions and therapeutic properties of chemical compounds

1. To alleviate pain without inducing sedation, analgesics are employed. Among these are acetaminophen,

morphine, and the opioid aspirin. They're effective because they block the nervous system's ability to process pain.

2. In order to combat bacterial infections, doctors turn to antibiotics. Penicillin, tetracycline, and erythromycin are just a few examples of antibiotics that can stop the spread of germs or even kill them outright. They work by inhibiting a particular bacterial process, such cell wall formation or protein synthesis, for example.
3. Depression and other mood disorders can be treated with antidepressants. Antidepressants like Prozac and Zoloft, known collectively as SSRIs, work by elevating brain serotonin levels to normalize emotional responses.
4. The effects of histamine, a substance generated in the body during an allergic reaction, can be mitigated using antihistamines. Itching, sneezing, and a runny nose are just some of the allergy symptoms they treat. Diphenhydramine and loratadine are two common antihistamines.
5. Antioxidants are chemicals that assist prevent oxidative stress and damage to cells produced by free radicals. Vitamins C and E, as well as beta-carotene, are all examples of antioxidants. Many illnesses, including cancer and heart disease, may benefit from them.
6. Heartburn and indigestion can be alleviated with the help of antacids, which are substances that work by neutralizing the acid produced by the stomach. Calcium carbonate and aluminum hydroxide are two of the more common types of antacids.
7. Diuretics are substances that stimulate the production of urine, which in turn aids in the elimination of excess fluid from the body. Conditions like excessive blood pressure, swelling, and heart failure are treated with them. Furosemide and hydrochlorothiazide are a couple of the most well-known diuretics.
8. Anti-inflammatory, immunosuppressive, and hormone-replacing capabilities are just a few of the many therapeutic applications for steroids. Examples are the anti-inflammatory effects of prednisone and the muscle-building effects of anabolic steroids.
9. The use of antipyretics to bring down a high temperature. Acetaminophen and ibuprofen are two of the most often used antipyretics. They are effective because they bring down the increased body temperature that results from a fever.
10. Anticoagulants are medications used to treat or prevent blood clots, such as those that cause a pulmonary embolism, a stroke, or deep vein thrombosis. Warfarin and heparin are two common types of anticoagulants.

Mechanisms of action of medicinal plants and herbs and how they interact with the human body.

Herbal remedies have been utilized for millennia as a means of combating illness and bolstering wellness. They're loaded with different bioactive substances that have different effects on the human body. Some of the most frequent ways in which herbs and plants used for medicine affect the human body are described below.

- Inflammation can be reduced thanks to the anti-inflammatory effect of numerous plants and herbs. Ginger, turmeric, and aloe vera are just a few examples. Inflammatory enzymes and molecule formation are both slowed by the chemicals found in these plants.
- Free radicals, which can produce oxidative stress, have been linked to cell damage and a number of diseases. Green tea, grapes, and berries are just a few examples of the many fruits and vegetables that contain antioxidants that can quench free radicals and prevent cellular harm.
- Plants and herbs with antibacterial activities are useful in the fight against bacteria, viruses, fungus, and other microorganisms. Natural antimicrobial chemicals, such those found in garlic and oregano, can prevent germs from multiplying.
- The ability to alleviate pain is just one of the many ways in which some plants and herbs can be classified as analgesics. Aspirin's main constituent, salicylic acid, is structurally related to salicin, which is found in willow bark.
- The body's ability to adapt to stressful situations and thrive is called an adaptogen's effect. Adaptogenic herbs like ginseng, ashwagandha, and rhodiola have been shown to increase the body's resistance to both mental and physical stress.
- Several plants and herbs have the ability to stimulate or depress the immune system, respectively. For instance, echinacea has been shown to strengthen the immune system and shorten the duration of cold and flu symptoms.
- Plants and herbs including garlic, hawthorn berry, and ginkgo biloba have long been recognized for their beneficial impact on cardiovascular health. They have the potential to reduce the risk of cardiovascular disease, increase blood flow, and lower blood pressure.
- Plants and herbs can regulate hormone levels and balance because they contain components that act on the body's endocrine system. Black cohosh, for instance, has been studied for its possible role in hormone regulation during menopause.
- Plants and herbs have long been used to aid digestion and reduce the discomfort of gastrointestinal problems. Symptoms of gas, indigestion, and nausea can be alleviated with the use of peppermint, chamomile, and ginger.
- It's crucial to keep in mind that the effects of medicinal plants and herbs can differ depending on the type of plant used, the method of preparation, the

amount taken, and the person taking it. While they may be helpful, people with preexisting problems or who are taking drugs should talk to their doctors before using them.

The effects of plants and medicinal herbs on immune system balance, inflammation, stress, etc.

The immune system, inflammation, stress, and other health issues may all be affected by plants and medicinal herbs, which have been utilized for ages in traditional medicine systems. Several plants and herbs have demonstrated potential results in scientific studies, albeit not all claims have been verified. This is not medical advise, and you should always check with your doctor before trying anything new, including herbal therapies.

1. Some plants and herbs may be able to aid in immune system regulation due to their alleged immune-modulating capabilities. Herbs and mushrooms like reishi, echinacea, ginseng, and astragalus are all good examples. It is believed that these compounds can improve immune function and could be employed to boost immunity.
2. Many diseases are linked to inflammation, especially when it persists over time. The anti-inflammatory effects of certain plants and herbs may be useful in alleviating inflammation. Commonly explored for their possible anti-inflammatory benefits are turmeric, ginger, Boswellia, and green tea. The body's ability to generate inflammatory chemicals may be hampered by these compounds.
3. Anxiety and stress: Adaptogenic herbs are thought to aid the body in dealing with stress and restoring equilibrium. The hypothalamic-pituitary-adrenal (HPA) axis is just one part of the stress response system that may be influenced by them. Commonly used adaptogens include licorice root, ashwagandha, rhodiola rosea, and holy basil. These herbs have the potential to aid with stress management, sleep, and overall mental health.
4. Antioxidant activity: Many plants and herbs are high in antioxidants, which neutralize free radicals and prevent cell damage. Blueberries, cranberries, green tea, chocolate, and spices like cinnamon and turmeric are all examples of foods high in antioxidants. Antioxidants may improve health and lower the risk of developing chronic diseases.
5. A healthy microbiome is associated with good gut health, and certain plants and herbs can have a beneficial effect on both. For instance, a varied gut flora is crucial for a healthy immune system, and probiotic-rich foods like yogurt and fermented vegetables can help foster this diversity. Peppermint, chamomile, and ginger are just few of the plants that may help calm an upset stomach.

Despite the promising results shown with the use of these plants and herbs, it is important to keep in mind that results will vary from person to person and that further study is required to completely understand their mechanisms of action and effectiveness. It is also important to check with a medical expert before adopting any new herbs into your routine because some of them may interfere with drugs or have side effects.

Synergy between compounds found in medicinal plants and herbs and how combination of compounds can increase efficacy

Synergy occurs when two or more active ingredients in a medicinal plant or herb work together to produce a greater therapeutic impact than either ingredient could produce alone. The term "synergistic effect" has become popular to describe this phenomena.

Alkaloids, flavonoids, terpenoids, phenolic compounds, and a plethora of others are only some of the bioactive components found in medicinal plants and herbs. Antioxidant, anti-inflammatory, antibacterial, analgesic, and anticancer effects are just some of the biological actions that may be exhibited by these substances.

A stronger effect can be achieved by combining various components from medicinal plants and herbs. This synergy can arise from several different sources:

1. By acting as a "potentiator," one drug increases the effectiveness of another molecule when administered together. Several methods exist for this to occur, including enhanced bioavailability, enhanced cellular absorption, and regulation of metabolic pathways.
2. There may be a more complete treatment effect if numerous routes or processes of a disease are targeted by different substances. This may be especially helpful in more complicated cases where several factors interact to cause illness.
3. Some chemicals can affect the pharmacokinetics of others by affecting their absorption, distribution, metabolism, or excretion. This can increase the combined drugs' effectiveness by increasing their bioavailability, lengthening their half-life, or decreasing their clearance.
4. Physiological responses can be amplified when numerous compounds engage with the same receptor or target site to increase binding affinity or activate different receptor subtypes.
5. It is also possible for chemicals to have antagonistic effects, albeit this is far less common. To obtain the intended therapeutic effect, it is crucial to think about the proportions and concentrations of the substances involved.

Herbal formulations, traditional preparations, and standardized extracts are only some of the methods that can be used to investigate the compound combination. Synergistic combinations can be found and their mechanisms of action better understood with the use of contemporary research methods such as high-throughput screening and computational modeling.

It's important to remember that mixing medicinal plant chemicals with conventional medications can have synergistic effects, which could improve treatment outcomes and decrease drug dosage needs. However, while combining multiple chemicals or therapies, it is crucial to think about possible interactions, contraindications, and safety considerations.

The potential for effective and holistic therapy methods for diverse health disorders is greatly enhanced by our growing knowledge of, and ability to harness, the synergy between chemicals found in medicinal plants and herbs.

Conclusion

In conclusion, the use of herbs and other botanicals for therapeutic purposes is what is meant by the term "herbal apothecary." Herbal medicine is the practice of preparing and using herbal treatments to improve health. Alternatives to conventional medicine such as herbal apothecaries have been used for ages in many civilizations across the globe.

Leaves, flowers, roots, and bark can all be used to create effective herbal treatments. These plants have medicinal value because of the large variety of bioactive substances they contain, including alkaloids, flavonoids, and essential oils. To that end, herbalists and other practitioners of herbal medicine have honed their skills in herb identification, harvesting, and preparation.

The holistic approach taken by a herbal apothecary is an advantage. Instead of simply masking symptoms, many herbal treatments seek to get to the root of the problem. They are thought to complement the body's inherent mechanisms for maintaining health and restoring equilibrium. Herbal remedies are often reported to have less adverse effects than medicines, and to be less harsh on the body overall.

Herbal apothecaries stock cures for many different health issues, such as those related to the digestive system, the respiratory system, the skin, anxiety, and insomnia. They are highly adaptable and can be utilized in a variety of ways, including as teas, tinctures, capsules, lotions, and essential oils.

Although herbal apothecary has its place in health and wellbeing, it is not a substitute for conventional medical care. Before adding herbal medicines into your healthcare practice, it is recommended that you speak with a certified herbalist, naturopathic doctor, or healthcare practitioner, especially if you have any pre-existing medical issues or are taking any pharmaceuticals.

Herbal apothecary provides an alternative and supplementary method of therapy that makes use of the long history of herbalism. It can help those who are looking for complementary or alternative remedies for their health problems by tapping into the healing potential of plants.

BOOK 2: BASIC HERBAL REMEDIES AND ADVANCED HERBAL REMEDIES

For generations, people have turned to herbal medicines for a more holistic and natural approach to health and wellbeing. Plants' leaves, roots, blossoms, and seeds are used to treat illness and restore health in these practices. There are two types of herbal treatments: the fundamentals and the more complex.

Basic Herbal Remedies:

Common plants and herbs have been used medicinally for centuries, both for common diseases and for maintaining overall health and fitness. Many people take use of these remedies as part of their regular routine because of how convenient they are. When used properly, most common herbal medicines are not only effective but also safe.

Advanced Herbal Remedies:

The utilization of specific plants or herbal formulations for increasingly complex health issues is at the heart of advanced herbal therapies. These treatments sometimes call for a more advanced knowledge of herbal medicine and use a synergy of herbs to treat specific diseases or long-term disorders. It is possible to combine cutting-edge herbal medicines with standard medical care, but doing so requires caution and the oversight of a medical professional.

However, before beginning any new herbal regimen, it is recommended that you speak with a healthcare practitioner or a certified herbalist, especially if you have preexisting health concerns, are taking drugs, are pregnant or nursing, or have any other reason to be cautious. They can tailor their recommendations to your individual needs and check that the herbs you're taking are safe.

Chapter 1:
Herbal Remedies For Common Ailments

Traditional herbal medicine has been used for millennia to treat a wide variety of health issues. Here are some herbal remedies that have traditionally been used for common ailments, though it is vital to visit a healthcare expert for accurate diagnosis and treatment.

1. Tea made from chamomile flowers has been used for centuries to help people relax and get to sleep.
2. Indigestion, gas, and nausea are among symptoms that peppermint tea or oil might alleviate.
3. Ginger is a popular remedy for nausea, motion sickness, and gastrointestinal distress. It can be brewed into tea, sprinkled over food, or taken as a pill.
4. As an immune system booster, echinacea may shorten the length and intensity of cold and flu symptoms. You can get it in capsules, tinctures, and a variety of teas.
5. Essential oil of lavender is popular for its sedative properties. Inhaling it, rubbing it into your skin, or soaking in a bath with it are all effective ways to calm down and unwind.
6. Garlic: Research suggests that garlic may help keep your heart healthy and prevent infections. It's a supplement that can be sprinkled on food or swallowed whole.
7. Curcumin, a chemical found in turmeric, is what gives it its anti-inflammatory effects. It has the potential to improve joint health and aid in the treatment of illnesses like arthritis. You can either put turmeric in your food or take it orally.
8. St. John's Wort is a plant that has been studied for its possible antidepressant benefits and is used by many. However, it is important to talk to a doctor before using it because of possible drug interactions.
9. The valerian root is a popular natural cure for sleeplessness and other sleep-related problems. It can be taken orally as a supplement or brewed into tea.
10. The topical use of aloe vera gel, which has anti-inflammatory and antimicrobial characteristics, can help relieve minor burns, skin irritations, and wounds.

Always check with your doctor before using a herbal remedy, especially if you have a preexisting disease or are already taking medicine, as there may be negative interactions with your current regimen.

Chapter 2:
Preparation Of Basic Herbal Remedies

Health and wellness have been supported by herbal therapies for millennia. For serious problems, it is best to see a doctor, but many common herbal treatments can be made at home. To assist you in making some common herbal treatments, here is a quick reference:

Herbal Infusions/Teas:

- Select the herb(s) you want to use based on its intended purpose. To unwind, try chamomile, and ease your stomach with peppermint.
- One to two teaspoons of dried herb, or two to four teaspoons of fresh herb, should be infused in boiling water.
- Put a lid on it and let it sit for 10 to 15 minutes to steep.
- You can now drink your herbal tea after straining the infusion. Honey may be added for taste if desired.

Herbal Tinctures:

- Herbal tinctures are extracts that have been concentrated using a solvent like alcohol or glycerin.
- The dried herb should be chopped or ground into a fine powder.
- Put the herb in a glass jar and fill it up to about two-thirds full.
- Vegetable glycerin or alcohol (vodka or brandy) can be poured over the herb to completely submerge it.
- Keep the jar well sealed and shake it every day for four to six weeks in a cool, dark spot.
- Once the liquid has steeped for the required amount of time, filter it using cheesecloth or a fine mesh strainer.
- Place the tincture in dark glass containers fitted with droppers.

Herbal Poultices:

- Herbal poultices are used topically for the treatment of skin diseases, inflammation, and pain.
- Based on their characteristics, select the herb(s) to use. For minor skin irritations and bruising, try using comfrey or plantain.
- Make a paste by combining the fresh herb(s) with a pinch of salt and a bit of boiling water.
- The infected area should be painted with the herbal paste.
- Leave the poultice on for 20 to 30 minutes with a clean bandage or towel covering it.
- Rinse the area gently with warm water after removing the poultice.

Herbal Salves:

- Salve applications help speed wound healing and relieve itching and discomfort.
- In a double boiler, combine 1 part beeswax with 4 parts carrier oil (such olive oil or coconut oil).

- Put in the necessary amount of dried herbs and mix thoroughly.
- Take it off the fire and let it cool a little before transferring to storage containers.
- Before securing the containers, make sure the salve has cooled and solidified fully.

Always make sure you know the recommended dosage, any side effects, and other details about a plant before using it. Consult a skilled herbalist or doctor if you have any doubts or if your health issue is severe.

Chapter 3:
Exotic Medicinal Plants

Medicinal plants native to locations outside of the typical range of well-known medicinal plants are considered exotic. The civilizations who cultivate these plants have often found special uses for their chemical components and traditional medicinal applications. Some exotic examples of therapeutic plants are as follows:

1. South Asian in origin, turmeric (Curcuma longa) is a perennial herb. Curcumin, found in the plant's rhizomes, is a powerful anti-inflammatory and antioxidant. In traditional medicine, turmeric is used to cure a wide range of diseases, including gastrointestinal issues, joint pain, and skin problems.
2. Withania somnifera (Ashwagandha): Ashwagandha is an adaptogenic herb native to India, but also found in the Middle East and some areas of Africa. It has a long history of usage in Ayurvedic medicine, where it is said to increase energy and resilience to stress. Ashwagandha has been studied for its potential to treat anxiety, depression, and inflammatory disorders.
3. Lepidium meyenii (Maca): Maca is a type of root crop that grows wild in the Peruvian Andes. Historically, it has been employed as an aphrodisiac and energy booster. Maca is a nutrient powerhouse, boasting high concentrations of B vitamins, minerals, and amino acids; it has also been shown to improve fertility, hormone balance, and libido.
4. Centella asiatica, more commonly known as gotu kola, is a Southeast Asian perennial plant. As a potential memory booster and wound healer, it has a long history of usage in both Ayurvedic and traditional Chinese medicine. Many people take gotu kola to enhance their memory, calm their nerves, and maintain healthy skin.
5. The Amazon rainforest and other portions of Central and South America are home to the woody vine known as cat's claw (Uncaria tomentosa). Native American communities have relied on it for millennia as an immune system booster and inflammation fighter. Antioxidant, antibacterial, and anti-inflammatory effects have been attributed to cat's claw.
6. Originally from Central and South America, the tropical fruit tree known as graviola (Annona muricata) is also known by its common name, soursop. The leaves, seeds, and fruit of the plant are all utilized in alternative medical practices. People have speculated that graviola has the ability to fight cancer, bacteria, and parasites.
7. Native to the South Pacific, kava (Piper methysticum) has long been valued for the calming and anxiety-relieving benefits it can have. Kava is a plant whose root is used to make a drink that is said to have calming and bonding

> effects on its consumers. It's worth noting, though, that kava may have unintended consequences and drug interactions.

Because of the risk of drug interactions and adverse effects, it's best to check with your doctor before using any unusual medicinal plants.

Chapter 4:
Extracts Of Medicinal Plants

The extract of aloe vera has healing and soothing effects. Its extract is frequently applied topically to heal burns, cuts, and soothe irritated skin. Consuming it orally may also improve digestive health and reduce inflammation.

Curcumin, which is found in turmeric, is a compound with strong anti-inflammatory and antioxidant properties. Extracts of the spice turmeric are used to aid in healing and prevent inflammation in the body.

As an extract, echinacea has been shown to strengthen the immune system. The immune system is bolstered and cold and flu symptoms are mitigated thanks to this extract. There's some speculation that it can reduce inflammation and kill bacteria, too.

Ginger has been used for centuries to aid digestion and calm nausea thanks to the extraction of its root. Ginger extract is commonly used for its ability to ease nausea, aid digestion, and lessen inflammation. Possible immune-enhancing and anti-oxidant properties.

The leaves of the Chinese tree Ginkgo biloba are used to make an extract known as ginkgo biloba. It is commonly used to boost mental acuity, memory, and general brain health. It's possible that ginkgo extract's antioxidant properties and ability to boost circulation are related.

Milk thistle is a plant that has been used for centuries to aid the liver. Silimarin, the extract of the plant, is anti-inflammatory and rich in antioxidants. It's meant to help the liver cleanse itself and protect the liver's cells from harm.

Extract of saw palmetto is gathered from the fruit of the saw palmetto tree. It's typically prescribed for men with benign prostatic hyperplasia to improve prostate health (BPH). Possible aid in alleviating BPH-related urinary symptoms.

Ginseng Extract: Ginseng is a well-known medicinal plant that aids the body in adjusting to stress. Ginseng extract has been studied for its potential to increase stamina, improve memory, and strengthen the immune system. It also has the potential to be an antioxidant.

Chapter 5:
Herbal Remedies For Complex Diseases

Acne

Devil's Club herb, Witch hazel, and sage can be used.

Acne happens when the sebaceous glands get infected, and as a result, shoots out painful bumps—what we all call "pimples" Acne affects all age groups and can appear on any part of the body.

Witch Hazel Toner

Ingredients:

- 3 Tablespoons of Rosemary oil
- 1 Cup of witch hazel

Tools Needed:

- Colored glass bottle (dark)
- Cotton (cosmetic pad)

Instructions:

1. Set all ingredients into a dark-colored glass bottle and shake.
2. Prepare a cotton cloth, dip this in the mixture, and apply it on the affected surface every morning and evening until the acne disappears from your skin.

Sage-Chamomile Gel

Ingredients:

- 3 Teaspoons of powdered sage leaf
- 1 Cup of water
- 3 Teaspoons of chamomile
- ¼ Cup of aloe vera gel

Tools Needed:

- Saucepan
- Cheesecloth
- Glass Jar
- Cotton

Instructions:

1. Set the saucepan on medium heat, add the sage leaf, chamomile, and water. Let it simmer, then get it off the heat when it reduces by half.
2. Let it cool for 3 minutes.
3. Prepare a cheesecloth, use it to cover the edge of the funnel, then pour all the mixture to the last drop into a bowl through the funnel.
4. Set all ingredients into a dark-colored glass bottle
5. Pour into the jar and store in a fridge.
6. Every morning and evening, dip the cotton into the mixture and apply it to the affected skin.

Allergies

Dong Quai

For well over a thousand years, it has been used to cure a wide variety of illnesses.

Mint

Herbal teas and spices are made from dried plants that have medicinal properties.

Rooibos

It's a common ingredient in brews said to treat a wide range of illnesses.

Goldenrod

Widely employed as a treatment for numerous illnesses.

Spirulina

It's a type of protein- and vitamin-packed blue-green algae.

Anti-Inflammatory

Burdock

Roots and leaves are both consumed and applied to the body. Do not use if you are pregnant or nursing.

Devil's Claw

Teas and boosters contain it, whereas poultices put it to use externally. Any pregnant or potentially pregnant adult female should avoid using this product.

Echinacea

Use the powdered, dried, or chewed roots topically or internally.

Chamomile

It is commonly used as a sleep-inducing tea.

Paud'arco

It is extensively used for a wide range of situations.

Antibacterial

Poke

The Native Americans have long relied on this plant for both food and medicine, despite the fact that some of its constituents are exceedingly harmful to cattle and people.

White Pine

Native Americans have traditionally used several parts of plants, including the inner bark, young shoots, twigs, pitch, and plants.

Slippery Elm

Native Americans made extensive use of this tree in their culture.

Wild Yam

Food and medicine are often used interchangeably.

Antimicrobial

Yellowroot and Laurel Sumac Malosma

The Chumash dried the fruits and mashed them to make flour while they used the bark of the roots to prepare herbal tea, which they used for treating dysentery.

Antioxidant

Ginkgo Biloba

It is one among the oldest trees still standing and has been utilized for both culinary and medicinal purposes.

Grapefruit

Internal problems are treated using seeds, pulp, and the inner peel.

Olive Oil

Past harvest of the tree for use in food and medicinal.

Sarsaparilla

It has been utilized for centuries in numerous medicinal preparations.

Schisandra

One variety of shrub with numerous medical use.

Spirulina

It's a type of protein- and vitamin-packed blue-green algae.

Willow, White

Willow tree bark has been used for hundreds of years.

Anxiety

Alfalfa

Today, alfalfa is most a cultivated plant, but you can find it growing wild just about anywhere in North America.

To use it, of course, you can add alfalfa sprouts to your salads and other dishes. But you can also get a tea using its dried leaves or crushed seeds. Use one teaspoon of your choice. Allow the leaves to steep for 10 to 15 minutes. The seeds need to boil for up to 30 minutes.

Stinging Nettles

This herb grows naturally throughout the United States.

Fresh or dried leaves are best to use to remedy anxiety and fatigue. They should come from the top of the plant, which is non-flowering. Use them daily as an infusion. Apply one teaspoon for each cup of water. Steep this for five to 20 minutes. You may also cook them as if they were greens.

Passionflower

There are just about 400 known species of passionflower. Several studies suggest that certain species may have the ability to relieve anxiety. One species is found in Missouri, while others are native to Arizona, Florida, and Texas.

To use it, all you need to do is make tea from all parts of the dried plant except the root. Use one teaspoon for the dried herb and two teaspoons; if you use the fresh flowers, crush and steep them for six to 10 minutes. Drink this as necessary.

Asthma

Common Milkweed herb; Skunk Cabbage herb; Smooth Upland Sumac herb; Trumpet Honeysuckle herb, Ginkgo-Thyme are often used.

This is after there is a blockage in the bronchial tubes in the lungs, thereby resulting in breathing shortage and difficulty when anything offensive is inhaled.

Ginkgo-Thyme Tea

Ingredients:

- Water to boil, 2 cups
- 1 1/2 teaspoons of Ginkgo Biloba extract
- Dried thyme, 2 teaspoons

Tools Needed:

- Large mug
- Boiling water

Instructions:

1. Add the dried herbs to the water in a big mug.

2. Tea should be steamed for at least 13 minutes.
3. Tea should be served and savored at your leisure.

Mint-Rosemary Vapor Treatment

Ingredients:

- 8 mugs of boiling water (not boiling)
- Two cups' worth of chopped mint leaves
- Fresh rosemary leaves, 1 cup, chopped

Tools Needed:

- 1 Large shallow bowl
- 1 Large towel

Instructions:

4. Get a big bowl, put the fresh mint and rosemary leaves in it, add the other ingredients, including the water, place it on a table and sit facing the mixture.
5. Get a big towel to cover your head and the bowl and inhale the steam coming from the herb.
6. Stop after the water stops steaming only.
7. Do this regularly until you notice some significant changes.

Conclusion

In conclusion, herbal remedies offer a natural and complementary approach to healthcare. Basic herbal remedies can be easily incorporated into daily life to support overall well-being, while advanced herbal remedies require a deeper understanding and expertise in herbal medicine. When used appropriately and under the guidance of a healthcare professional, herbal remedies can be a valuable tool for promoting health and addressing various health concerns.

BOOK 3: MEDICINAL PLANT FROM A TO D

MEDICINAL PLANTS LIST

- Aloe Vera (Aloe vera)
- Angelica (Angelica archangelica)
- Arnica (Arnica montana)
- Ash Trees (Fraxinus sp.)
- Ashwagandha (Withania somnifera)
- Astragalus (Astragalus propinquus)
- Balsam Poplar (Populus balsamifera)
- Barberry (Berberis sp.)
- Bay Laurel (Laurus nobilis)
- Bee Balm (Monarda sp.)
- Beech Tree (Fagus sp.)
- Belladonna (Atropa belladonna)
- Birch Tree (Betula sp.)
- Black Cohosh (Actaea racemosa)
- Black-Eyed Susan (Rudbeckia hirta)
- Black Walnut (Juglans nigra)
- Blessed Thistle (Cnicus benedictus)
- Blue Vervain (Verbena hastata)
- Borage (Borago officinalis)
- Burdock (Arctium lappa)
- Calendula (Calendula officinalis)
- California Poppy (Eschscholzia californica)
- Cayenne (Capsicum annuum)
- Chickweed (Stellaria media)
- Clover, Red (Trifolium pratense)
- Comfrey (Symphytum officinale)
- Cornflower (Centaurea cyanus)
- Chamomile (Matricaria recutita and Anthemis nobilis)

- Crampbark (Viburnum opulus)
- Cranberry (Vaccinium macrocarpon)
- Daisy (Bellis perennis)
- Dandelion (Taraxacum officinale)
- Echinacea (Echinacea purpurea)
- Elecampane (Inula helenium)
- Elderberry (Sambucus nigra)
- Eucalyptus (Eucalyptus sp.)
- Evening Primrose (Oenothera biennis)
- Feverfew (Tanacetum parthenium)
- Flaxseed (Linum usitatissimum)
- Foxglove (Digitalis lanata)
- Garlic (Allium sativum)
- Ginger (Zingiber officinale)
- Ginko (Ginkgo biloba)
- Ginseng (Panax sp.)
- Goldenseal (Hydrastis canadensis)
- Ground Ivy (Glechoma hederacea)
- Hawthorn (Crataegus sp.)
- Hazelnut Tree (Corylus sp.)
- Herb Robert (Geranium robertianum)
- Horehound (Marrubium vulgare)
- Horse Chestnut (Aesculus hippocastanum)
- Hollyhock (Alcea rosea)
- Hophornbean Tree (Ostrya virginiana)
- Horsetail (Equisetum arvense)
- Hyssop (Hyssopus officinalis)
- Jasmine (Jasminum officinale)
- Jewelweed (Impatiens capensis)
- Joe Pye Weed (Eutrochium sp.)
- Lady's Slipper Orchid (Cypripedium parviflorum)
- Lavender (Lavandula angustifolia)
- Lemon (Citrus limon)

- Lemongrass (Cymbopogon flexuosus)
- Lemon Balm (Melissa officinalis)
- Licorice Root (Glycyrrhiza glabra)
- Linden (Tilia cordata)
- Lotus (Nelumbo nucifera)
- Maple Tree (Acer sp.)
- Marsh Mallow (Althaea officinalis)
- Milk Thistle (Silybum marianum)
- Mint (Mentha sp.)
- Motherwort (Leonurus cardiaca)
- Mugwort (Artemisia vulgaris)
- Mullein (Verbascum thapsus)
- Nettle, Stinging (Urtica dioica)
- Oregano (Origanum vulgare)
- Passionflower (Passiflora)
- Pine Tree (Pinus sp.)
- Pineapple Weed (Matricaria discoidea)
- Plantain (Plantago lanceolata)
- Queen Anne's Lace (Daucus carota)
- Rose (Rosa sp.)
- Rosemary (Rosmarinus officinalis)
- Sage (Salvia officinalis)
- Saint John's Wort (Hypericum perforatum)
- Sea Buckthorn (Hippophae rhamnoides)
- Skullcap (Scutellaria sp.)
- Slippery Elm (Ulmus Rubra)
- Staghorn Sumac *(Rhus typhina)*
- Tea Tree (Melaleuca alternifolia)
- Thyme (Thymus vulgaris)
- Tulsi (Ocimum tenuiflorum)
- Turmeric (Curcuma longa)
- Watercress (Nasturtium officinale)
- Witch Hazel (Hamamelis virginiana)
- Yarrow (Achillea millefolium)

- Yellow Dock (Rumex crispus)
- Valerian (Valeriana officinalis)
- Veronica (Veronica officinalis)
- Violets (Viola sp.)
- Wild lettuce *(Lactuca virosa)*
- Willow (Salix sp.)
- Wintergreen (Gaultheria procumben

ALOE VERA (ALOE VERA)

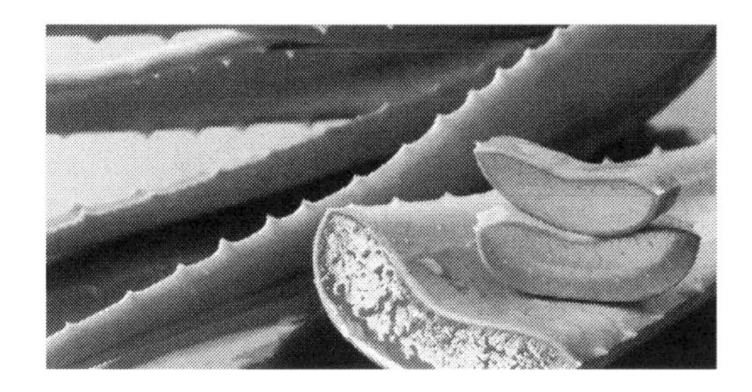

Aloe vera, renowned for its diverse healing properties, is a versatile plant found in various regions. It's a hardy succulent that thrives both indoors as a common houseplant in colder areas and outdoors in arid desert climates.Healing Properties and Cutaneous ApplicationsThe plant is highly valued for its nutrient-rich gel extracted from its fleshy leaves. Numerous studies affirm its efficacy in treating a wide array of skin issues. This includes its ability to alleviate conditions such as psoriasis, dandruff, and minor skin irritations like small cuts, burns, and abrasions.Role in Skin Protection Aloe vera's soothing and moisturizing properties make it a widely used natural remedy for sun-related damage and potentially even for managing side effects of cancer radiation therapy. Its capability to shield against UV damage renders it a valuable ally in skincare and skin protection. Internal Use and Potential RisksHistorically, aloe vera juice has been consumed internally as a remedy for constipation. However, recent research highlights potential risks associated with its internal consumption, revealing potentially excessive laxative effects and other complications. Presently, internal use is not recommended.

Cultivation and Domestic Usage

Cultivating aloe vera is relatively simple, requiring minimal care. Having a few plants on hand ensures easy access to its beneficial gel. This gel can be utilized to craft homemade facial creams and sanitizing gels, showcasing its versatility not only in skincare but also in everyday hygiene.

Aloe vera, with its blend of healing properties and diverse applications, stands as a revered natural resource catering to a wide spectrum of health and wellness needs

ANGELICA (ANGELICA ARCHANGELICA)

Angelica, renowned for its historical use in medicinal remedies since medieval times, is commonly found as a perennial in many gardens. While primarily grown today for its ornamental blossoms, its health properties are equally notable.

Research indicates Angelica's potential in addressing various health issues, such as malaria, anemia, fever, and arthritis. It also carries significance in gynecology by aiding in initiating menstrual cycles, though some regions utilize Angelica for its abortion-related attributes.

Historically, Angelica has been utilized for numerous other ailments, including digestive discomforts like heartburn and flatulence, along with alleviating anxiety. It's commonly brewed as an herbal infusion or applied as a salve, with caution advised, particularly during pregnancy.

BENEFITS OF ANGELICA

Addresses heartburn, intestinal gas, and appetite loss.

Enhances libido and promotes increased urine output.

Eases nerve and joint discomfort when used topically.

Reduces nicotine withdrawal symptoms when utilized in aromatherapy

ARNICA (ARNICA MONTANA & A. CHAMISSONIS)

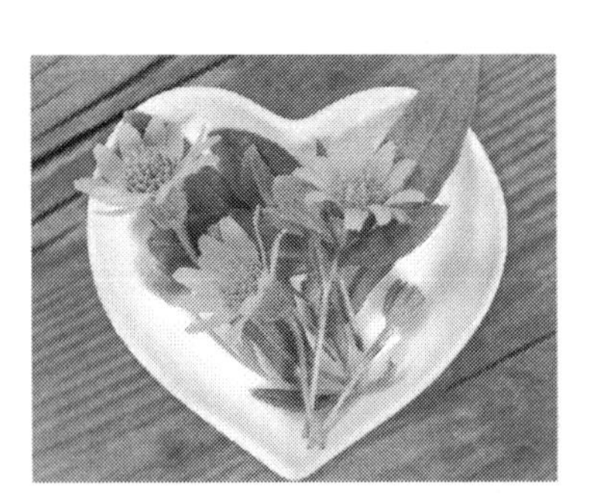

L'arnica, a robust perennial plant, thrives in temperate climates and withstands low temperatures and frost. During the summer, its daisy-like flowers bloom, offering not only a decorative touch but also medicinal value. It's best to gather the flowers right after blooming and let them air dry for a period.

Topical use of arnica provides several therapeutic benefits. Commonly associated with creams and ointments available in stores, it's equally possible to produce them independently using garden-grown flowers. Personally, we prepare arnica oils and ointments to treat bruises, muscle strains, joint pains, and provide effective relief for minor burns.

The key benefits of arnica include alleviating muscle pains and joint inflammations, aiding in reducing bruises, swelling, and post-injury pain, as well as offering valuable support in the healing of wounds, especially those linked to minor traumas. Additionally, it's known to provide relief from skin irritations such as dermatitis, eczema, and insect bites.

The safety of using arnica is associated with topical application, strictly avoiding oral ingestion as arnica extracts could be toxic if ingested. The best methods of use are through creams, ointments, or oils, always being mindful of concentrations to prevent adverse reactions. It's important to conduct a skin sensitivity test on a small area before widespread use and consult a healthcare professional for any queries or concerns regarding the use of arnica, particularly when combined with other treatments or medication.

ASH TREES (FRAXINUS SP.)

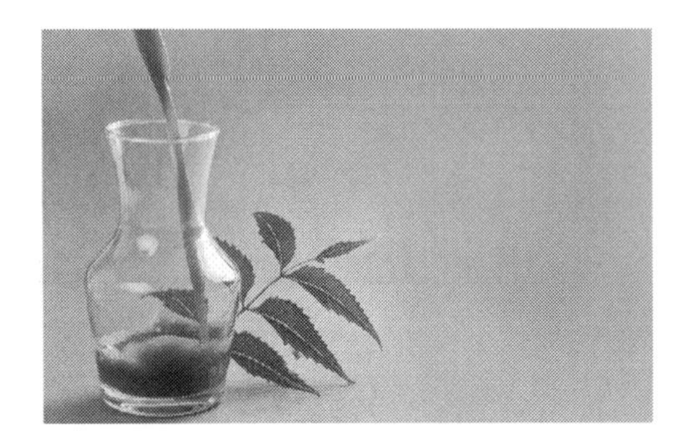

The history of ash trees in Native American medicinal practices spans generations. These grand trees, often soaring up to 30 meters tall and thriving for well over a century, add a touch of elegance to the landscape with their blossoms blooming from April through May. Recognizable by their light grey bark and large leaves composed of four to eight lance-shaped leaflets, ash trees have long been esteemed for their therapeutic qualities.

Although their medicinal usage has declined over time, ash trees still harbor a wealth of potential benefits. Native Americans regarded these trees as possessing profound healing attributes, believing them to be a remedy for snake bites, with each part of the tree serving a distinct purpose.

Contemporary research validates some of these traditional uses, confirming the efficacy of ash trees as a laxative and anti-inflammatory agent, particularly in easing symptoms of arthritis and gout. The bark of white ash trees has been utilized to address dysmenorrhea and to treat skin sores, lice, and itchiness (Source).

However, the imminent threat posed by the Emerald Ash Borer presents a grave risk to these trees, potentially driving them toward extinction within a few decades. Thus, the conservation of healthy ash trees in their natural habitat becomes paramount.

BENEFITS OF ASH TREES:

Ingesting parts of the ash tree, due to its diuretic properties, aids in reducing cellulite.

Topical application of ash tree derivatives helps alleviate swelling caused by arthritis and rheumatism.

The tree's wood is highly esteemed in various industries, used in crafting sports equipment, tool handles, and furniture owing to its resilience and durability.

ASHWAGANDHA (WITHANIA SOMNIFERA)

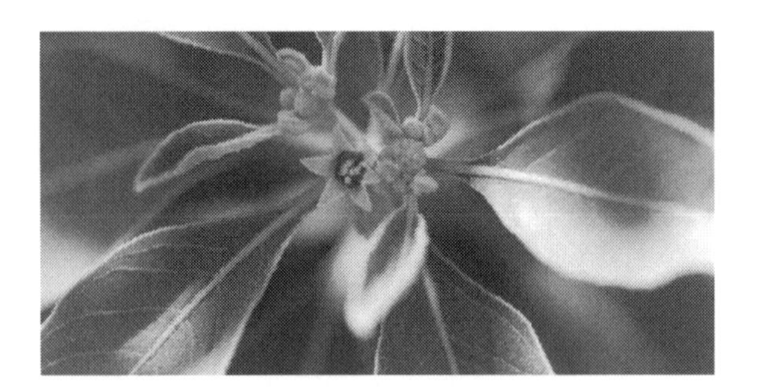

Ashwagandha, a native herb originating from India and Nepal, has gradually become a prominent fixture in backyard cultivation due to its adaptability, flourishing in diverse conditions and persisting as a perennial plant up to zone six. Even though it's considered a perennial, within our zone 4 Vermont garden, we treat it as an annual, ensuring we harvest its roots before the initial frost sets in. What's particularly intriguing about Ashwagandha is its dual usability, with both its leaves and roots offering significant value.

Numerous studies have shed light on this ancient herb's potential in enhancing cognitive function and aiding in memory retention. It exhibits promising attributes in treating neurodegenerative conditions, such as Alzheimer's disease, and its anti-inflammatory properties render it a valuable ally in the management of arthritis (studies).

Ashwagandha's documented attributes, with a history spanning over 3,000 years, underscore its efficacy in stress reduction and enhancement of concentration. Recent studies even suggest its potential in addressing depression (study).

ASHWAGANDHA BENEFITS:

Beyond its established properties, Ashwagandha's dual utility proves to be an invaluable resource. Its leaves and roots both play distinctive roles. The leaves, rich in bioactive compounds, contribute to stress relief, offering adaptogenic properties and aiding in cognitive function. Meanwhile, the roots, known for their potency, serve in reducing inflammation, boosting the immune system, and supporting adrenal health. This comprehensive utilization of both leaves and roots amplifies the diverse therapeutic potential of this ancient herb.

ASTRAGALUS (ASTRAGALUS PROPINQUUS)

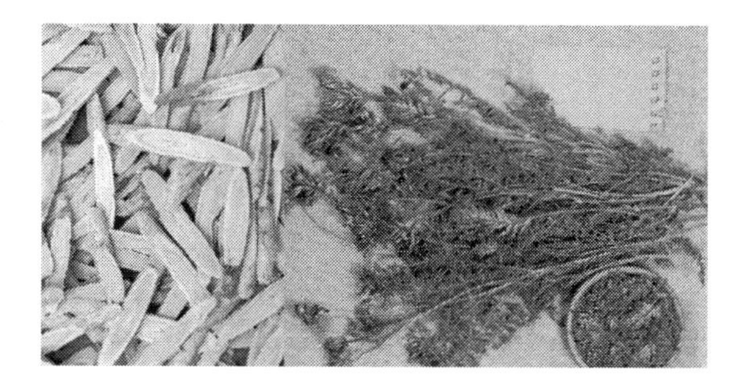

Astragalus, the herbaceous perennial originating from China, stands proudly, reaching heights of about four feet, adorned with charming, petite, yellow blossoms that grace gardens from the heat of midsummer well into the waning days of fall. While traditionally thriving in zones 6 to 11 as a reliable perennial, recent winters in our zone 4 garden have showcased its resilience, hinting at potential adaptability even in colder regions.

It's a patient gardener's endeavor; Astragalus requires two years of cultivation to yield a rootstock potent enough for medicinal purposes, somewhat hindering its suitability for annual growth.

The rich tapestry of Astragalus's ancient medicinal heritage unfolds through numerous studies. Research backs its capacity to guard the body against threats of cancer and diabetes, underscoring its formidable anti-aging properties (Studies).

The essence of this medicinal herb lies in fortifying and supporting the immune system, acting as a bastion against common colds and infections. Moreover, its anti-inflammatory attributes render it a valuable ally in managing minor wound care.

ASTRAGALUS BENEFITS:
Astragalus extends a spectrum of benefits beyond the well-known. Its role transcends the traditional realm of cold prevention and common diseases. It's a robust contender in the arena of stress reduction and disease prevention, a stalwart safeguard for maintaining overall well-being. Not confined to fending off common colds, Astragalus demonstrates promise in diabetes management by regulating blood sugar levels. Additionally, it exhibits potential in minimizing allergy symptoms, particularly for individuals grappling with hay fever or allergic rhinitis.

Yet, Astragalus's story doesn't end there. Unveiling layers of therapeutic potency, its adaptogenic traits aid the body in managing stress, fortifying resilience against a myriad of stressors while nurturing vitality. Its impact on cardiovascular health is noteworthy, potentially assisting in reducing cholesterol levels and fortifying heart health. With its antioxidant properties, it contributes to cellular health, potentially alleviating oxidative stress and preserving overall wellness.

This comprehensive array of Astragalus's potential applications epitomizes its holistic support for health and well-being. Be it as a guardian of immune function, a protector against diseases, or an assistant in managing allergies and stress, Astragalus embodies a comprehensive botanical resource.

BALSAM POPLAR (POPULUS BALSAMIFERA)

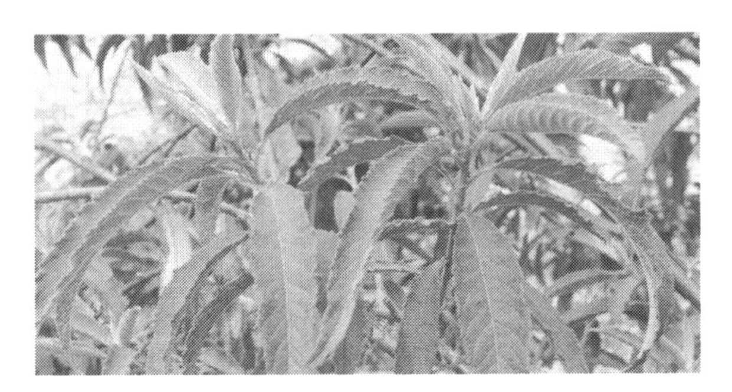

Balsam Poplar, a prominent North American native tree species, exhibits diverse cultivars and numerous hybrids, known for its rapid growth and towering heights, often exceeding 50 feet. Thriving in warm climates with moist soil conditions, these trees typically have a lifespan of at least 50 years.

Studies highlight the potential health benefits of Balsam Poplar, particularly in weight loss and diabetes management. Research indicates its significant impact on inhibiting adipogenesis, suggesting promising anti-obesity properties. Moreover, it shows potential in antidiabetic therapies. (Studies)

The medicinal properties of Balsam Poplar and other Poplar species are utilized as expectorants to alleviate chest congestion. Extracts from the buds are transformed into ointments and salves effective in treating skin conditions such as sores, rashes, and even frostbite. Applying Balsam Poplar ointment within the nostrils is known to relieve congestion caused by colds and bronchitis.

BALSAM POPLAR BENEFITS

Treats sores, wounds, and arthritis effectively when used as a salve.
Application of the salve aids in alleviating sprains or muscle pains.
Eases coughing and chest congestion, acting as a natural remedy.
Exhibits properties beneficial in managing fevers.
Provides relief from menstrual cramps.

Additionally, the bark of Balsam Poplar has been historically used in traditional medicine, recognized for its therapeutic properties in alleviating various ailments, including headaches, sore muscles, and respiratory issues.

BEE BALM (MONARDA SP.)

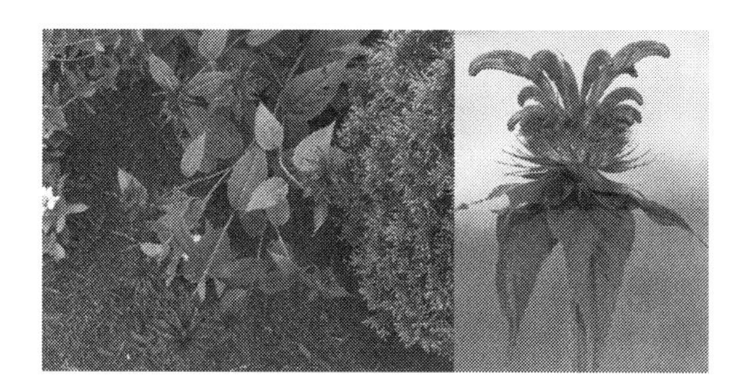

Bee balm, a member of the mint family, showcases a vibrant spectrum from bright reds to gentle pinks and whites. This perennial herb typically grows up to three feet in height and thrives best in well-drained soil under full sunlight.

Historically, bee balm has served dual roles in traditional herbal medicine and the culinary domain. Its leaves are used as a seasoning, similar to oregano, while its flowers make a delightful and aromatic tea.

Research supports the traditional applications of bee balm, underscoring its antimicrobial, antibacterial, antiviral, and antispasmodic properties. Furthermore, it demonstrates a potential in reducing insomnia. (Studies)

Crafted into an herbal infusion, bee balm serves as a potent remedy for various cold symptoms, effectively addressing congestion, headaches, and sore throats. Inhaling steam infused with bee balm aids in sinus relief.

BEE BALM BENEFITS

Eases the discomfort from bee stings and bug bites.
Alleviates anxiety and stress.
Provides relief from upset stomachs, gas, and nausea.
Treats sore throats and mouth sores.

Extending its medicinal qualities, bee balm extracts exhibit anti-inflammatory traits, often used in addressing skin conditions like eczema and minor burns. Its calming effects and aroma are harnessed in aromatherapy, proving effective in relaxing the mind and reducing nervous tension. Besides, bee balm contains antioxidants that are beneficial in reducing inflammation and promoting overall health.

BARBERRY (BERBERIS SP.)

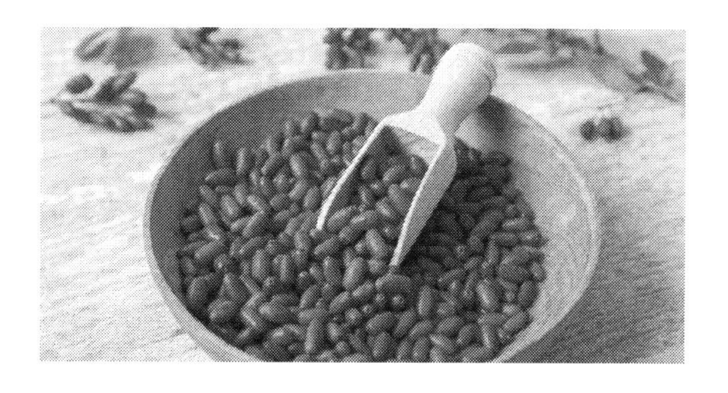

Barberry, a deciduous shrub requiring minimal upkeep, adapts exceptionally well to most garden environments. With over 400 species, the diversity includes the invasive Japanese Barberry and the more domesticated European Barberry, known for its culinary and medicinal use.Thriving in full sunlight and well-draining soil, Barberry varieties have a natural tendency to spread through bird-dispersed seeds, often found in the wild.Research highlights the significant medicinal benefits of Barberry.

With anti-inflammatory properties, it's employed in treating various ailments such as liver disease, gallbladder pain, gallstones, and urinary tract infections. (Studies)For centuries, Barberry has served as a pivotal element in traditional medicine, addressing digestive issues and infections. Rich in diverse antioxidants, it demonstrates potential in managing conditions like diabetes and oral infections.In culinary practices, European Barberry is often utilized in dried forms, much like raisins or currants, added to rice dishes or crafted into simple jams and jellies.

BARBERRY BENEFITSAids in managing digestive problems like diarrhea, constipation, and heartburn.Treats skin conditions such as acne, eczema, and minor wounds.Alleviates the pain and redness of canker sores.Shows promise in reducing blood sugar levels for individuals with diabetes.

Moreover, the plant's extracts have historical applications in holistic medicine for easing sore throats and managing respiratory conditions. The bark and roots, packed with berberine, an active compound, are known for their antimicrobial and antimycotic properties, aiding in treating fungal and bacterial infections.

BAY LAUREL (LAURUS NOBILIS)

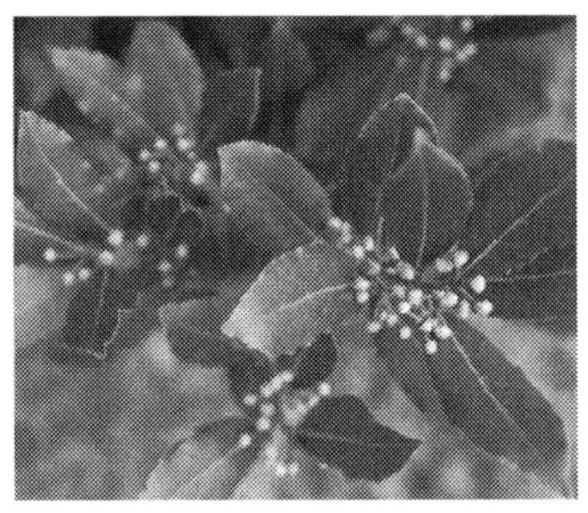

Bay Laurel, an evergreen belonging to the Lauraceae family, boasts fragrant leaves and finds its prominence in both culinary and medicinal spheres. While thriving in USDA zone eight and above under full sunlight, these resilient trees can be successfully cultivated indoors with enriched compost-laden soil.Research indicates the robust medicinal qualities of bay laurel. Known for its antibacterial, immune-stimulating, and antifungal properties, it stands as a healing aid for wounds and an agent in fighting infections. (Studies)

The leaves of the bay laurel tree, known for their savory essence, are both culinary and medicinally valuable. Employed in soups and stews, both fresh and dried leaves offer unique flavor profiles. When dried, the leaves intensify in flavor and are perfect for brewing herbal teas, addressing upper respiratory infections or soothing upset stomachs.In traditional wisdom, placing a bay leaf in pantry staples like flour, rice, or pasta keeps pests at bay, especially deterring weevils.

BAY LAUREL BENEFITSHistorically recognized in addressing various types of cancer.Eases upper respiratory tract issues.Alleviates arthritis discomforts.Calms stomach aches and stimulates appetite.Soothes ear infections when used as ear drops.

Moreover, extracts from bay laurel have been attributed to reducing fever and acting as an anti-inflammatory agent, aiding in various health conditions, including skin irritations and insect bites. The plant's aromatic oil is believed to possess stress-relieving qualities, often incorporated in aromatherapy practices for relaxation and mental well-being.

BEECH TREE (FAGUS SP)

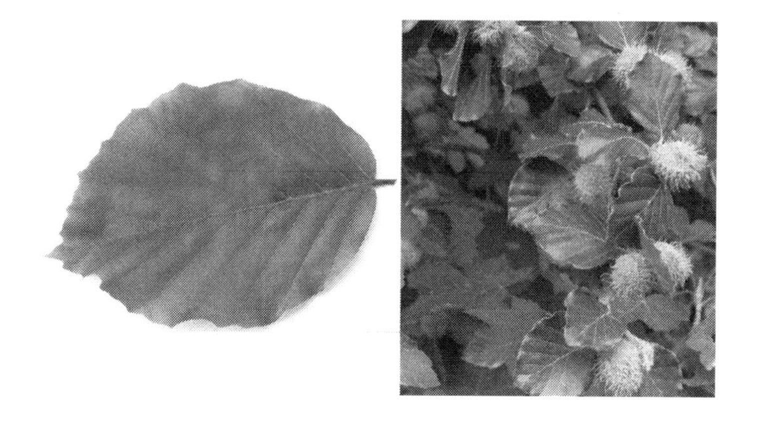

The American beech tree stands out with its smooth, grey bark, easily recognizable amidst forests. These grand trees soar to towering heights of up to 80 feet and require a well-thought-out choice of location—moist, well-draining soil—for optimal growth, thriving for an impressive lifespan of 200-300 years.

Numerous studies highlight the formidable medicinal potential of beech trees, attributing them with robust antiviral, antimicrobial, and antibacterial properties. Delving into the bark's properties, it showcases an ability to scavenge free radicals and exhibits efficacy against various strains of Candida, including E. coli. (Studies)Both the leaves and bark boast remarkable medicinal attributes. The bark is celebrated for its antacid, antiseptic, expectorant, and antibacterial qualities. Internally, it serves as a remedy for toothaches and aids in clearing congestion.During the fall, the beech trees yield beechnuts, known for their rich and buttery taste reminiscent of pinenuts. Moreover, these trees belong to the selection of over 20 species that can be tapped for syrup, producing a luscious syrup with delightful butterscotch notes.

Remarkably, beech trees host the growth of lion's mane mushrooms, renowned for their edible and medicinal qualities. These mushrooms have been scientifically linked to enhancing focus and reducing cognitive decline.

BEECH TREE BENEFITS

Regulates the digestive system, offering relief and balance.

Eases headaches and minor pain issues when utilized as a poultice or salve.

Neutralizes free radicals associated with the development of cancer.

Enhances kidney function and encourages urination when prepared as a decoctio

In addition, beech leaves, when brewed into a tea, provide astringent properties, aiding in managing skin conditions, and their extract has been historically used to promote healthy hair growth. The rich tannins in the leaves and bark are known for their antifungal and antibacterial actions, beneficial for skin-related ailments and minor wounds.

BELLADONNA (ATROPA BELLADONNA)

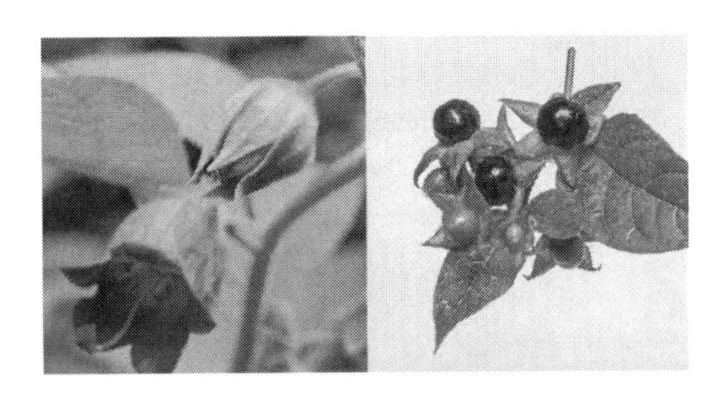

Belladonna, commonly known as Deadly Nightshade, is a hardy, perennial woody shrub native to Europe, introduced to North America by European colonists. It thrives in zones five through nine, requiring well-drained soil and full to partial sunlight.

It's crucial to approach Belladonna with caution due to its well-documented poisonous nature. Every part of the plant, including its berry-like fruits, harbors potentially lethal toxins. Although it might not be fatal, it induces hallucinations and delirium. Antidotes have been developed, but the dangers remain significant.

Interestingly, Belladonna-induced hallucinations have been linked to the myth of witches riding broomsticks, as Belladonna salve can elevate the heartbeat and provoke flying-like hallucinations.

In the pursuit of herbal knowledge, old Medieval herbals often depicted Belladonna's potential medicinal value, sparking interest in its use. However, historical texts might not always provide accurate information. Belladonna's extreme toxicity likely led to fatal outcomes when used in the Middle Ages.

Scientific studies indicate that Belladonna could have potential medicinal applications, particularly in treating peptic ulcers and pain relief. Nonetheless, the risks associated with its use far outweigh any potential benefits, considering the availability of numerous other effective medicinal plants without the same hazards.

While frequently mentioned in old herbals, it serves more as a warning due to its extreme toxicity. Even with precise dosing, I do not advocate its use for any purpose, as even topical applications can be toxic.

BELLADONNA BENEFITS

None significant enough to justify the substantial risks associated with this potentially deadly toxic plant.

TREE (BETULA SP.)

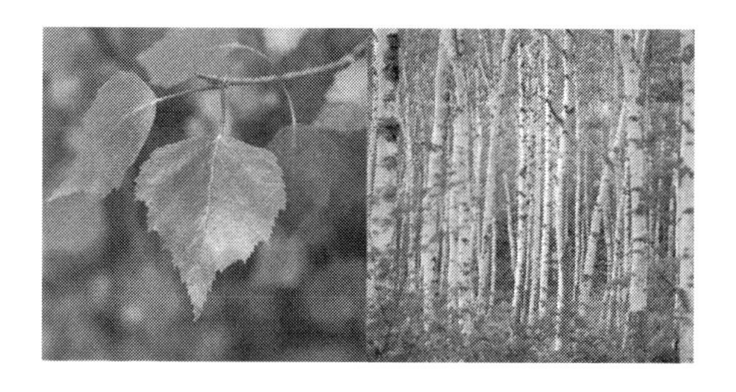

Birch trees flourish primarily in cooler climates and are known for their distinctive, light-colored peeling bark. These trees are prized for their diverse uses and the potential health benefits they offer.

Research suggests that Birch trees harbor therapeutic properties, particularly in treating degenerative joint diseases. Their bark and leaves contain compounds that exhibit anti-inflammatory, antimicrobial, antiviral, and antioxidant qualities, making them valuable in herbal medicine.

Birch contains salicylate, akin to aspirin, making it a natural pain reliever effective against arthritis, inflammation, and muscle pain. It's also believed to aid in reducing fevers. Birch sap itself holds medicinal promise and is used to produce various forms like birch syrup and birch beer.

Additionally, Birch trees play host to several medicinal mushrooms believed to derive their potency from the tree. Species like Chaga, birch polypore, and tinder polypore, growing in symbiosis with Birch, have been used in traditional medicine for their unique healing properties.

The benefits of Birch trees span a broad spectrum. They aid in treating skin disorders such as eczema, combating urinary tract infections and cystitis, soothing symptoms of arthritis and gout, and even assisting in reducing cellulite. Always exercise caution and seek professional advice when considering the use of plants for medicinal purposes.

BLACK COHOSH (ACTAEA RACEMOSA)

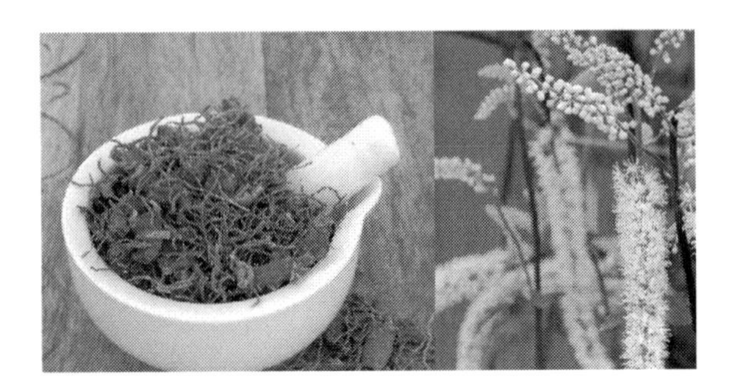

Black Cohosh, an indigenous medicinal herb found in select regions of North America, stands as an herbaceous perennial, often attaining heights of up to four feet and spreading approximately 22 inches in width.

Known colloquially as bugbane within horticultural circles, this botanical gem showcases clusters of creamy to white-hued blossoms adorning wand-like stems, gracing gardens with their presence from May through July, particularly thriving in shaded environments.

Renowned for its efficacy in mitigating menopausal discomforts, Black Cohosh has garnered attention for its ability to address a spectrum of symptoms, including but not limited to hot flashes, night sweats, vaginal dryness, tinnitus, vertigo, as well as psychological manifestations like nervousness and irritability. Impressively, its usage has been notably free from documented adverse side effects.

Amidst our lush garden, where it thrives harmoniously alongside the blackcurrant, Black Cohosh emerges as a natural, nurturing ally, offering solace and support for a variety of menopausal challenges.

BENEFITS OF BLACK COHOSH:

Aids in mitigating the intensity and frequency of hot flashes and night sweats, providing much-needed relief during menopausal transitions.
Exhibits promise in alleviating symptoms related to premenstrual syndrome and menstrual pain, contributing to a more comfortable menstrual experience.
Demonstrates potential in reducing inflammatory responses associated with conditions such as osteoarthritis and rheumatoid arthritis, hinting at its broader spectrum of benefits beyond menopausal concerns.

BLACK-EYED SUSAN (RUDBECKIA HIRTA)

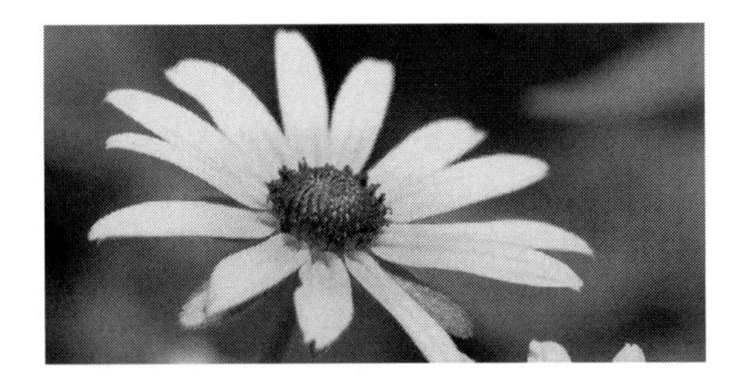

Thriving predominantly in central and eastern regions of North America, the majestic Black Walnut trees stand among native flora like Sugar Maples and Hickory, flourishing for up to an impressive 200 years. Their grandeur extends up to 100 feet with sprawling canopies that define the landscapes they grace. However, it's important to note that these trees contain juglone, a chemical emitted by their roots as a defense mechanism against neighboring plant competition. This compound, while fostering the tree's growth, can be toxic to surrounding vegetation and, for some individuals, may induce reactions when incorporated into remedies involving Black Walnut nuts and husks.

Renowned for their array of medicinal properties, Black Walnuts boast antimicrobial, anti-inflammatory, and antioxidant attributes, promising potential benefits across various health concerns.

One exceptional aspect of Black Walnuts lies in the green hulls enveloping their nuts, representing one of the scarce sources of terrestrial iodine. These hulls undergo processing to produce Black Walnut tinctures and powders, frequently employed as iodine supplements and for combating intestinal parasites in both human and animal healthcare.

EXPANDED BLACK WALNUT BENEFITS:

Effectively combats food-borne illnesses such as Listeria, Salmonella, and E. coli, showcasing its antimicrobial prowess.
Demonstrates potential in aiding weight loss efforts, possibly attributed to its compounds and effects on metabolic processes.
Exhibits promising abilities in eradicating Candida strains and other fungal infections, contributing to overall health and wellness.
Mildly acts as a laxative, fostering healthy bile flow and supporting gastrointestinal health while gently aiding in digestion.

BLACK WALNUT (JUGLANS NIGRA)

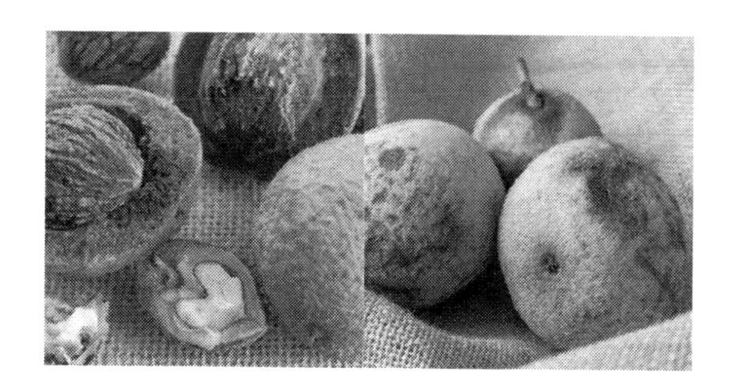

Black Walnut trees are prevalent in central and eastern North America, coexisting with native trees like Sugar Maples and Hickory. These long-lived trees, with a lifespan of up to 200 years, exhibit an expansive canopy, often reaching heights of 100 feet. However, it's crucial to note that Black Walnuts contain juglone, a chemical primarily produced by their roots to inhibit nearby plant competition. This compound is toxic to neighboring plants, effectively excluding competitors in the tree's vicinity. Although the nuts and nut husks, which are utilized for medicinal purposes, contain small amounts of juglone, some individuals may experience reactions when using remedies involving Black Walnuts.

Research suggests that Black Walnut offers multiple medicinal properties, including antimicrobial, anti-inflammatory, and antioxidant effects, rendering it potentially useful for addressing various health issues.

An intriguing aspect of Black Walnuts is the green hulls surrounding the nuts, which serve as one of the few terrestrial sources of iodine. These hulls are processed to create Black Walnut tincture and powder, commonly used as an iodine supplement and for the treatment of intestinal parasites in both humans and animals.

BLACK WALNUT BENEFITS

Effective against food-borne illnesses like Listeria, Salmonella, and E. coli.
May contribute to weight loss.
Shows promise in eliminating Candida strains and other fungal infections.
Exhibits a mild laxative effect while promoting healthy bile flow.

BLESSED THISTLE (CNICUS BENEDICTUS)

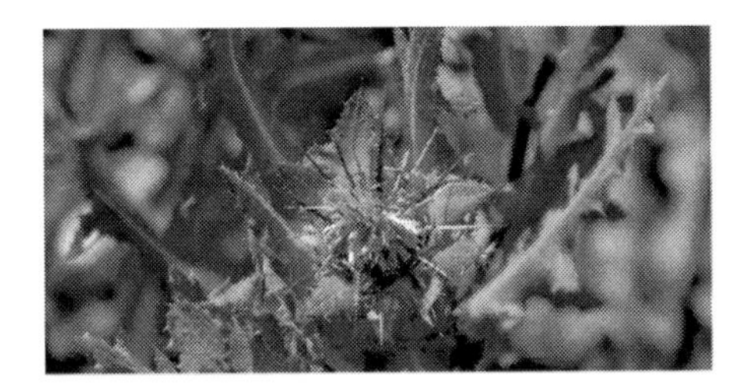

Black Walnut trees are prevalent in central and eastern North America, coexisting with native trees like Sugar Maples and Hickory and boasting a lifespan of up to 200 years. They are known for their expansive canopies, stretching up to 100 feet. However, it's essential to understand that Black Walnuts contain juglone, a chemical produced by the roots to deter nearby plant competition. This compound can be toxic to other plants and may cause reactions in some individuals when used in remedies involving Black Walnut nuts and husks.

Research indicates that Black Walnuts possess various medicinal properties, including antimicrobial, anti-inflammatory, and antioxidant qualities, making them potentially beneficial for a range of health issues.

One unique feature of Black Walnuts is the green hulls surrounding the nuts, which serve as one of the few terrestrial sources of iodine. These hulls are processed into Black Walnut tincture and powder, often used as an iodine supplement and to combat intestinal parasites in both humans and animals.

BLACK WALNUT BENEFITS

Effective against food-borne illnesses like Listeria, Salmonella, and E. coli.
May contribute to weight loss.
Shows promise in eliminating Candida strains and other fungal infections.
Exhibits a mild laxative effect while promoting healthy bile flow.

BLUE VERVAIN (VERBENA HASTATA)

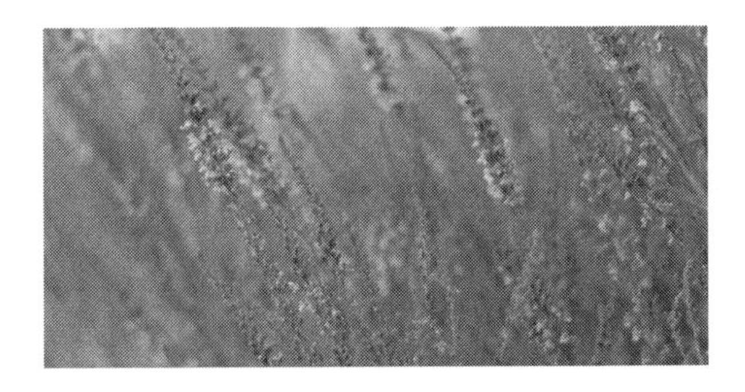

Blue Vervain, native to North American ecosystems, thrives elegantly in damp meadows and areas along streams, boasting clusters of vibrant bluish-purple flowers that adorn its stem from midsummer through early autumn. Thriving best under abundant sunlight and moist but non-swampy soil, this wildflower reveals various medicinal properties that have made it a cherished herb in natural remedies. Its applications extend to addressing an array of ailments, notably providing relief from anxiety, depression, menstrual irregularities, abdominal concerns, and aiding in better sleep patterns.

Delving deeper into its therapeutic qualities, Blue Vervain is noted for its remarkable pain-relieving attributes and its capacity as an anti-inflammatory agent, validated by research findings. Its potential in treating and safeguarding against ulcers underscores its significance in herbal medicine.

Internal use of Blue Vervain extends its remedial applications to alleviating symptoms of depression, fevers, coughs, cramps, and headaches. Externally, this plant proves effective when utilized as a poultice or salve for treating skin conditions such as acne, ulcers, and minor cuts. However, while its benefits are profound, it's vital to exercise caution in consumption as overindulgence could interfere with blood pressure medication or hormone therapy.

BLUE VERVAIN BENEFITS
Relief from pain and inflammation.
Management of premenstrual syndrome.
Treatment of ulcers.
Alleviation of symptoms associated with anxiety and depression.

BORAGE (BORAGO OFFICINALIS)

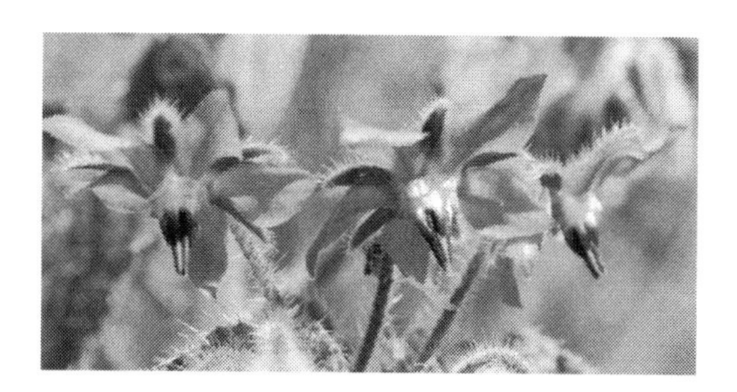

Borage, scientifically known as Borago officinalis, is a flowering plant native to the Mediterranean region and widely cultivated for both culinary and medicinal purposes. It's a herbaceous annual plant characterized by its vibrant star-shaped blue flowers and bristly leaves.

The plant is famed for its culinary uses, with its edible flowers and leaves often added to salads, soups, or used as a garnish to add a mild cucumber-like flavor to dishes. Rich in nutrients like vitamins and gamma-linolenic acid, borage is prized for its health benefits.

Medicinally, borage has been traditionally used to alleviate various conditions, thanks to its anti-inflammatory and antioxidant properties. It's often prepared as an herbal tea or used in supplements to support heart health, reduce inflammation, and alleviate symptoms associated with skin conditions.

Beyond its health uses, borage is also appreciated by gardeners as it's known to attract pollinators like bees, contributing to the overall health of garden ecosystems.

BORAGO OFFICINALIS BENEFITS
Aids in reducing inflammation.
Supports heart health.

Alleviates symptoms of skin conditions.
Attracts pollinators, supporting garden biodiversity.

BURDOCK (ARCTIUM LAPPA)

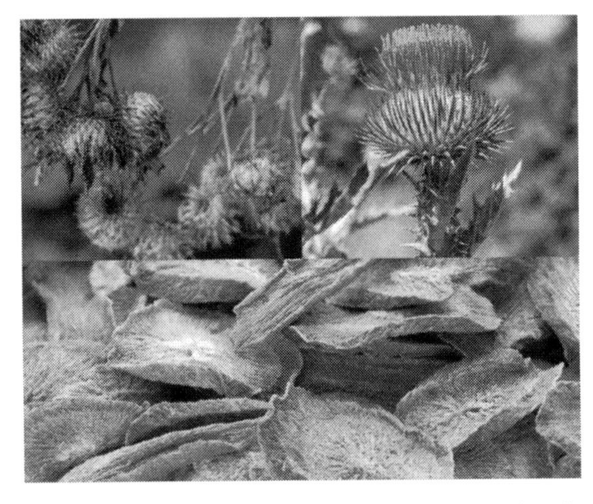

Burdock, also known as Arctium lappa, is a herb with a long history and a range of potential health benefits. The plant, native to Europe and Asia, is recognized for its large leaves and purple flowers.

Health Benefits of Burdock:

Detoxification: Burdock root is thought to have detoxifying properties, aiding in cleansing the blood and eliminating toxins from the body.

Skin Health: Traditionally used for skin conditions like acne, eczema, and psoriasis, burdock is believed to possess anti-inflammatory and antibacterial properties beneficial for skin health.

Antioxidant Content: Rich in antioxidants, burdock helps combat free radicals, potentially reducing oxidative stress in the body.

Digestive Health: Burdock root's prebiotic properties may support beneficial gut bacteria, aiding digestion and improving gut health.

Blood Sugar Regulation: Some studies suggest compounds in burdock may help regulate blood sugar levels, potentially benefiting individuals with diabetes or insulin resistance.

Culinary and Usage:
Edible Roots: The roots can be eaten raw or cooked, commonly used in various dishes.
Herbal Tea: Burdock root is frequently used to make herbal tea, offering a convenient way to enjoy its potential benefits.
Precautions:

While burdock offers potential health benefits, it's important to be cautious:

Allergies: Some individuals may be allergic to burdock, especially if they have allergies to plants in the Asteraceae family.
Medication Interactions: Consult a healthcare professional, especially if taking medications or having specific health concerns.

Burdock's origins trace back to Europe and Asia, but its popularity has spread globally due to its historical medicinal use and culinary value. Today, it remains a subject of interest for those seeking natural health and wellness alternatives.

CALENDULA (CALENDULA OFFICINALIS)

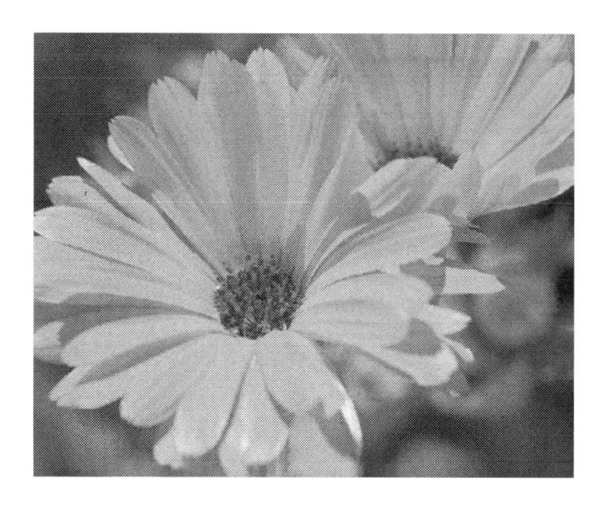

Calendula, scientifically known as Calendula officinalis, is a vibrant and versatile herb renowned for its historical significance and numerous potential benefits. Native to the Mediterranean region, this plant has a rich tapestry of uses in traditional medicine, skincare, and culinary applications.

Origins:

Mediterranean Roots: Calendula has ancient origins in Mediterranean countries like Greece, Egypt, and Spain, where it was highly valued for its therapeutic properties and ornamental beauty.

Historical Uses: Throughout history, Calendula has been utilized for various purposes, including treating wounds, soothing skin irritations, and even as a culinary ingredient.

Health Benefits of Calendula:

Skin Healing: Its anti-inflammatory and antiseptic properties make it a common ingredient in ointments, creams, and salves, aiding in wound healing, relieving skin conditions, and potentially reducing inflammation.

Antioxidant Rich: Calendula is packed with antioxidants, which are believed to help combat free radicals and reduce oxidative stress.

Oral Health: Some studies suggest that Calendula may have benefits for oral health, such as reducing plaque and gingivitis.

Digestive Support: Traditionally, Calendula has been used to soothe digestive issues, although more research is needed in this area.

Culinary and Usage:
Edible Petals: The vibrant petals can be used to add color to salads, soups, and other dishes, offering a mild, peppery taste.
Infusions: Calendula flowers are used to make teas or infusions that are believed to carry over some of its potential health benefits.
Precautions:
Allergies: Individuals with allergies to plants in the Asteraceae family might be sensitive to Calendula.
Pregnancy and Nursing: Consult a healthcare professional before using Calendula products during pregnancy or while nursing.

Calendula's versatility, from herbal remedies to culinary enhancements, continues to make it a popular choice for those seeking natural solutions for health and wellness. Its rich history and potential benefits contribute to its ongoing significance in modern times.

CALIFORNIA POPPY (ESCHSCHOLZIA CALIFORNICA)

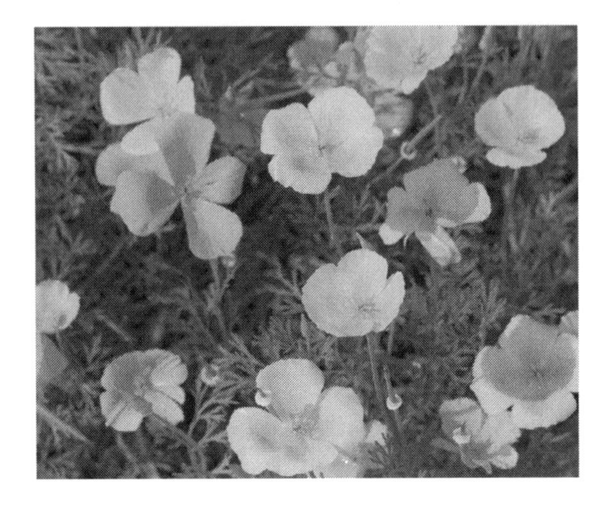

The California Poppy, scientifically known as Eschscholzia californica, is a vibrant and iconic wildflower native to the western United States and northern Mexico. Renowned for its stunning blooms, this plant has historical, cultural, and potential health benefits.

Origins and Cultural Significance:

Native to Western North America: The California Poppy thrives in regions with well-drained, sandy soil, particularly in California, where it holds the title of the state flower.

Cultural Symbolism: Beyond its natural beauty, the California Poppy holds cultural significance. It's seen as a symbol of resilience, freedom, and the pioneering spirit of the American West.

Health Benefits and Traditional Uses:

Relaxation and Sleep Aid: The California Poppy has been historically used by some Native American tribes as a mild sedative to promote relaxation and aid sleep.

Pain Relief: Traditionally, it was used for its potential analgesic properties, believed to alleviate various types of pain.

Anxiety and Nervousness: In herbal medicine, it's believed to have calming effects and has been used to reduce anxiety and nervousness.

Modern Usage:
Herbal Supplements: California Poppy is available in various forms, including tinctures, teas, and capsules, often marketed for relaxation and sleep support.
Precautions:

Interaction with Medications: If taking medications or with existing health conditions, it's advisable to consult a healthcare professional before using California Poppy supplements.

Pregnancy and Nursing: Pregnant or nursing individuals should consult a healthcare provider before using this herb.

The California Poppy's cultural significance and historical use in traditional medicine have contributed to its ongoing interest and exploration for its potential health benefits. As with any herbal remedy, caution and professional guidance are recommended for safe and effective use.

CAYENNE (CAPSICUM ANNUUM)

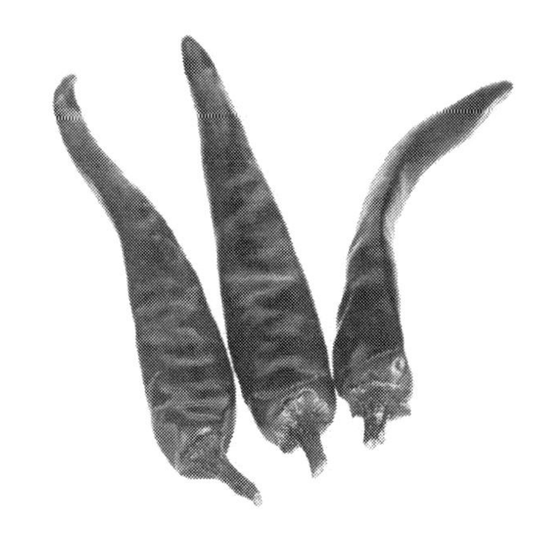

Cayenne, derived from the Capsicum annuum plant, is a fiery chili pepper with a rich history and a range of potential health benefits. Its origins lie in Central and South America, but it's cultivated and enjoyed worldwide.

Origins and History:

Central and South American Roots: Capsicum annuum, the plant from which cayenne peppers come, is native to the Americas and has been cultivated for thousands of years.

Historical Uses: Cayenne has been a part of traditional medicine in various cultures. The pepper was used to aid digestion, relieve pain, and even as a topical application for its warming properties.

Health Benefits of Cayenne:

Pain Relief: Capsaicin, the active compound in cayenne, is known for its potential to reduce pain. It's often used in topical creams for arthritis and muscle pain.

Metabolism and Weight Management: Some studies suggest that cayenne may slightly increase metabolism and help with weight management.

Digestive Health: Cayenne peppers are believed to have digestive benefits, potentially aiding in reducing stomach issues and improving digestion.

Heart Health: Research indicates that the consumption of cayenne may have positive effects on heart health by reducing cholesterol and improving circulation.

Culinary and Usage:

Spice in Cuisine: Cayenne peppers are a popular spice used to add heat and flavor to a wide range of dishes.

Capsaicin Creams: Topical creams containing capsaicin from cayenne are used for pain relief.

Precautions:

Spicy Sensitivity: Some individuals may be sensitive to the heat of cayenne, causing stomach irritation or exacerbating heartburn.

Interaction with Medications: Consult a healthcare professional, especially if using medications, to avoid potential interactions.

Cayenne's versatility, both as a culinary spice and a potential natural remedy, continues to pique interest for its range of health benefits. As with any potent ingredient, understanding its potential effects and consulting a professional for guidance on its use is advisable.

CHICKWEED (STELLARIA MEDIA)

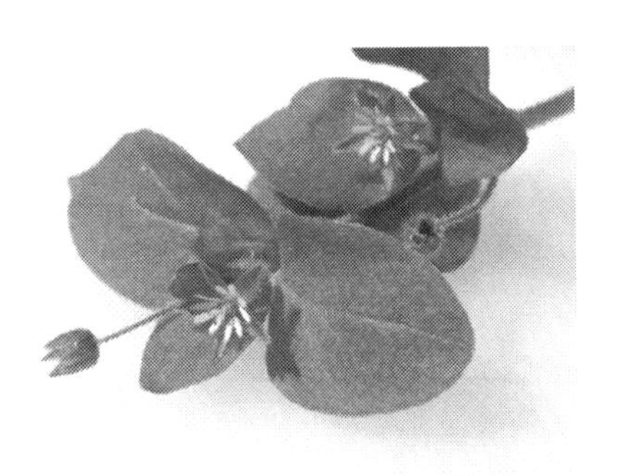

Chickweed, scientifically known as Stellaria media, is a delicate yet resilient herb that holds a history of traditional use and potential health benefits. Native to Europe but now widespread globally, it's recognized for both its culinary and medicinal applications.

Origins and Traditional Uses:

European Roots: Originating in Europe, chickweed has been utilized for centuries in traditional European herbal medicine for various ailments.

Historical Significance: Chickweed was historically used as a culinary herb and for its potential health benefits, ranging from skin issues to digestive troubles.

Health Benefits of Chickweed:

Skin Health: Chickweed has been used topically to soothe minor skin irritations like rashes, eczema, and minor burns due to its potential anti-inflammatory and cooling properties.

Nutrient Content: It's a source of vitamins and minerals, potentially providing nutritional support.

Digestive Aid: Traditionally, chickweed has been used to support digestive health, believed to have mild laxative properties.

Anti-Inflammatory: Its constituents are believed to possess anti-inflammatory properties that may aid in reducing inflammation.

Culinary and Usage:

Edible Greens: Chickweed leaves and stems can be eaten raw in salads or cooked as a nutritious addition to soups and stir-fries.

Topical Applications: In herbal remedies, chickweed is often used in ointments and salves for skin conditions.

Precautions:

Allergies: Individuals with allergies to plants in the Caryophyllaceae family may have sensitivities to chickweed.

Pregnancy and Nursing: Pregnant or nursing individuals should consult a healthcare provider before using chickweed products.

Chickweed's long-standing use in traditional medicine and its nutritional content make it a herb of interest for those exploring natural remedies and wholesome culinary additions. However, as with any herbal remedy, consulting a professional for guidance on usage is prudent.

CLOVER, RED (TRIFOLIUM PRATENSE)

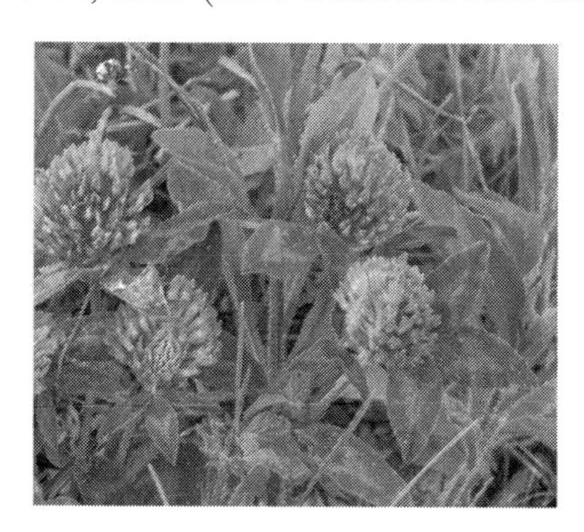

Red clover, scientifically known as Trifolium pratense, is a perennial herb that holds both historical significance and potential health benefits. Originating in Europe and Asia, it has spread globally and is revered for various applications in traditional medicine and nutrition.

Origins and Traditional Uses:

European and Asian Origins: Red clover's use dates back centuries in European and Asian traditional medicine for its potential health properties.

Historical Significance: It was historically used to address a range of conditions, from skin problems to respiratory issues and women's health concerns.

Health Benefits of Red Clover:

Isoflavones: Red clover contains isoflavones, plant-based compounds with estrogen-like effects that may help ease menopausal symptoms and support women's health.

Antioxidants: The herb is rich in antioxidants, which may help combat free radicals and reduce oxidative stress in the body.

Skin Health: It's been used topically in traditional medicine for skin conditions, such as eczema and psoriasis, due to its potential anti-inflammatory properties.

Bone Health: Some research suggests red clover may have a positive effect on bone density, potentially supporting bone health.

Culinary and Usage:

Herbal Teas: Red clover is often used to brew herbal teas, offering a convenient way to potentially benefit from its properties.

Supplements: It's available in supplement form, like capsules or extracts, for those seeking a more concentrated intake.

Precautions:

Hormonal Effects: Due to its estrogen-like effects, individuals with hormone-sensitive conditions or those on hormone-related medications should use red clover cautiously and consult a healthcare provider.

Pregnancy and Nursing: Pregnant or nursing individuals should consult a healthcare professional before using red clover.

Red clover's historical use and potential health benefits continue to make it a subject of interest for those exploring natural remedies and holistic wellness. As with any herbal remedy, consulting a healthcare provider for guidance on its usage is recommended.

COMFREY (SYMPHYTUM OFFICINALE)

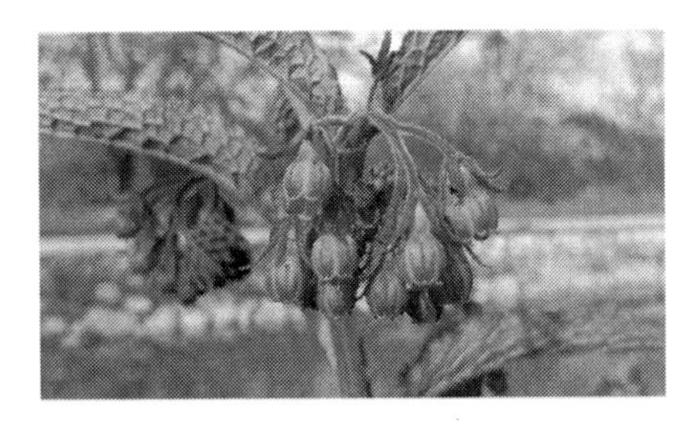

Comfrey, scientifically known as Symphytum officinale, is a herb highly regarded in traditional herbal medicine for its potential health benefits. However, it's also important to note its associated controversies and precautions.

Origins and Traditional Uses:

European Roots: Comfrey has historical roots in Europe, where it was utilized in traditional herbal remedies for various health concerns.

Historical Significance: It was commonly used topically to promote healing of bruises, sprains, and minor wounds due to its purported anti-inflammatory and tissue-repairing properties.

Health Benefits and Controversies:

Healing Properties: Comfrey was historically used for its potential to aid in the healing of minor wounds and skin irritations.

Hepatotoxic Alkaloids: Concerns arose regarding the presence of pyrrolizidine alkaloids, compounds found in some species of comfrey, which may be toxic to the liver if consumed in large amounts or for extended periods.

Culinary and Usage:

Topical Applications: Comfrey leaves were often used to create ointments or poultices for external use on the skin.

Precautions:

Internal Use Concerns: Due to the potential presence of toxic alkaloids, internal consumption of comfrey is discouraged, especially for prolonged periods or in large quantities.

Pregnancy and Nursing: Pregnant or nursing individuals should avoid using comfrey due to its potential risks.

Given the controversies around its safety, it's essential to approach the use of comfrey cautiously. While it holds historical significance in traditional medicine, the potential risks associated with its internal use have led to advisories to avoid consumption and focus on safer alternatives for health and wellness. Consulting a healthcare professional before using comfrey is highly recommended.

CORNFLOWER (CENTAUREA CYANUS)

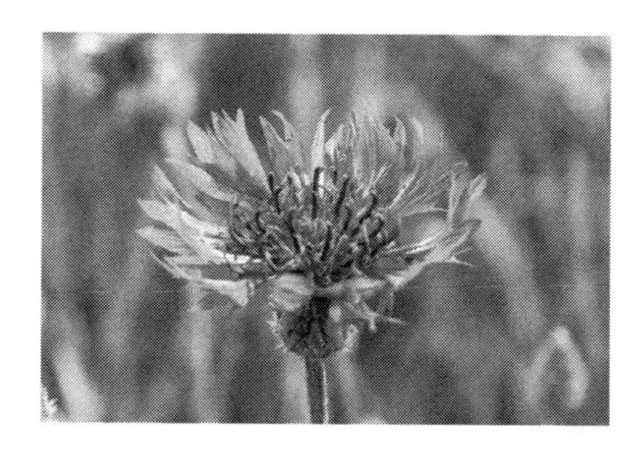

Cornflower, scientifically known as Centaurea cyanus, is an enchanting flowering plant that boasts both aesthetic charm and potential health benefits. Originally native to Europe, it's widely appreciated for its beauty and has found its way into various applications.

Origins and Cultural Significance:

European Origins: Cornflower's natural habitat was predominantly in Europe, where it was loved for its vibrant blue blooms.

Symbolism and Use: Historically, it was used in herbal medicine and often held symbolic significance, featuring in art and literature.

Health Benefits and Usage:

Anti-Inflammatory Properties: Cornflower has been used in traditional medicine for its potential anti-inflammatory effects, often employed in herbal remedies.

Eye Health: In some cultures, cornflower tea was used to soothe tired or irritated eyes due to its believed properties to reduce inflammation.

Culinary and Cultural Use:

Edible Petals: The petals are sometimes used as a colorful addition to salads or herbal teas, adding aesthetic appeal.

Modern Applications:

Herbal Teas and Supplements: Cornflower is used in herbal teas or supplements, often appreciated for its potential health benefits.

Precautions:

Allergy Concerns: Individuals with allergies to plants in the Asteraceae family, like daisies or ragweed, might have sensitivities to cornflower.

Pregnancy and Nursing: As with any herbal remedy, pregnant or nursing individuals should consult a healthcare professional before using cornflower products.

Cornflower's visual allure and potential health benefits continue to make it a source of interest for those exploring natural remedies and seeking a touch of beauty in their culinary and wellness pursuits. However, caution and professional advice are advisable before using it, especially for those with specific health conditions or concerns.

CHAMOMILE (MATRICARIA RECUTITA AND ANTHEMIS NOBILIS)

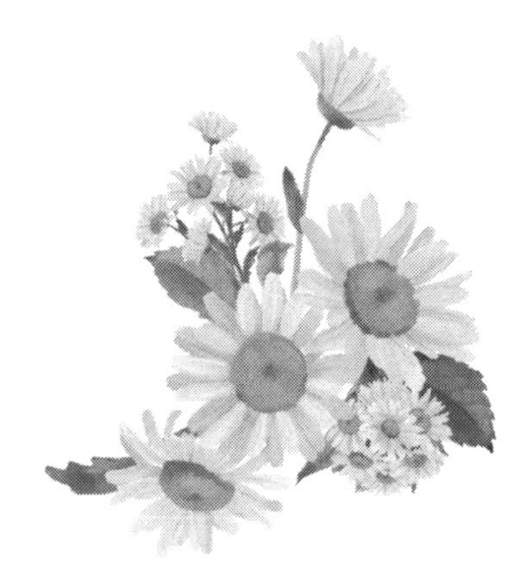

Chamomile, encompassing Matricaria recutita and Anthemis nobilis, is a herb treasured for its soothing properties and historical significance in various cultures. Both types—Matricaria recutita and Anthemis nobilis—belong to the chamomile family and are used similarly in herbal medicine and tea.

Origins and Traditional Uses:

European and Mediterranean Roots: Chamomile has a long history in European and Mediterranean regions, where it was revered for its potential health benefits.

Herbal Medicine: It was traditionally used for its calming and soothing properties, often in teas and topical applications for skin and digestive issues.

Health Benefits:

Relaxation and Sleep: Chamomile is celebrated for its calming effects, believed to aid in relaxation and promote better sleep.

Digestive Health: It's used to soothe digestive discomfort, potentially helping with issues like bloating and indigestion.

Skin Care: Topically, it's used in various forms to alleviate skin irritations due to its potential anti-inflammatory properties.

Culinary and Usage:

Herbal Teas: Chamomile is most commonly consumed as a soothing herbal tea appreciated for its calming effects.

Topical Applications: It's used in creams, ointments, and essential oils for skin care and aromatherapy.

Precautions:

Allergic Reactions: Individuals with allergies to plants in the Asteraceae family might have sensitivities to chamomile.

Pregnancy and Nursing: Pregnant or nursing individuals should consult a healthcare professional before using chamomile products.

Chamomile's gentle nature and potential health benefits have made it a beloved herb in traditional and modern wellness practices. However, as with any remedy, it's advisable to seek guidance from a healthcare professional, especially when incorporating it into your routine, to ensure it aligns with your individual health needs.

CRAMP BARK (VIBURNUM OPULUS)

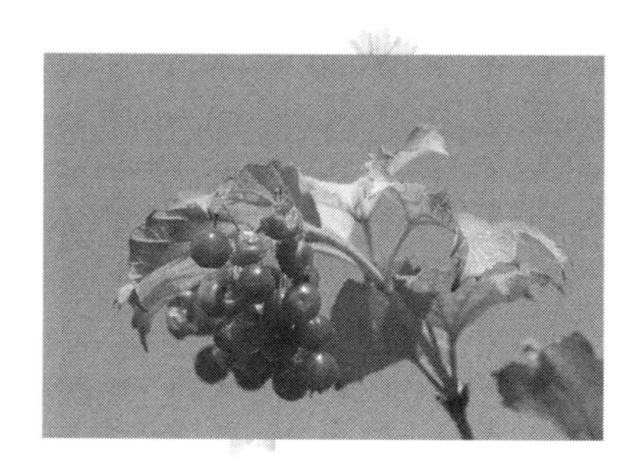

Cramp bark, scientifically known as Viburnum opulus, is a flowering shrub appreciated for its historical use in traditional medicine, particularly for its potential in addressing muscle cramps and various health issues.

Origins and Traditional Uses:

Native to Europe and Northern America: Cramp bark is indigenous to Europe and Northern America and has been utilized for centuries in traditional healing practices.

Historical Significance: The bark of this shrub was historically used by various indigenous communities for addressing menstrual cramps, muscle spasms, and certain health issues.

Health Benefits:

Muscle Relaxant: Cramp bark is reputed for its potential muscle-relaxing properties, particularly beneficial for menstrual cramps and muscle spasms.

Urinary Health: It has been used traditionally to support urinary health and address related discomfort.

Modern Usage:

Herbal Supplements: Cramp bark is available in various forms such as tinctures, capsules, or teas, often taken for its potential health benefits.

Precautions:

Pregnancy and Nursing: Pregnant or nursing individuals should consult a healthcare professional before using cramp bark.

Allergic Reactions: Individuals with allergies to plants in the Viburnum family may have sensitivities to cramp bark.

The historical significance of cramp bark in addressing muscle-related discomfort and its modern applications as a potential remedy make it a subject of interest for those seeking natural solutions for muscle cramps and related issues. As with any herbal remedy, consulting a healthcare professional is recommended before use, especially for individuals with specific health conditions or concerns.

CRANBERRY (VACCINIUM MACROCARPON)

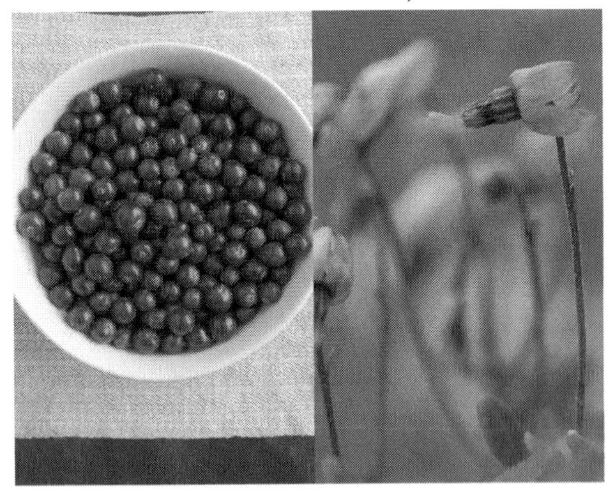

Cranberries, scientifically known as Vaccinium macrocarpon, are vibrant and tangy fruits that are celebrated for their distinctive taste and potential health benefits. These berries have a rich history and are widely recognized for their contribution to both culinary delights and potential wellness advantages.

Origins and Culinary Use:

Native to North America: Cranberries have their origins in North America, where they've been utilized by Native American tribes for their nutritional and medicinal properties.

Culinary Delights: These tart berries are commonly used in various culinary creations, from sauces and jams to baked goods, owing to their unique flavor.

Health Benefits:

Urinary Tract Health: Cranberries are popularly associated with potentially preventing urinary tract infections (UTIs) due to certain compounds that may inhibit the adherence of bacteria to the urinary tract walls.

Antioxidant Rich: They are packed with antioxidants, which help combat free radicals and reduce oxidative stress.

Heart Health: Some research suggests that cranberries might contribute to heart health by potentially reducing the risk of cardiovascular diseases.

Modern Usage:

Cranberry Products: These include juices, supplements, and dried fruits, often marketed for their potential health benefits, particularly for urinary health.

Precautions:

Interaction with Medications: Consult a healthcare professional, especially if on medications, as cranberry products might interact with certain drugs.

Allergic Reactions: Individuals with allergies to similar berries should use cranberry products cautiously.

The unique tang and potential health benefits of cranberries, particularly in maintaining urinary health, continue to make them a popular choice. While they're generally safe and nutritious, it's wise to seek guidance from a healthcare provider, especially if incorporating cranberry products into your routine or if you have specific health conditions.

DAISY (BELLIS SP.)

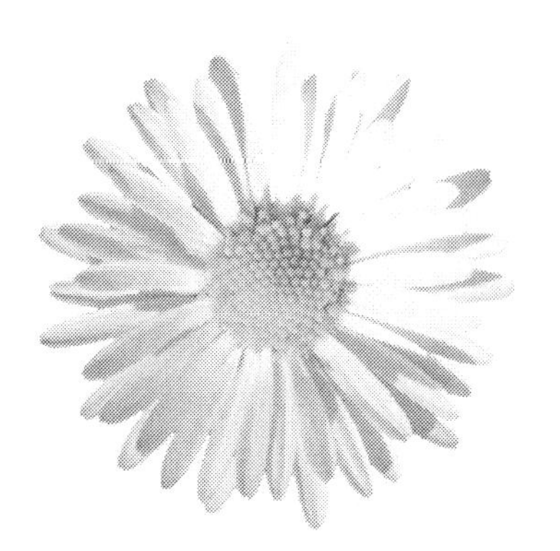

The daisy, belonging to the Bellis species, is a charming and widespread flowering plant that holds both cultural symbolism and some historical significance in traditional medicine.

Cultural Significance:

Symbol of Innocence and Purity: The daisy, with its delicate white petals surrounding a sunny yellow center, often symbolizes innocence, purity, and simplicity.

Folklore and Literature: The daisy has appeared in various folklore and literature, often representing themes of beauty and youth.

Traditional Uses:

Limited Medicinal Use: Historically, the daisy has had limited use in traditional medicine, primarily for minor issues like coughs or digestive troubles.

Topical Applications: In some traditional practices, daisy flowers were used topically for minor skin irritations.

Modern Context:Ornamental Purposes: Daisies are commonly grown in gardens and landscapes for their aesthetic appeal.

Limited Medicinal Use: In modern times, while not extensively used for medicinal purposes, some herbalists may still utilize daisy preparations for minor ailments.

Precautions:

Allergic Reactions: Individuals with known allergies to plants in the Asteraceae family, to which daisies belong, should be cautious.

Pregnancy and Nursing: Pregnant or nursing individuals should consult a healthcare professional before using daisy preparations.

The daisy's symbolism and cultural significance, combined with its limited historical use in traditional medicine, make it more of an ornamental flower than a major player in herbal remedies. While it may offer mild benefits, it's essential to approach its use with caution and, as always, consult a healthcare professional for guidance.

DANDELION (TARAXACUM OFFICINALE)

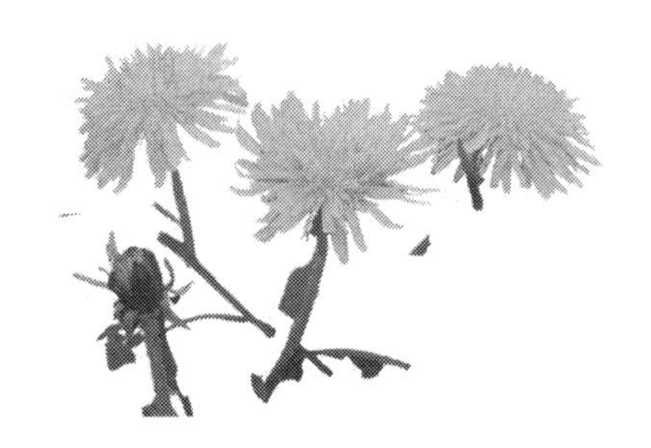

Dandelion, scientifically known as Taraxacum officinale, is a versatile herb that's often considered a weed but boasts a range of potential health benefits. Despite its reputation as a garden nuisance, this herbaceous plant has a rich history and a variety of uses in traditional medicine and culinary applications.

Origins and Traditional Uses:

Global Distribution: Dandelions are found worldwide, flourishing in various climates and soil types.

Historical Medicinal Use: For centuries, dandelions have been utilized in traditional medicine for their potential health benefits, particularly for digestive issues, liver health, and as a diuretic.

Health Benefits:

Nutrient-Rich: Dandelion greens are packed with vitamins, minerals, and antioxidants, potentially supporting overall health.

Digestive Aid: Dandelion root and leaves have been used traditionally to aid digestion and stimulate appetite.

Liver Support: Some research suggests dandelion may aid liver health by increasing bile production and promoting detoxification

Culinary and Modern Usage:

Culinary Applications: Dandelion leaves, flowers, and roots are used in salads, teas, and even as an ingredient in certain recipes.

Herbal Supplements: Dandelion is available in supplement form, such as capsules or teas, often used for its potential health benefits.

Precautions:

Allergic Reactions: Individuals with allergies to plants like ragweed, marigolds, or daisies may have sensitivities to dandelions

Interaction with Medications: Consult a healthcare professional, especially if on medications, as dandelion supplements might interact with certain drugs.

Dandelion's versatile nature, from a garden weed to a potential health ally, makes it a subject of interest for those exploring natural remedies and nutritious culinary additions.

However, it's crucial to consult a healthcare professional, particularly when incorporating it into your routine or if you have specific health concerns or conditions.

BOOK 4: MEDICINAL PLANT FROM E TO M

ELECAMPANE (INULA HELENIUM)

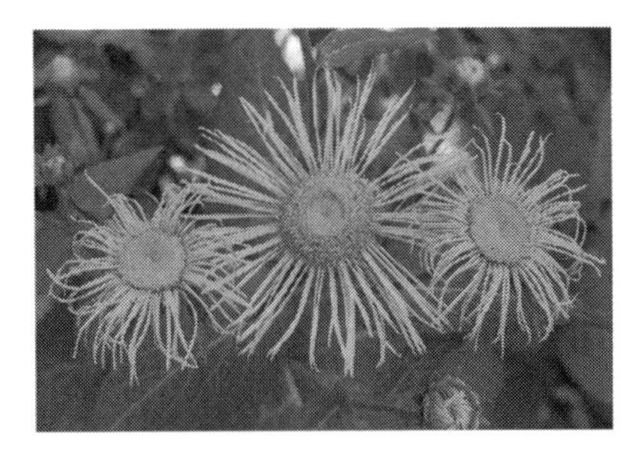

Elecampane, scientifically known as Inula helenium, is an herb esteemed for its historical use in traditional medicine and potential health benefits. This plant has a storied past and is celebrated for its various medicinal properties.

Origins and Traditional Uses

European Origins: Elecampane is native to Europe and parts of Asia, where it has been used in traditional herbal medicine for centuries.

Historical Significance: It was historically valued for its potential as a respiratory aid and for digestive health, among other medicinal purposes.

Health Benefits:

Respiratory Health: Elecampane was commonly used to address respiratory issues, such as coughs, bronchitis, and asthma, owing to its potential expectorant and soothing properties.

Digestive Support: Some traditional uses included elecampane for digestive complaints, believed to aid in indigestion and stimulate appetite.

Culinary and Usage:

Herbal Preparations: Elecampane roots were utilized in various herbal remedies, often in teas, tinctures, or extracts.

Precautions:

Allergic Reactions: Individuals with known allergies to plants in the Asteraceae family, which includes daisies, marigolds, and sunflowers, may have sensitivities to elecampane.

Pregnancy and Nursing: Pregnant or nursing individuals should consult a healthcare professional before using elecampane.

Elecampane's historical prominence in traditional medicine for respiratory and digestive issues continues to make it a subject of interest for those seeking natural remedies. However, due to its potential interactions and individual health considerations, it's advisable to seek guidance from a healthcare professional before using elecampane, especially if you have specific health concerns or conditions.

EUCALYPTUS (EUCALYPTUS SP.)

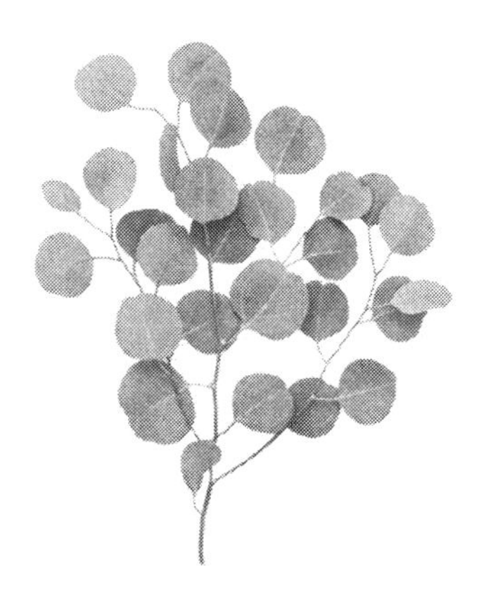

Eucalyptus, from the Eucalyptus genus, is a diverse group of flowering trees and shrubs known for their aromatic leaves and potential health benefits. Native to Australia, these trees are globally recognized and widely used in various forms for their medicinal properties.

Origins and Traditional Uses:

Australian Origins: Eucalyptus trees are primarily native to Australia, where they've been used for centuries by Indigenous Australians for their healing properties.

Traditional Medicine: Eucalyptus has been used in traditional medicine to relieve symptoms of coughs, colds, and respiratory issues due to its potential decongestant and expectorant properties.

Health Benefits:

Respiratory Aid: Eucalyptus is known for its ability to alleviate respiratory issues, including congestion, coughs, and sinus problems, owing to its menthol-like properties

Antiseptic and Anti-inflammatory: Its oil is appreciated for its potential antiseptic and anti-inflammatory effects, often used in topical applications for skin irritations or in aromatherapy.

Modern Usage:

Aromatherapy: Eucalyptus oil is widely used in aromatherapy, providing a refreshing and invigorating scent.

Topical Applications: Eucalyptus oil is found in ointments, balms, and chest rubs for its potential respiratory and soothing properties.

Precautions:

Caution with Undiluted Oil: Direct application of undiluted eucalyptus oil to the skin can cause irritation. It's recommended to dilute it before use.

Avoid Ingestion: Eucalyptus oil should not be ingested as it can be toxic.

Eucalyptus's refreshing scent and potential health benefits make it a popular choice for various applications, especially in respiratory and aromatherapy contexts. However, it's crucial to use it safely and in recommended forms, and consulting a healthcare professional before use is advisable, especially for those with specific health conditions.

EVENING PRIMROSE (OENOTHERA BIENNIS)

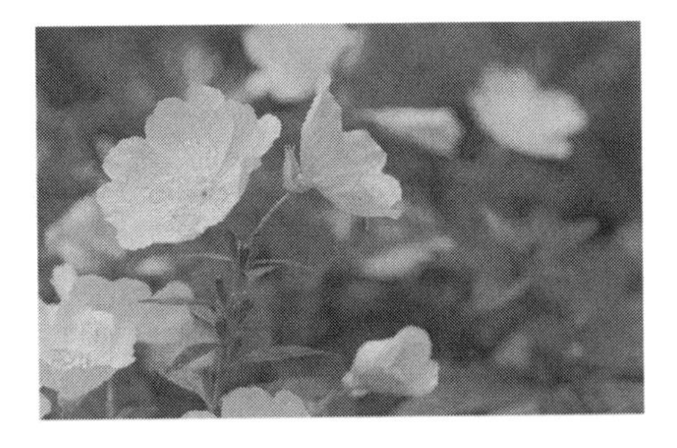

Evening primrose, scientifically known as Oenothera biennis, is a flowering plant highly regarded for its oil, derived from its seeds, and recognized for its potential health benefits, particularly in skincare and women's health.

Origins and Traditional Uses

Native to North America: Evening primrose is indigenous to North America, and historically, various Native American tribes used it for its nutritional and healing properties

Traditional Medicine: The oil extracted from evening primrose seeds has been traditionally used to address various conditions, including skin irritations and women's health issues.

Health Benefits:

Skin Health: Evening primrose oil is rich in gamma-linolenic acid (GLA), an omega-6 fatty acid believed to have anti-inflammatory properties, potentially benefiting skin health, especially for conditions like eczema.

Women's Health: It's been used for menstrual discomfort, menopausal symptoms, and certain hormonal imbalances due to its perceived hormone-balancing properties.

Modern Usage:

Supplements and Topical Applications: Evening primrose oil is available in supplement form, like capsules, and used in skincare products such as creams and lotions.

Precautions:

Allergic Reactions: Individuals with allergies to plants in the Onagraceae family may have sensitivities to evening primrose.

Pregnancy and Nursing: Pregnant or nursing individuals should consult a healthcare professional before using evening primrose.

Evening primrose's oil, particularly prized for its potential benefits in skincare and women's health, continues to be a subject of interest for those exploring natural remedies. However, as with any supplement or herbal remedy, it's wise to seek guidance from a healthcare professional, especially if you have specific health conditions or concerns.

FEVERFEW (TANACETUM PARTHENIUM)

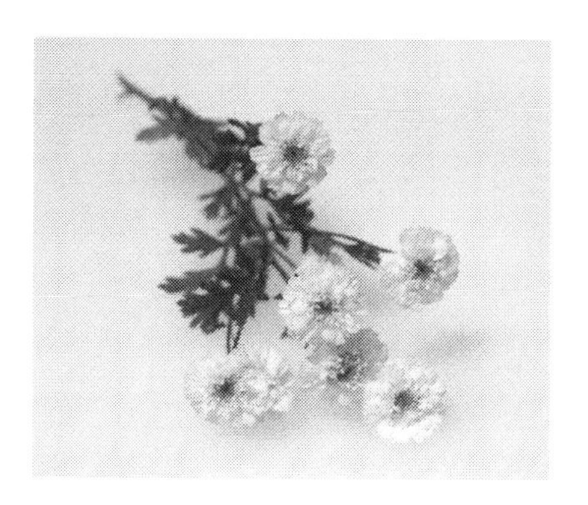

Feverfew, scientifically known as Tanacetum parthenium, is an herb renowned for its historical significance in traditional medicine, especially for its potential in managing headaches and certain health conditions.

Origins and Traditional Uses:

European Origins: Feverfew is native to Europe and has been utilized for centuries in traditional herbal medicine.

Historical Significance: It was historically used to manage fevers and various ailments, particularly for its potential in reducing the frequency and severity of headaches, including migraines.

Health Benefits:

Headache Relief: Feverfew is known for its potential to reduce the frequency and intensity of headaches, particularly migraines.

Anti-inflammatory Properties: It's believed to possess anti-inflammatory effects, potentially contributing to its headache-relief properties.

Modern Usage:

Supplements: Feverfew is available in various forms, such as capsules or tablets, often used by those seeking natural remedies for headaches.

Precautions:

Pregnancy and Nursing: Pregnant or nursing individuals should consult a healthcare professional before using feverfew.

Allergic Reactions: Some individuals may have sensitivities or allergies to feverfew, particularly if allergic to plants in the Asteraceae family.

Feverfew's historical use in managing headaches and its potential anti-inflammatory properties make it a subject of interest for those exploring natural remedies. However, consulting a healthcare professional before using feverfew, especially for individuals with specific health conditions, is advisable to ensure its compatibility with individual health needs.

FLAXSEED (LINUM USITATISSIMUM)

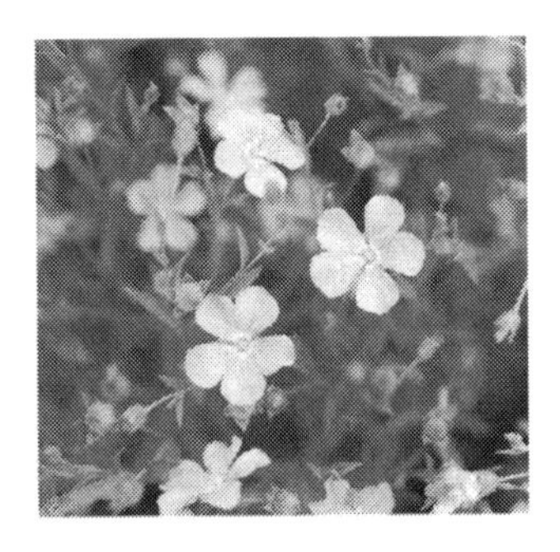

Flaxseed, derived from the plant Linum usitatissimum, is a tiny yet powerful seed known for its nutritional richness and potential health benefits. These seeds have gained popularity for their versatility in culinary use and their significant nutrient content.

Origins and Nutritional Profile:

Cultivated Worldwide: Flaxseed has been cultivated globally for centuries, primarily for its seeds, which are rich in omega-3 fatty acids, lignans, and fiber.

Nutritional Powerhouse: They are renowned for their high content of alpha-linolenic acid (ALA), an omega-3 fatty acid, as well as fiber and lignans, which possess antioxidant properties.

Health Benefits:

Heart Health: The omega-3 fatty acids in flaxseeds are associated with potentially reducing the risk of heart disease and improving cholesterol levels.

Digestive Health: Flaxseeds are a good source of soluble and insoluble fiber, aiding digestion and potentially relieving constipation.

Anti-Inflammatory and Antioxidant Properties: Lignans found in flaxseeds are known for their potential anti-inflammatory and antioxidant effects.

Culinary and Usage:

Flaxseed Oil and Ground Seeds: They can be used in various ways, from adding ground seeds to smoothies, cereals, or baked goods to using flaxseed oil in salad dressings or as a supplement.

Precautions:

Potential Allergies: Some individuals may have allergic reactions to flaxseeds.

Digestive Sensitivities: Starting with small amounts of flaxseeds and gradually increasing intake can prevent digestive discomfort.

Flaxseeds' nutrient richness and potential health benefits make them a popular choice for those seeking natural sources of essential fatty acids and other nutrients. However, as with any new addition to your diet, it's recommended to start with small amounts and consult a healthcare professional, especially if you have specific health conditions or concerns.

FOXGLOVE (DIGITALIS LANATA)

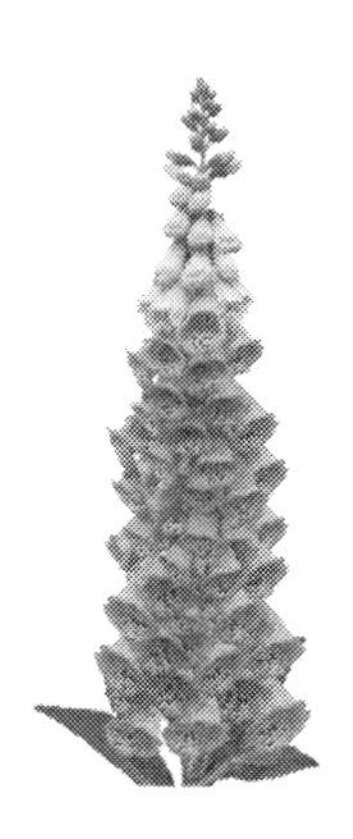

Foxglove, scientifically known as Digitalis lanata, is a strikingly beautiful yet potentially toxic plant with significant historical use in medicine. It's acclaimed for its active compounds and its role in the development of a critical medication.

Origins and Traditional Uses:

Native to Europe: Foxglove is native to Europe and has a long history of use in traditional herbal medicine.

Historical Significance: It was used in traditional medicine, primarily for its potential effects on the heart and as a diuretic.

Medicinal Significance:

Digitalis Compounds: Foxglove contains compounds called cardiac glycosides, particularly digitoxin and digoxin, known for their potential impact on heart function.

Cardiovascular Medicine: Extracts from foxglove plants were historically used and served as the basis for the development of medications to treat heart conditions, particularly congestive heart failure.

Precautions and Toxicity:

Toxicity Risk: All parts of the foxglove plant are considered highly toxic if ingested, potentially leading to severe health issues, including heart irregularities.

Medical Use vs. Home Consumption: Medications derived from foxglove are carefully dosed and prescribed by healthcare professionals. Home consumption or use is strongly discouraged due to the high toxicity levels.

The historical significance of foxglove in the development of heart medications highlights its critical role in modern medicine. However, due to its extreme toxicity, the utilization of foxglove or its derivatives should strictly be under medical supervision, and any use or consumption by individuals without professional guidance is strongly advised against.

GARLIC (ALLIUM SATIVUM)

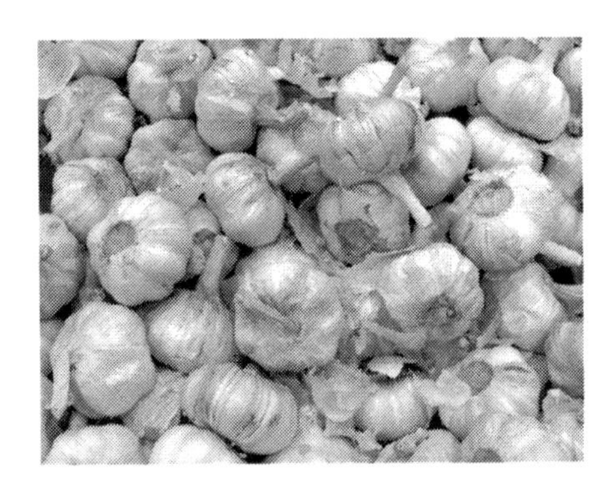

Garlic, scientifically known as Allium sativum, is a pungent and versatile herb renowned for both its culinary uses and potential health benefits. It's celebrated worldwide for its distinct flavor and numerous medicinal properties.

Origins and Nutritional Profile:

Ancient Origins: Garlic has a history dating back thousands of years and is believed to have originated in Central Asia.

Nutrient-Rich: It contains various vitamins and minerals such as manganese, vitamin B6, vitamin C, selenium, and fiber.

Health Benefits:

Heart Health: Garlic is associated with potential benefits for heart health, including reducing cholesterol levels and blood pressure.

Antibacterial and Antiviral Properties: It's believed to have natural antimicrobial properties, potentially aiding in fighting infections.

Antioxidant Effects: Garlic contains antioxidants that combat free radicals and reduce oxidative stress in the body.

Culinary and Usage:

Culinary Applications: Widely used in cooking to add flavor to various dishes, from savory meals to sauces and dressings

Supplements: Garlic supplements are available, often taken for their potential health benefits, particularly for heart health.

Precautions:

Possible Interactions: Garlic supplements might interact with certain medications, especially blood thinners. Consult a healthcare professional if using medications.

Breath and Body Odor: The strong odor of garlic can cause breath and body odor.

Garlic's flavorful addition to cuisines and its potential health benefits make it a popular choice for those seeking natural remedies and flavorful cooking ingredients. However, it's crucial to be aware of potential interactions with medications and to consult a healthcare professional, especially for individuals with specific health conditions or concerns.

GINGER (ZINGIBER OFFICINALE)

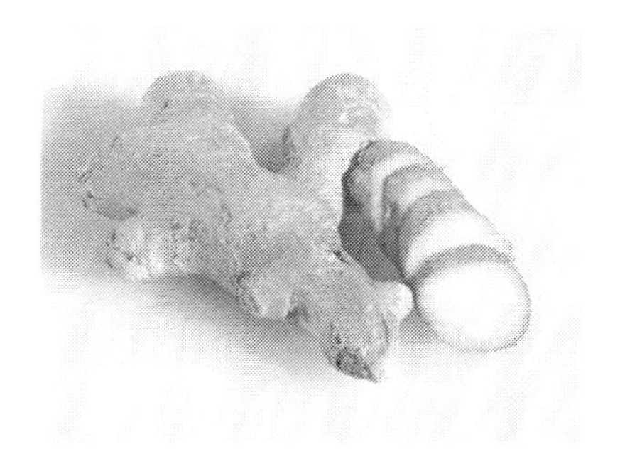

Ginger, scientifically known as Zingiber officinale, is a versatile and widely used herb celebrated for its culinary significance and potential health benefits. Its distinct taste and medicinal properties have made it a favorite in both traditional and modern practices.

Origins and Culinary Use:

Tropical Origins: Ginger originates from Southeast Asia and has been cultivated for over 3,000 years for its culinary and medicinal purposcs.

Flavorful Spice: It's renowned for its unique, pungent flavor and is a staple in various cuisines, adding warmth and depth to dishes.

Health Benefits:

Digestive Aid: Ginger is well-known for its potential to ease digestive discomfort, including nausea, indigestion, and motion sickness.

Anti-inflammatory and Antioxidant Properties: It contains gingerol, a bioactive compound believed to possess anti-inflammatory and antioxidant effects.

Pain Relief: Some studies suggest ginger may help alleviate muscle and joint pain due to its anti-inflammatory properties.

Culinary and Usage:

Culinary Spice: Used fresh, dried, or as a powder in a wide array of dishes, from savory meals to teas and desserts.

Herbal Remedies: Ginger is used in various forms such as teas, tinctures, and capsules for its potential health benefits.

Precautions:

Blood-Thinning Effect: Ginger may act as a blood thinner, so individuals on blood-thinning medications should consult a healthcare professional before using it regularly.

Pregnancy and Nursing: Pregnant or nursing individuals should consult a healthcare provider before using ginger supplements or consuming it in large amounts.

Ginger's distinctive flavor and potential health benefits, particularly in aiding digestion and reducing inflammation, continue to make it a popular choice in both culinary and medicinal practices. However, it's advisable to seek guidance from a healthcare professional, especially for those with specific health conditions or concerns before using it extensively.

GINKGO (GINKGO BILOBA)

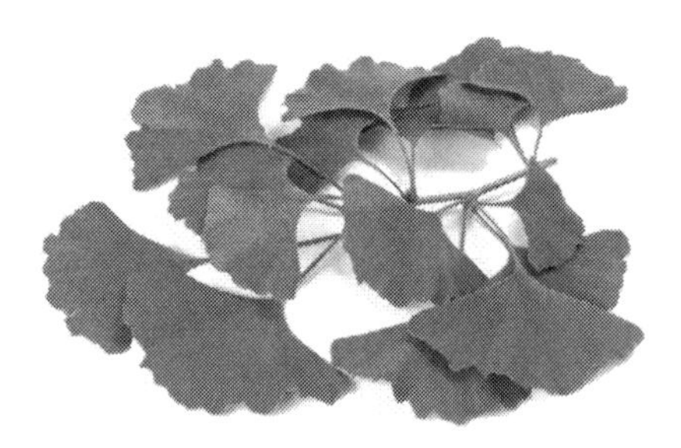

Ginkgo, scientifically known as Ginkgo biloba, is a unique and ancient tree species revered for its potential medicinal properties, particularly in supporting cognitive health and overall well-being.

Origins and Medicinal Significance:

Ancient Roots: Ginkgo is a living fossil, dating back to prehistoric times, and is native to China. It has a rich history in traditional Chinese medicine.

Medicinal Use: Ginkgo leaves and seeds have been used for various medicinal purposes, especially in aiding memory and cognitive function.

Health Benefits:

Cognitive Support: Ginkgo is associated with potential benefits in supporting cognitive function, memory, and mental clarity, especially in aging populations.

Antioxidant Properties: The leaves contain flavonoids and terpenoids, known for their potential antioxidant effects, which help combat free radicals

Circulatory Health: It's believed to improve blood circulation, potentially benefiting various bodily functions.

Modern Usage:

Supplements: Ginkgo supplements, available in various forms like capsules or extracts, are often used for their potential cognitive and overall health benefits.

Precautions:

Interactions with Medications: Ginkgo may interact with certain medications, especially blood thinners. Consult a healthcare professional, especially if taking medications

Allergic Reactions: Some individuals may have sensitivities or allergies to ginkgo.

Ginkgo's historical significance and potential benefits in cognitive health continue to make it a subject of interest for those seeking natural remedies to support memory and overall well-being. However, due to potential interactions and individual health considerations, consulting a healthcare professional before using ginkgo supplements is advisable, particularly for individuals with specific health conditions or concerns.

GINSENG (PANAX SP.)

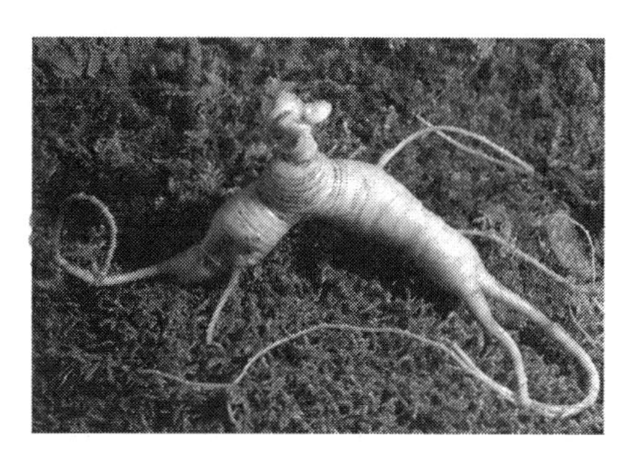

Ginseng, encompassing various species of the Panax genus, is a highly esteemed herb known for its potential health benefits and adaptogenic properties. It's deeply rooted in traditional medicine and is renowned for its contributions to overall wellness.

Origins and Cultural Significance:

Eastern Origins: Ginseng has been used for centuries in traditional Eastern medicine, particularly in China and Korea.

Cultural Importance: It's highly regarded in traditional practices for its potential to improve overall health and vitality.

Health Benefits:

Adaptogenic Properties: Ginseng is believed to possess adaptogenic qualities, potentially aiding the body in adapting to stress and promoting overall well-being.

Energy and Cognitive Function: It's associated with potential benefits in enhancing energy levels, mental alertness, and cognitive function.

Immune Support: Some research suggests it may have immune-boosting effects.

Varieties and Usage:

Asian and American Ginseng: Both are utilized for their potential health benefits, with Asian ginseng (Panax ginseng) often associated with more stimulating effects and American ginseng (Panax quinquefolius) considered milder.

Supplements and Teas: Ginseng is available in various forms, such as capsules, powders, teas, and extracts, taken for its potential health benefits.

Precautions

Interaction with Medications: Ginseng might interact with certain medications. Consult a healthcare professional, especially if on medications.

Individual Sensitivities: Some individuals may experience side effects like insomnia, headaches, or digestive issues.

Ginseng's long-standing reputation for its potential in enhancing vitality and overall health continues to make it a subject of interest for those seeking natural remedies to support well-being. However, due to its potential interactions and individual health considerations, it's advisable to consult a healthcare professional before using ginseng supplements, particularly for those with specific health conditions or concerns.

GOLDENSEAL (HYDRASTIS CANADENSIS)

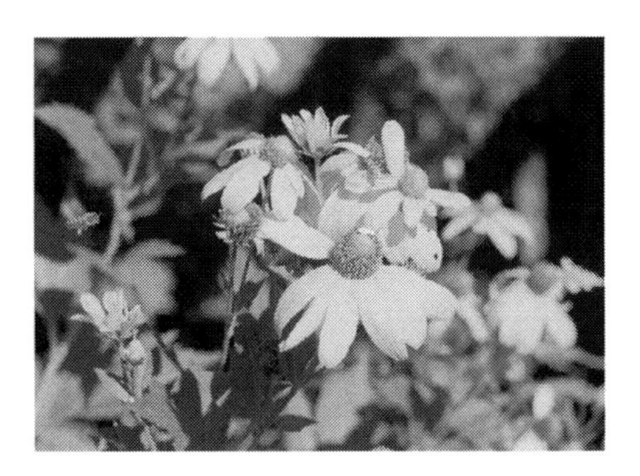

Goldenseal, scientifically known as Hydrastis canadensis, is an herb native to North America highly esteemed for its historical use in traditional medicine and potential health benefits. It's recognized for its active compounds and applications in wellness.

Origins and Traditional Uses:

North American Roots: Goldenseal is indigenous to the eastern United States and Canada, historically used by Native American tribes for various medicinal purposes.

Historical Significance: It was used traditionally for its potential antibacterial and anti-inflammatory properties.

Health Benefits:

Antibacterial Properties: Goldenseal contains berberine, a compound believed to have antimicrobial effects, potentially supporting immune health and fighting infections.

Digestive Aid: It's associated with potential benefits in supporting digestive health, aiding issues like diarrhea and stomach discomfort.

Modern Usage:

Herbal Supplements: Goldenseal supplements, often available in various forms like capsules or tinctures, are used for their potential health benefits.

Precautions:

Pregnancy and Nursing: Pregnant or nursing individuals should consult a healthcare professional before using goldenseal.

Allergic Reactions: Some individuals may have sensitivities or allergies to goldenseal.

Goldenseal's historical use in traditional medicine for its potential antibacterial and digestive support properties continues to spark interest in modern herbal remedies. Yet, due to individual health considerations and its potential interactions, consulting a healthcare professional before using goldenseal supplements is advisable, especially for individuals with specific health conditions or concerns.

GROUND IVY (GLECHOMA HEDERACEA)

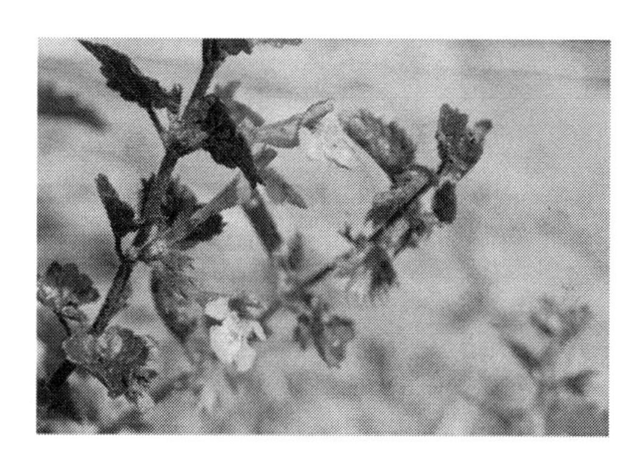

Ground ivy, scientifically known as Glechoma hederacea, is an herbaceous plant appreciated for its historical use in herbal medicine and its wide-ranging properties.

Origins and Traditional Uses:

Native to Europe and Asia: Ground ivy is indigenous to Europe and Asia and has been used historically in herbal medicine.

Medicinal Significance: It was traditionally utilized for various purposes, including as a mild astringent and for its potential to alleviate mild respiratory or digestive discomfort.

Healh Benefits:

Anti-inflammatory and Astringent Properties: Ground ivy is believed to possess mild anti-inflammatory and astringent effects, potentially aiding in minor health issues.

Digestive and Respiratory Support: It was historically used to relieve mild digestive complaints and soothe minor respiratory irritations.

Modern Usage:

Limited Commercial Use: Ground ivy is less commonly used in modern herbal remedies but may still be employed in certain formulations.

Precautions:

Allergic Reactions: Some individuals may have sensitivities or allergies to ground ivy or plants in the mint family, to which it belongs.

Ground ivy's historical significance in traditional medicine and its mild properties for addressing minor health discomfort make it an herb of interest. However, its limited modern usage and individual sensitivities warrant caution, and consulting a healthcare professional before using ground ivy is advisable, especially for individuals with specific health conditions or concerns.

HAWTHORN (CRATAEGUS SP.)

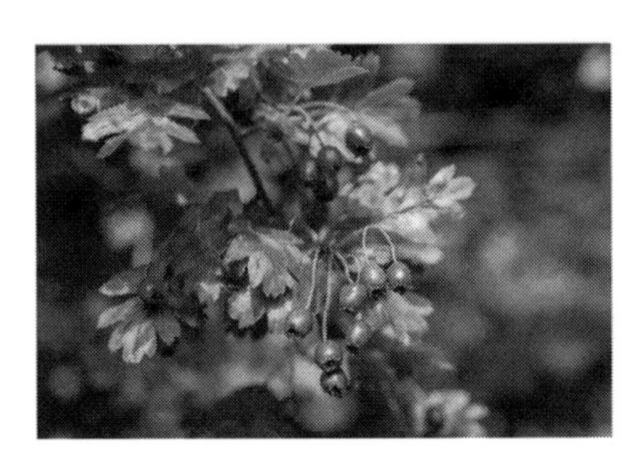

Hawthorn, encompassing various species within the Crataegus genus, is a flowering shrub highly regarded for its historical use in traditional medicine and its potential cardiovascular benefits.

Origins and Traditional Uses:

Global Distribution: Hawthorn is native to many regions worldwide, including North America, Europe, and Asia, and has been used in traditional herbal medicine for centuries.

Historical Significance: It was traditionally used for various cardiovascular conditions, including as a tonic for the heart.

Health Benefits

Heart Health: Hawthorn is associated with potential benefits in supporting heart health, particularly for conditions like congestive heart failure and high blood pressure.

Antioxidant Properties: It contains flavonoids and other compounds believed to have antioxidant effects, combating free radicals in the body.

Modern Usage:

Herbal Supplements: Hawthorn supplements, available in various forms like capsules, extracts, and teas, are often used for their potential cardiovascular benefits.

Precautions:

Interaction with Medications: Hawthorn supplements may interact with certain heart medications. Consult a healthcare professional, especially if on medications.

Allergic Reactions: Some individuals may have sensitivities or allergies to hawthorn.

Hawthorn's historical use in supporting heart health and its potential cardiovascular benefits continue to make it a subject of interest for those exploring natural remedies. However, due to potential interactions and individual health considerations, it's advisable to consult a healthcare professional before using hawthorn supplements, especially for individuals with specific health conditions or concerns.

HERB ROBERT (GERANIUM ROBERTIANUM)

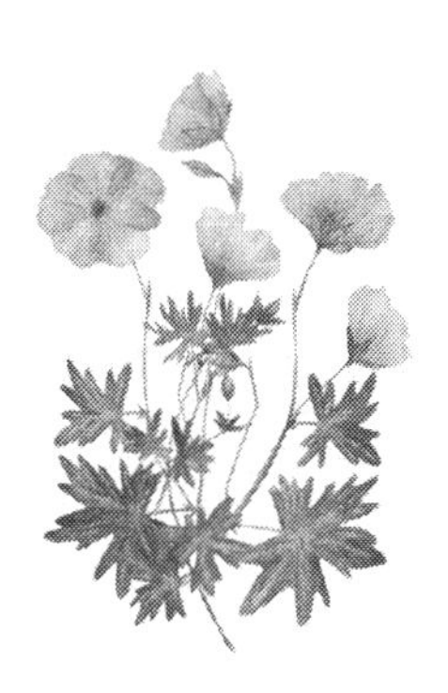

Herb Robert, scientifically known as Geranium robertianum, is a delicate flowering plant celebrated for its historical use in traditional medicine and its potential health properties.

Origins and Traditional Uses:

Native to Europe and Asia: Herb Robert is indigenous to Europe and parts of Asia, where it has been historically utilized in herbal medicine.

Medicinal Significance: It was traditionally used for various health issues, including as a mild astringent and for its potential to address minor ailments.

Health Benefits:

Antioxidant Properties: Herb Robert is believed to contain antioxidants that combat free radicals and support overall health

Potential Anti-inflammatory Effects: It's associated with mild anti-inflammatory properties, aiding in soothing minor discomfort.

Modern Usage:

Limited Commercial Use: While Herb Robert was historically used in herbal remedies, its use in modern practices is less widespread.

Precautions:

Allergic Reactions: Some individuals may have sensitivities or allergies to Herb Robert or plants in the geranium family.

Herb Robert's historical significance in traditional medicine and its mild health properties continue to pique interest. However, its limited modern usage and individual sensitivities warrant caution, and consulting a healthcare professional before using Herb Robert is advisable, especially for individuals with specific health conditions or concerns.

HOREHOUND (MARRUBIUM VULGARE)

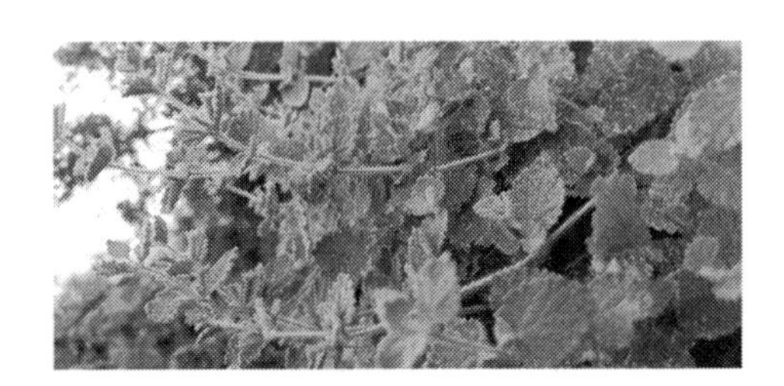

Horehound, scientifically known as Marrubium vulgare, is an herb highly regarded for its historical use in traditional medicine and its potential health benefits, especially in addressing respiratory issues and digestive discomfort.

Origins and Traditional Uses:

Native to Europe and Asia: Horehound is indigenous to Europe and parts of Asia and has been historically utilized in herbal medicine.

Medicinal Significance: It was traditionally used for various purposes, particularly for respiratory ailments and as a mild expectorant.

Health Benefits:

Respiratory Support: Horehound is associated with potential benefits in managing coughs, throat irritation, and other respiratory issues due to its expectorant properties.

Digestive Aid: It was used traditionally to alleviate minor digestive discomfort and as a mild laxative.

Modern Usage:

Herbal Preparations: Horehound is used in various forms such as teas, syrups, lozenges, and extracts for its potential health benefits.

Precautions:

Pregnancy and Nursing: Pregnant or nursing individuals should consult a healthcare professional before using horehound.

Allergic Reactions: Some individuals may have sensitivities or allergies to horehound.

Horehound's historical significance in addressing respiratory and digestive issues continues to make it an herb of interest. However, as with any herbal remedy, consulting a healthcare professional before using horehound, especially for individuals with specific health conditions or concerns, is advisable.

HORSE CHESTNUT (AESCULUS HIPPOCASTANUM)

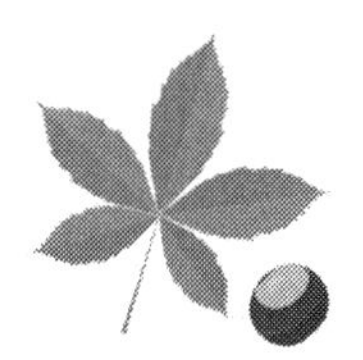

Horse chestnut, scientifically known as Aesculus hippocastanum, is a majestic tree admired for its seeds and bark, often valued for their potential medicinal properties and historical uses.

Origins and Traditional Uses:

Native to the Balkans: Horse chestnut trees are indigenous to the Balkan Peninsula in Southeast Europe.

Medicinal Significance: The seeds and bark were traditionally used in herbal medicine for various conditions, particularly to address issues related to blood circulation and swelling.

Health Benefits:

Vein Health: Horse chestnut seeds are associated with potential benefits for venous conditions, such as chronic venous insufficiency and varicose veins.

Anti-inflammatory Effects: The seeds contain a compound called aescin, believed to have anti-inflammatory properties.

Modern Usage:

Topical Applications: Horse chestnut seed extract is often used in topical creams or ointments for vein-related issues.

Supplements: Horse chestnut supplements are available in various forms, but their use should be under professional guidance due to potential toxicity in raw seeds.

Precautions:

Toxicity of Raw Seeds: Raw horse chestnut seeds are toxic and should not be consumed. Extracts and supplements are processed to remove the toxic component.

Interaction with Medications: Horse chestnut supplements may interact with certain medications. Consult a healthcare professional, especially if on medications.

Horse chestnut's historical significance in addressing venous conditions and its potential anti-inflammatory effects make it a subject of interest in modern herbal remedies. However, it's crucial to use processed forms under professional guidance due to the toxicity of raw seeds and potential interactions, especially for individuals with specific health conditions or concerns.

HOLLYHOCK (ALCEA ROSEA)

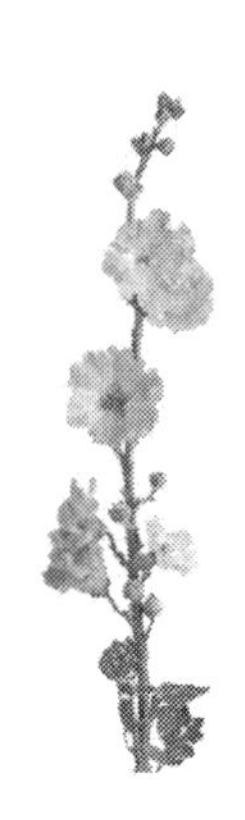

Hollyhock, scientifically known as Alcea rosea, is a flowering plant highly esteemed for its ornamental value in gardens and its historical use in traditional medicine for its potential health properties.

Origins and Traditional Uses:

Cultivated Ornamental Plant: Hollyhock is a flowering plant cultivated primarily for its beauty and tall, showy flowers that come in various colors.

Historical Medicinal Use: It was historically used in traditional herbal medicine, particularly for minor ailments and skin conditions.

Health Benefits:

Mild Medicinal Properties: Hollyhock was traditionally used for its mild expectorant and demulcent properties, potentially aiding in soothing coughs and mild respiratory discomfort.

Topical Applications: The flowers and leaves were utilized in poultices or creams for skin irritations and minor wounds.

Modern Usage:

Limited Medicinal Use: While hollyhock was historically used in herbal remedies, its modern usage is less widespread for medicinal purposes.

Precautions:

Allergic Reactions: Some individuals may have sensitivities or allergies to hollyhock.

Hollyhock's historical significance in traditional medicine, particularly for minor respiratory and skin issues, continues to reflect its mild medicinal properties. However, its limited modern usage and individual sensitivities warrant caution, and consulting a healthcare professional before using hollyhock for medicinal purposes is advisable, especially for individuals with specific health conditions or concerns.

HOPHORNBEAM TREE (OSTRYA VIRGINIANA)

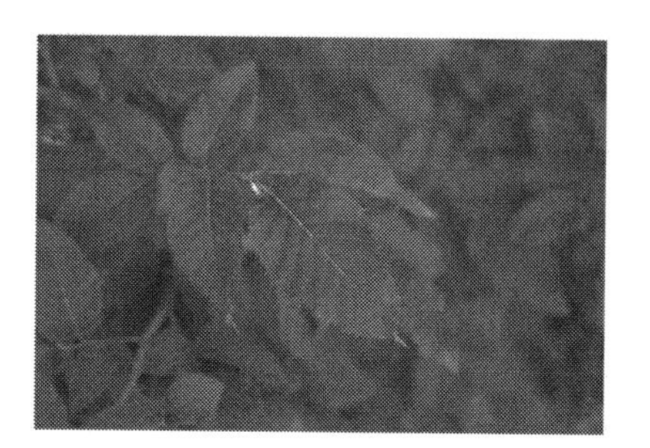

The Hop Hornbeam tree, scientifically known as Ostrya virginiana, is a deciduous tree native to North America. It's characterized by its unique appearance and various practical and ecological attributes.

Tree Characteristics and Appearance:

Native Habitat: The Hop Hornbeam is indigenous to eastern North America and is commonly found in regions across the United States and Canada.

Distinct Bark and Leaves: It features bark that peels or shreds, resembling a hop vine, thus lending it the "Hop" in its name. Its leaves are finely serrated and reminiscent of birch leaves.

Practical and Ecological Uses:

Durable Wood: The tree yields hard and durable wood used in making tool handles, furniture, and other wooden items due to its toughness.

Wildlife Support: Its seeds serve as a food source for various wildlife, contributing to the local ecosystem.

Landscaping and Ornamental Value:

Aesthetic Appeal: The Hop Hornbeam is appreciated in landscaping for its attractive appearance, particularly its bark, and is occasionally used in garden designs.

Moderate Shade Provider: While not primarily planted for shade, it can offer reasonable shade in suitable conditions.

Conservation Significance:

Native Preservation: Conservation efforts often focus on preserving native tree species like the Hop Hornbeam due to their ecological importance and contribution to local biodiversity.

The Hop Hornbeam tree is notable for its durable wood, wildlife support, and ornamental value in landscaping. As a native tree, it plays a role in supporting local ecosystems, making its preservation and conservation significant in maintaining biodiversity.

HORSETAIL (EQUISETUM ARVENSE)

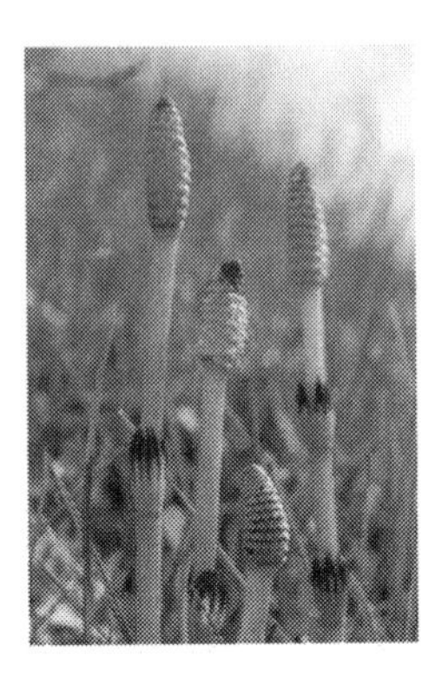

Horsetail, scientifically known as Equisetum arvense, is a unique perennial plant celebrated for its historical medicinal use and its distinct appearance resembling the tail of a horse.

Origins and Traditional Uses:

Global Distribution: Horsetail is found worldwide, primarily in moist environments, and has a long history of use in traditional herbal medicine.

Medicinal Significance: It was traditionally used for various purposes, including as a diuretic and to address mild edema and urinary issues.

Health Benefits:

Silica Content: Horsetail contains silica, which is believed to contribute to its potential benefits for skin, hair, and nail health.

Mild Diuretic and Anti-inflammatory Effects: It's associated with potential mild diuretic properties and mild anti-inflammatory effects.

Modern Usage:

Herbal Supplements: Horsetail supplements are available in various forms, such as capsules or teas, and are used for their potential health benefits.

Precautions:

Thiaminase Content: Prolonged excessive use of horsetail can lead to thiamine deficiency. Controlled consumption is advised.

Pregnancy and Nursing: Pregnant or nursing individuals should consult a healthcare professional before using horsetail.

Horsetail's historical significance in traditional medicine and its potential benefits for skin, hair, and mild urinary issues continue to make it a subject of interest for those exploring natural remedies. However, due to potential interactions and individual health considerations, consulting a healthcare professional before using horsetail supplements is advisable, especially for individuals with specific health conditions or concerns.

HYSSOP (HYSSOPUS OFFICINALIS)

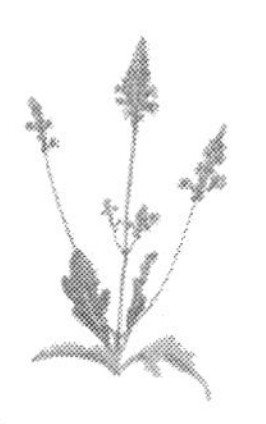

Hyssop, scientifically known as Hyssopus officinalis, is an aromatic herb highly valued for its historical significance in herbal medicine, culinary uses, and ceremonial practices

Origins and Traditional Uses:

Mediterranean Origins: Hyssop is native to the Mediterranean region and has a history dating back to ancient times in various cultures.

Medicinal Significance: It was traditionally used for its potential medicinal properties, particularly in aiding respiratory issues and digestive discomfort.

Health Benefits:

Respiratory Support: Hyssop is associated with potential benefits in addressing coughs, congestion, and mild respiratory discomfort due to its expectorant properties.

Antioxidant and Anti-inflammatory Effects: It contains compounds believed to possess antioxidant and anti-inflammatory properties, contributing to its potential health benefits.

Culinary and Ceremonial Uses:

Culinary Herb: Hyssop's aromatic leaves have been used in culinary applications, particularly in seasoning and flavoring dishes.

Ceremonial and Spiritual Significance: It has been historically used in various cultures for ceremonial and symbolic purposes.

Precautions:

Pregnancy and Nursing: Pregnant or nursing individuals should consult a healthcare professional before using hyssop.

Allergic Reactions: Some individuals may have sensitivities or allergies to hyssop.

Hyssop's historical significance in addressing respiratory and digestive issues, its culinary uses, and its ceremonial value continue to make it an herb of interest. However, consulting a healthcare professional before using hyssop, especially for individuals with specific health conditions or concerns, is advisable due to potential interactions and individual sensitivities.

JASMINE (JASMINUM OFFICINALE)

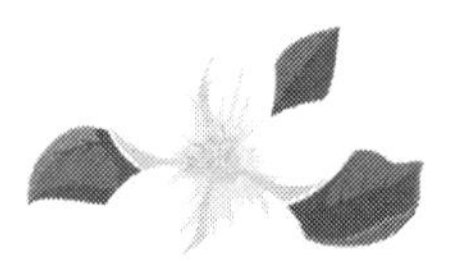

Jasmine, scientifically known as Jasminum officinale, is a fragrant flowering plant revered for its exquisite scent and diverse applications in various cultural and practical contexts.

Origins and Characteristics:

Geographical Roots: Jasmine is native to regions in Asia, particularly China and Persia, but is cultivated in various parts of the world.

Aromatic Flowers: Known for its delicate white flowers that emit a sweet, intoxicating fragrance.

Practical and Cultural Significance:

Fragrance Production: Jasmine's flowers are often used in perfumery and aromatherapy due to their captivating scent.

Tea Production: Jasmine blossoms are sometimes added to teas, infusing them with their aromatic essence.

Symbolism and Traditions: In many cultures, jasmine is associated with love, sensuality, purity, and grace, often used in weddings and ceremonies.

Health Benefits:

Aromatherapy: Jasmine's aroma is believed to have a calming effect, aiding in stress reduction and promoting relaxation.

Skin and Hair Care: Jasmine oil is used in skincare for its potential to nourish and revitalize skin and hair.

Precautions:

Allergies: Some individuals may have sensitivities or allergies to jasmine, particularly when used in essential oils.

Pregnancy and Nursing: Pregnant or nursing individuals should consult a healthcare professional before using jasmine, especially in concentrated forms like essential oils.

Jasmine's captivating fragrance, symbolic significance, and potential health benefits in aromatherapy and skincare continue to make it a beloved and versatile plant. However, for those with specific health conditions or concerns, consulting a healthcare professional before using jasmine, particularly in concentrated forms, is advisable.

JEWELWEED (IMPATIENS CAPENSIS)

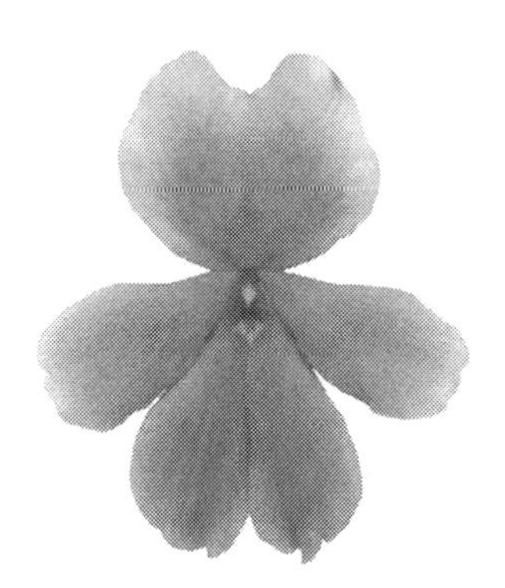

Jewelweed, scientifically known as Impatiens capensis, is a plant native to North America, celebrated for its vibrant appearance and historical use in traditional medicine, particularly for its potential to alleviate skin irritations

Origins and Characteristics:

North American Native: Jewelweed thrives in damp, shaded areas, commonly found near streams or in woodland environments across North America.

Distinct Appearance: Recognizable by its unique trumpet-shaped flowers in shades of orange or yellow and its explosive seed pods that burst upon touch, dispersing seeds.

Traditional Uses:

Skin Remedies: Jewelweed has a historical reputation as a natural remedy for various skin irritations, particularly for rashes and itching, and is often associated with relieving discomfort caused by poison ivy.

Topical Application: Traditionally, the plant's sap was applied topically to affected skin areas for its potential anti-inflammatory and soothing properties.

Precautions:

Limited Scientific Evidence: While it has been used in traditional medicine, scientific research validating its effectiveness is limited.

Possible Allergies: Individuals may exhibit sensitivities or allergies to jewelweed.

Jewelweed's historical use in alleviating skin irritations, notably reactions to poison ivy, continues to draw interest in natural remedies. However, due to the limited scientific evidence and potential individual sensitivities, consulting a healthcare professional before using jewelweed for skin issues is advisable, particularly for individuals with specific health conditions or concerns.

JOE PYE WEED (EUTROCHIUM SP.)

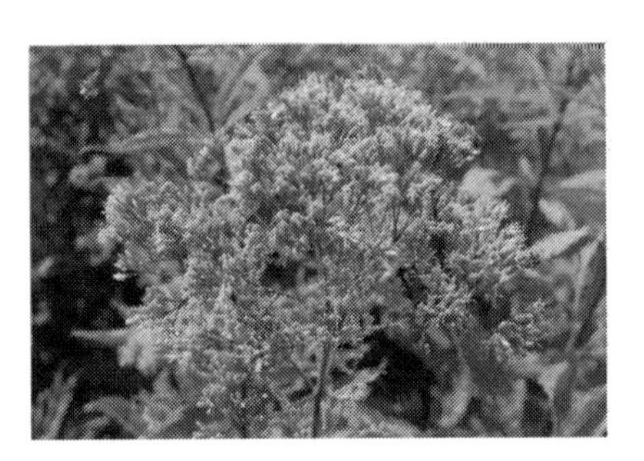

Joe Pye weed, belonging to the Eutrochium genus, is a native North American perennial plant celebrated for its ornamental beauty and historical use in traditional herbal medicine.

Origins and Characteristics:

Native to North America: Joe Pye weed is indigenous to North America and is found in various regions, often in moist or wet habitats.

Flowering Plant: Known for its clusters of pink or purple flowers, which bloom in late summer and attract butterflies and bees.

Traditional Uses:

Traditional Medicine: Historically, various Native American tribes used Joe Pye weed for medicinal purposes, including for conditions such as fevers and as a diuretic.

Potential Healing Properties: Its leaves and flowering tops were used in teas or tinctures for their potential medicinal benefits.

Modern Usage:

Ornamental Landscaping: Beyond its historical medicinal use, it's appreciated for its tall, showy flowers and is often included in gardens for its ornamental value.

Precautions:

Limited Scientific Validation: While it has historical use in traditional medicine, scientific evidence validating its medicinal properties is limited

Possible Allergies: Individuals may have sensitivities or allergies to Joe Pye weed.

Joe Pye weed's historical significance in traditional medicine and its ornamental value continue to capture interest. However, due to the limited scientific validation of its medicinal properties and potential individual sensitivities, consulting a healthcare professional before using Joe Pye weed for health purposes is advisable, especially for individuals with specific health conditions or concerns.

LADY SLIPPER ORCHIDS (CYPRIPEDIUM PARVIFLORUM)

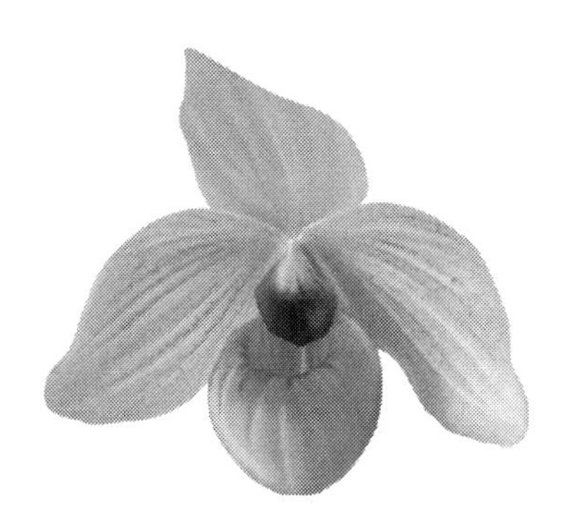

Lady's Slipper Orchids, specifically the Cypripedium parviflorum, are a distinctive group of orchids highly regarded for their unique appearance and occasional use in traditional medicine.

Characteristics and Habitat:

Native Orchids: Lady's Slipper Orchids are native to North America, known for their slipper-shaped pouch-like flowers in various colors.

Habitat: They often grow in wooded areas, preferring moist, shaded environments in regions across North America.

Traditional Uses:

Native American Medicine: Some indigenous tribes historically used these orchids in traditional medicine for various purposes, including as a mild sedative or to address nervousness.

Potential Medicinal Qualities: They were occasionally used for their potential benefits, although scientific validation is limited.

Conservation Status:

Protected Species: Lady's Slipper Orchids are often considered endangered or protected due to their sensitivity to habitat loss and overharvesting.

Precautions:

Conservation Concerns: Due to their protected status and potential ecological significance, caution should be taken in harvesting or using these orchids.

Lady's Slipper Orchids, such as the Cypripedium parviflorum, hold a historical place in traditional medicine among some indigenous groups. However, their protected status and limited scientific validation of their medicinal properties warrant careful consideration. It's crucial to be mindful of conservation efforts and legal regulations regarding these orchids, especially when considering their use for medicinal purposes.

LAVENDER (LAVANDULA ANGUSTIFOLIA)

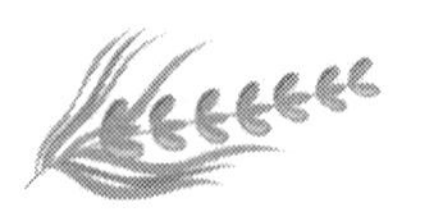

Lavender, scientifically known as Lavandula angustifolia, is a fragrant and versatile herb celebrated for its aromatic qualities, culinary uses, and therapeutic applications.

Origins and Characteristics:

Native to the Mediterranean: Lavender is indigenous to the Mediterranean region but is cultivated and appreciated globally.

Aromatic Features: Known for its sweet, floral scent, lavender boasts slender, aromatic purple-blue flowers.

Practical and Therapeutic Uses:

Aromatherapy: Lavender is a popular choice in aromatherapy for its calming and stress-relieving properties. Its scent is believed to promote relaxation.

Culinary Uses: The flowers are used in culinary applications, lending a delicate floral flavor to dishes, desserts, and beverages.

Therapeutic Benefits: Lavender oil is employed in skincare for its potential to soothe skin irritations and promote relaxation in massage oils.

Health Benefits:

Relaxation and Sleep Aid: Its aroma is associated with reducing stress and promoting better sleep quality.

Skincare: Lavender oil is used in skincare products for its potential anti-inflammatory and soothing effects on the skin.

Precautions:

Allergic Reactions: While rare, some individuals may have sensitivities or allergies to lavender.

Lavender's calming aroma and versatile applications in aromatherapy, culinary uses, and skincare continue to make it a popular herb. Its potential benefits in promoting relaxation and aiding skin health make it a beloved choice, though it's always wise to be cautious regarding individual sensitivities or allergies when using lavender products.

LEMON (CITRUS LIMON)

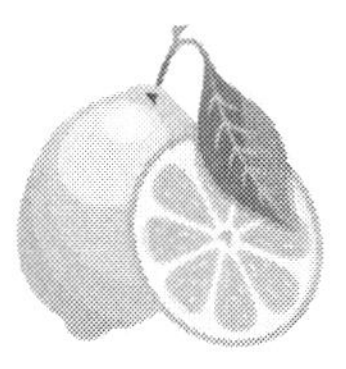

Lemon, scientifically known as Citrus limon, is a citrus fruit renowned for its bright, tangy flavor, versatility in culinary applications, and potential health benefits.

Characteristics and Origins:

Citrus Origin: Lemons are a type of citrus fruit, believed to have originated in South Asia, and are now cultivated in various parts of the world.

Tart Flavor: Lemons are prized for their distinctive sour taste, which adds zing to numerous dishes and beverages.

Culinary Uses:

Cooking and Baking: Lemons are a staple in cooking and baking, used to flavor dishes, dressings, desserts, and more.

Beverages: Lemon juice is a common ingredient in refreshing beverages like lemonade and is used to garnish cocktails and teas.

Health Benefits:

Vitamin C: Lemons are a rich source of vitamin C, known for its potential immune-boosting properties.

Antioxidants: They contain antioxidants that combat free radicals and may contribute to overall health.

Digestive Aid: Lemon juice is sometimes consumed with warm water in the morning and is believed to aid digestion.

Other Uses:

Cleaning: Lemon juice can be used as a natural cleaning agent due to its acidity and fresh scent.

Fragrance: Lemon's pleasant aroma is used in perfumes and household products.

Precautions:

Oral Health: Lemon's acidity can erode tooth enamel, so it's advisable to rinse your mouth with water after consuming lemon juice.

Lemons' versatility in the kitchen and their potential health benefits, particularly due to their high vitamin C content, make them a popular and valuable addition to various aspects of daily life. However, as with any food or ingredient, it's important to use them in moderation and be aware of any potential sensitivities or allergies.

LEMONGRASS (CYMBOPOGON FLEXUOSUS)

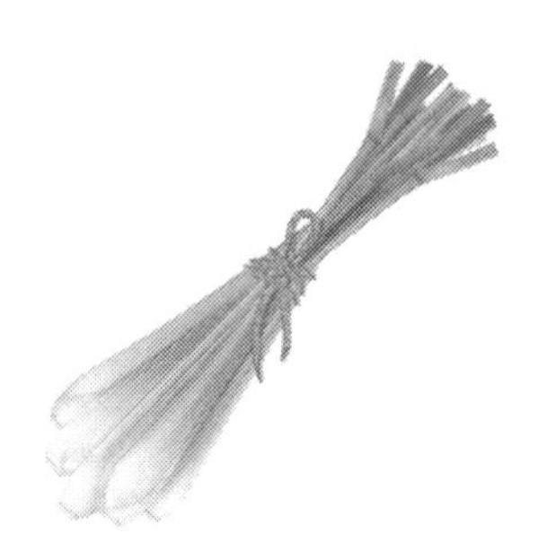

Lemongrass, scientifically known as Cymbopogon flexuosus, is a fragrant herb widely valued for its culinary, medicinal, and aromatic properties.

Characteristics and Origins:

Herbaceous Plant: Lemongrass is an herb known for its strong lemony aroma and is native to tropical regions in Asia.

Citrusy Flavor: It's recognized for its citrus-like flavor, adding a zesty and refreshing taste to dishes.

Culinary Uses:

Flavoring Agent: Often used in Asian cuisine, lemongrass adds a unique citrusy flavor to soups, curries, stir-fries, and teas.

Infusions and Marinades: Its stalks are used whole or crushed to infuse flavors into dishes and marinades.

Health Benefits:

Digestive Health: Lemongrass is believed to aid digestion and alleviate stomach discomfort.

Antioxidant Properties: It contains antioxidants that combat free radicals in the body.

Aromatic and Medicinal Uses:

Aromatherapy: Its scent is used in aromatherapy for its calming and stress-relieving properties.

Traditional Medicine: In some cultures, lemongrass is used for its potential in alleviating cold symptoms and as a mild sedative.

Precautions:

Allergic Reactions: Some individuals may have sensitivities or allergies to lemongrass.

Lemongrass's fresh, citrusy taste and aroma, along with its potential health benefits, make it a versatile herb in both culinary and medicinal practices. However, as with any herb or ingredient, it's important to be aware of individual sensitivities or allergies when using lemongrass.

LEMON BALM (MELISSA OFFICINALIS)

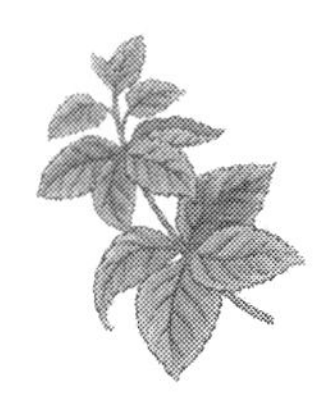

Lemon balm, scientifically known as Melissa officinalis, is a fragrant herb renowned for its lemony scent and a wide range of applications in culinary, medicinal, and aromatic practices.

Characteristics and Origins:

Herbaceous Plant: Lemon balm is a member of the mint family and is native to the eastern Mediterranean region.

Lemon-Like Aroma: It's prized for its strong, citrusy fragrance, similar to that of lemons.

Culinary Uses:

Flavoring: Lemon balm is used in culinary creations, including teas, salads, dressings, and as a seasoning for various dishes, imparting a subtle lemon flavor.

Infusions and Beverages: Its leaves are used to make refreshing herbal teas or infusions.

Medicinal Benefits:

Calming Properties: Lemon balm is associated with mild calming effects and is sometimes used to ease stress and promote relaxation.

Digestive Support: It's believed to aid in digestive discomfort and soothe mild stomach issues.

Aromatic and Herbal Uses:

Aromatherapy: Lemon balm's pleasant scent is used in aromatherapy for its potential calming and mood-enhancing effects.

Herbal Remedies: Traditionally, it's been used in herbal medicine for various minor ailments, including cold sores.

Precautions:

Allergies: Some individuals may have sensitivities or allergies to lemon balm.

Lemon balm's delightful lemony aroma, culinary versatility, and potential calming properties make it a popular herb in various applications. However, it's important to be mindful of individual sensitivities or allergies when using lemon balm for culinary or medicinal purposes.

LICORICE ROOT (GLYCYRRHIZA GLABRA)

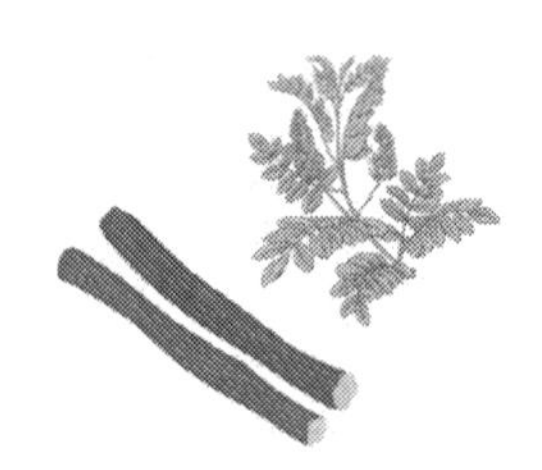

Licorice root, scientifically known as Glycyrrhiza glabra, is a herb highly esteemed for its distinct sweet flavor and diverse applications in traditional medicine, culinary uses, and confectionery.

Characteristics and Origins:

Herbaceous Plant: Licorice root is a perennial legume native to Southern Europe and parts of Asia.

Distinct Flavor: Known for its sweet and slightly woody taste, lending itself to a wide array of culinary and medicinal applications.

Culinary Uses:

Flavoring Agent: Used in cooking and confectionery to add a unique sweet taste, commonly found in candies, teas, and beverages.

Cultural Foods: Utilized in various traditional dishes and sweets across different cultures.

Medicinal Benefits:

Throat Soothing: Licorice root is often used to alleviate sore throats and coughs due to its potential soothing properties.

Digestive Aid: It's believed to aid in digestive discomfort and is sometimes used to support gastrointestinal health.

Health Precautions:

Blood Pressure: Long-term or excessive consumption may affect blood pressure due to compounds that mimic the effects of hormones.

Pregnancy and Health Conditions: Pregnant or nursing individuals and those with health conditions should use licorice root cautiously and consult a healthcare professional.

Herbal and Cultural Significance:

Traditional Medicine: In herbal medicine, it's employed for various purposes, including its potential for soothing respiratory and gastrointestinal issues.

Cultural Traditions: Licorice root is part of cultural traditions in both medicine and culinary practices across the globe.

Licorice root's unique sweet taste and potential health benefits make it a valuable ingredient in both culinary delights and traditional medicine. However, due to its effect on blood pressure and potential interactions, it's wise to use it in moderation and consult a healthcare professional, especially for individuals with specific health conditions or concerns.

LINDEN (TILIA SP.)

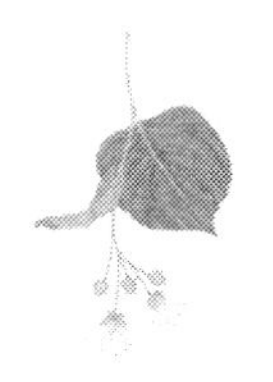

Linden, belonging to the Tilia genus, comprises several species of trees valued for their fragrant blossoms, which have been historically used for various purposes.

Characteristics and Origins:

Deciduous Trees: The Linden trees, also known as lime trees, produce fragrant and nectar-rich flowers.

Native to Europe: Commonly found in Europe and parts of North America, these trees are admired for their beauty and sweet-smelling blooms.

Culinary and Herbal Uses:

Teas and Infusions: The flowers are often used in herbal teas known for their calming and relaxing properties.

Flavoring: Linden flowers may be used as a flavoring agent in various culinary creations.

Medicinal Applications:

Relaxation and Sleep: Linden tea is believed to promote relaxation and aid in sleeping due to its mild sedative properties.

Respiratory Support: It's occasionally used to address minor respiratory discomfort.

Other Uses:

Honey Production: Linden trees produce nectar that bees use to create a light, fragrant honey highly esteemed for its flavor.

Woodwork: The wood of Linden trees is soft and easily worked, suitable for carving and used in certain crafts.

Precautions:

Allergic Reactions: Some individuals may have sensitivities or allergies to Linden flowers or products.

Linden's fragrant blossoms and their historical use in teas for relaxation and potential medicinal properties continue to make them a subject of interest. Yet, as with any natural remedy, it's essential to be aware of individual sensitivities or allergies when using Linden products.

LOTUS (NELUMBO NUCIFERA)

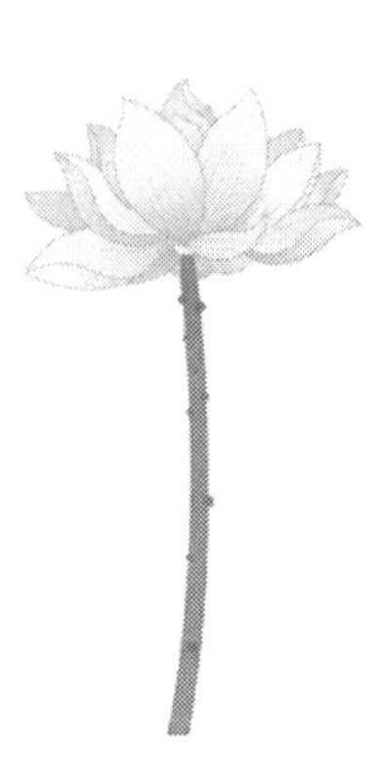

The lotus, scientifically known as Nelumbo nucifera, is an aquatic plant celebrated for its cultural significance, ornamental beauty, and potential medicinal applications.

Characteristics and Origins:

Aquatic Plant: Lotus plants are often found in ponds, lakes, and other shallow water bodies.

Cultural Significance: Revered in various cultures for its symbolic value, representing purity, enlightenment, and rebirth.

Ornamental Uses:

Aesthetic Beauty: The lotus is admired for its striking, large, and fragrant flowers that come in various colors, typically pink or white.

Landscaping: Often used decoratively in ponds or water gardens for its aesthetic appeal.

Medicinal Applications:

Traditional Medicine: Used in traditional medicine for various purposes, including digestive support and potential soothing effects.

Potential Health Benefits: Associated with properties that may aid in digestion and alleviate mild gastrointestinal discomfort.

Culinary Uses:

Edible Parts: Some parts of the lotus, like the seeds and rhizomes, are used in culinary dishes in certain cultures.

Nutritional Value: Lotus seeds are rich in nutrients and are used in both savory and sweet dishes.

Precautions:

Allergies: Individuals may have sensitivities or allergies to lotus or its parts.

Lotus' symbolic significance, ornamental beauty, and potential medicinal and culinary applications continue to make it a plant of interest. However, as with any plant or natural remedy, it's essential to be aware of individual sensitivities or allergies when using lotus in any form.

BOOK 5: MEDICINAL PLANT TO M FROM Z

MAPLE TREE (ACER SP.)

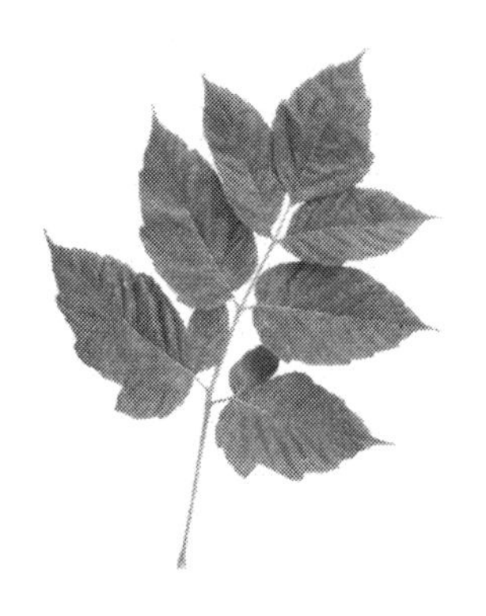

Maple trees, belonging to the Acer genus, are renowned for their diverse species, distinctive leaves, and the production of maple syrup.

Characteristics and Origins:

Diverse Genus: The Acer genus comprises various species of deciduous trees, known for their lobed leaves and beautiful foliage.

Global Distribution: Maple trees are native to Asia, Europe, and North America, and are prized for their ornamental and economic value.

Culinary Significance:

Maple Syrup: Extracted from the sap of certain maple species, especially in North America, it's a sweet syrup used as a topping or sweetener.

Edible Seeds: Some maple species have seeds, known as "helicopter seeds," that are edible and consumed in some cultures.

Wood and Ornamental Uses:

Woodwork: Maple wood is highly valued for its strength and used in furniture, flooring, and musical instruments.

Landscaping: Maple trees are planted for their beautiful foliage and are widely used in landscaping and as ornamental trees.

Medicinal and Cultural Significance:

Traditional Medicine: Some cultures use parts of the maple tree in herbal remedies for various purposes.

Symbolism: In several cultures, the maple tree holds symbolic value, representing strength, endurance, and generosity.

Precautions:

Allergies: Individuals may have sensitivities or allergies to certain parts of the maple tree, including the pollen or sap.

Maple trees' broad applications in producing syrup, woodwork, landscaping, and their cultural significance make them a valuable and esteemed tree. However, being mindful of individual sensitivities or allergies to its parts, especially in medicinal uses or interactions, is crucial when engaging with the maple tree.

MARSHMALLOW (ALTHAEA OFFICINALIS)

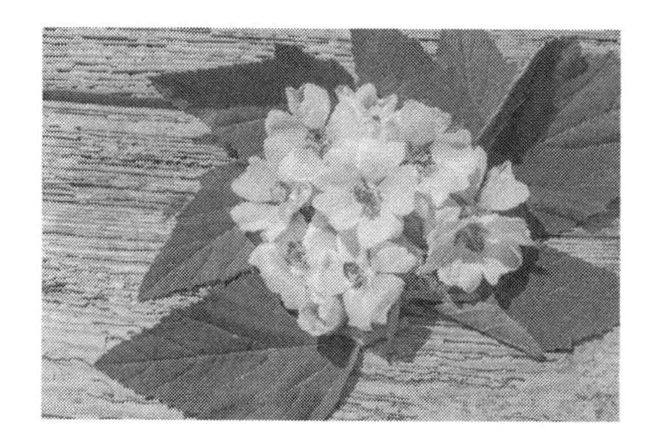

Marshmallow, scientifically known as Althaea officinalis, is an herb widely recognized for its historical use in traditional medicine, particularly for its potential soothing properties.

Origins and Characteristics:

Herbaceous Plant: Marshmallow is a perennial herb native to Europe and parts of Asia, found in damp, marshy areas.

Root and Leaves: Its roots and leaves are the parts commonly used for various purposes.

Medicinal Uses:

Respiratory Support: Marshmallow is believed to aid in addressing minor respiratory discomfort, such as soothing a cough or throat irritation.

Digestive Health: It's used to potentially alleviate mild stomach issues and to support gastrointestinal health.

External Applications:

Skin Soothing: Externally, marshmallow is used for its potential to soothe skin irritations and mild wounds.

Topical Preparations: Its extracts are sometimes included in ointments or creams for skin health.

Culinary and Historical Significance:

Culinary Ingredient: Historically, marshmallow sap was used to make a confectionery treat, although the modern version differs significantly.

Traditional Medicine: Marshmallow has been used for centuries in traditional herbal medicine.

Precautions:

Allergic Reactions: Some individuals may have sensitivities or allergies to marshmallow or its components.

Marshmallow's potential soothing properties for respiratory, digestive, and skin issues have contributed to its historical use in traditional medicine. However, as with any herb or remedy, being aware of individual sensitivities or allergies when using marshmallow for medicinal purposes is important.

MILK THISTLE (SILYBUM MARIANUM)

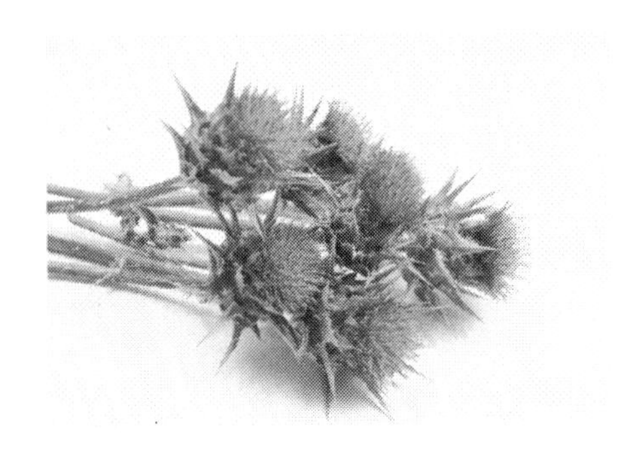

Milk thistle, scientifically known as Silybum marianum, is a flowering herb celebrated for its potential medicinal properties and historical use in promoting liver health.

Characteristics and Origins:

Flowering Herb: Milk thistle is recognized for its purple flowered heads and spiny leaves, commonly found in Mediterranean regions and now cultivated worldwide.

Medicinal Compounds: The seeds of milk thistle contain silymarin, a compound believed to offer various health benefits.

Medicinal Uses:

Liver Support: Silymarin is thought to have protective effects on the liver, potentially aiding in liver health and supporting its detoxification processes.

Antioxidant Properties: It's known for its potential antioxidant effects, combating free radicals in the body.

Health Benefits:

Digestive Support: Milk thistle may aid in mild digestive discomfort, promoting digestive health.

Skin Health: It's occasionally used in skincare products for its potential to promote skin health.

Hrbal Preparations:

Supplements: Milk thistle is available in various forms, including capsules and extracts, for its potential health benefits.

Teas and Tinctures: Herbal teas and tinctures are made from milk thistle seeds and used in natural remedies.

Precautions:

Potential Interactions: It's advisable to consult a healthcare professional before using milk thistle, especially if taking medications or for individuals with specific health conditions.

Milk thistle's potential benefits for liver health and its antioxidant properties have contributed to its widespread use in natural remedies. As with any supplement or herbal remedy, consulting a healthcare professional before use is recommended, particularly for individuals with specific health concerns or those taking medications.

MINT (MENTHA SP.)

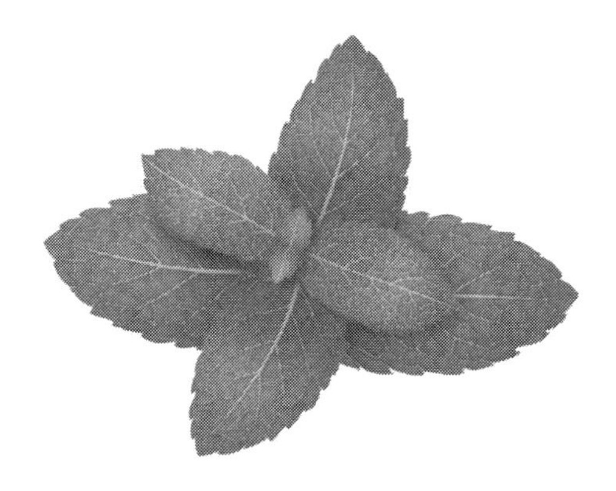

Mint, belonging to the Mentha genus, comprises various aromatic herbs appreciated for their refreshing scent and diverse culinary, medicinal, and aromatic applications.

Characteristics and Origins:

Aromatic Herbs: Mint includes different species like peppermint and spearmint, known for their distinctive aroma and taste.

Global Distribution: Found across the globe, mint thrives in various climates and is cultivated in both culinary and medicinal contexts.

Culinary Uses:Flavoring: Mint is widely used to add a fresh taste to various dishes, beverages, salads, and desserts.

Teas and Infusions: Its leaves are steeped in hot water to create mint teas, known for their refreshing taste.

Medicinal Applications:

Digestive Support: Mint is believed to aid in digestion and is used to address mild stomach discomfort.

Respiratory Benefits: Menthol in mint provides a cooling sensation and may help ease breathing.

Aromatic and Culinary Significance:

Aromatherapy: Mint's scent is used in aromatherapy for its potential to uplift mood and promote alertness.

Cultural Significance: Mint has cultural significance in various traditions and is valued for its versatility in both sweet and savory dishes.

Precautions:

Potential Allergies: Some individuals may have sensitivities or allergies to mint.

Mint's versatility in culinary, medicinal, and aromatic applications, along with its refreshing flavor and aroma, make it a widely cherished herb. However, being mindful of individual sensitivities or allergies to mint is essential when using it in various forms.

MOTHERWORT (LEONURUS CARDIACA)

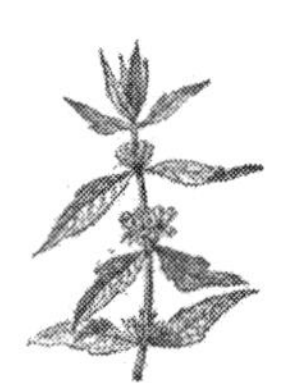

Motherwort, scientifically known as Leonurus cardiaca, is an herb highly valued in traditional medicine for its potential medicinal properties and historical use in supporting various aspects of health.

Origins and Characteristics:

Herbaceous Plant: Motherwort is a perennial herb native to Europe and Asia, now cultivated in various regions across the globe.

Distinctive Leaves: Its leaves are deeply lobed and have a serrated edge, and it produces small pink or white flowers.

Medicinal Uses:

Cardiovascular Support: Motherwort is known for its potential to support heart health and aid in mild heart-related discomfort.

Calming Properties: It's often used for its potential to promote relaxation and ease nervousness or stress.

Women's Health:

Menstrual Support: Motherwort has been historically used to address menstrual discomfort and support women's health.

Labor and Childbirth: In some traditional practices, it's believed to aid in labor and childbirth.

Preparations:

Teas and Tinctures: Motherwort is commonly prepared as teas or tinctures to harness its potential benefits.

Herbal Supplements: It's available in various forms, including capsules and liquid extracts.

Precautions:

Pregnancy: Pregnant individuals should use motherwort cautiously and only under the guidance of a healthcare professional due to its historical use in childbirth-related practices.

Motherwort's potential to support heart health, ease stress, and its historical application in women's health make it a valuable herb in traditional medicine. However, caution and consultation with a healthcare professional, especially for pregnant individuals, are advised before using motherwort for specific health concerns.

MUGWORT (ARTEMISIA VULGARIS)

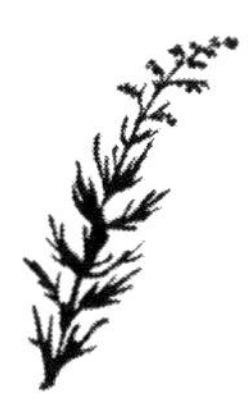

Mugwort, scientifically known as Artemisia vulgaris, is an herb with a rich history in traditional medicine, culinary uses, and cultural practices

Characteristics and Origins:

Aromatic Herb: Mugwort is a perennial plant known for its slightly bitter taste and strong aroma.

Global Distribution: Found in many parts of the world, Mugwort thrives in various climates and is cultivated for multiple purposes.

Medicinal and Culinary Uses:

Traditional Medicine: Mugwort has been used in traditional herbal medicine for a wide range of health issues, from digestion to promoting menstruation.

Culinary Applications: In some cultures, its leaves are used sparingly as a seasoning or to flavor certain dishes.

Ritual and Cultural Significance:

Cultural Practices: Mugwort has been used in various cultural and spiritual practices for its supposed cleansing and protective properties.

Traditional Remedies: It's believed to promote dreams and aid in sleep in some traditional practices.

Precautions:

Allergic Reactions: Some individuals may have sensitivities or allergies to Mugwort.

Mugwort's diverse uses in traditional medicine, culinary practices, and cultural traditions make it a herb of significant interest. However, due to potential individual sensitivities or allergies, cautious use is advisable, especially in medicinal or culinary applications.

MULLEIN (VERBASCUM THAPSUS)

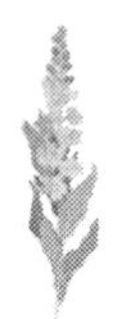

Mullein, scientifically known as Verbascum thapsus, is a biennial herb highly regarded for its historical use in herbal medicine and various practical applications.

Characteristics and Origins:

Herbaceous Plant: Mullein is recognized by its tall stature, soft fuzzy leaves, and distinctive flowering stalks.

Native Origins: Originally native to Europe and Asia, it's now found in various regions globally.

Medicinal Uses:

Respiratory Support: Mullein has been historically used to address respiratory discomfort, such as coughs or mild lung issues.

Topical Remedies: Its leaves are occasionally used in oils or ointments for skin conditions or ear discomfort.

Practical Applications:

Candlewicks: Dried mullein stems were traditionally used as candlewicks due to their absorbent nature.

Landscaping: Mullein's tall, striking appearance often makes it a choice for garden or landscaping aesthetics.

Preparations:

Teas and Tinctures: Mullein leaves are used to create herbal teas or tinctures to harness its potential health benefits.

Herbal Supplements: It's available in various forms, such as capsules or liquid extracts.

Precautions:

Allergies: Some individuals may have sensitivities or allergies to mullein.

Mullein's historical significance in herbal remedies, practical applications, and its distinctive appearance continue to make it a herb of interest. However, as with any herb, it's essential to be mindful of individual sensitivities or allergies when using mullein for medicinal or other purposes.

NETTLE, STINGING (URTICA DIOICA)

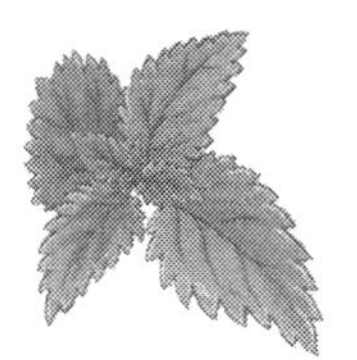

Stinging nettle, scientifically known as Urtica dioica, is a perennial herb known for its stinging hairs on its leaves and stems, and it's valued for its diverse culinary, medicinal, and even textile uses.

Characteristics and Origins:

Stinging Hairs: The hairs on the leaves and stems release chemicals that can cause skin irritation upon contact.

Global Distribution: Found in various regions worldwide, including North America, Europe, Asia, and Africa.

Culinary and Nutritional Uses:

Edible Leaves: Despite the stinging hairs, when cooked or dried, the leaves are used in teas, soups, or as a leafy green vegetable.

Nutritional Value: Rich in vitamins, minerals, and antioxidants, nettles are valued for their nutritional content.

Medicinal Applications:

Anti-inflammatory: Nettles are used in traditional herbal medicine for their potential anti-inflammatory properties.

Diuretic Effects: They're believed to have mild diuretic effects, aiding in eliminating excess water from the body.

Textile and Practical Uses

Fiber Production: Historically, nettles were used to produce a strong and durable fiber for textiles.

Gardening and Composting: Nettle plants are occasionally used in gardening or composting for their nutrient-rich properties.

Precautions:

Skin Irritation: The stinging hairs can cause skin irritation upon contact, so handling nettles with care is advised. Stinging nettles' multifaceted uses in culinary, medicinal, and textile applications, despite their stinging nature, make them a versatile and valuable herb. When using nettles for culinary or medicinal purposes, precautions to avoid skin irritation from the stinging hairs are crucial.

OREGANO (ORIGANUM VULGARE)

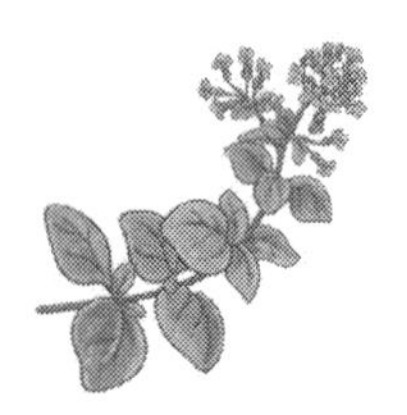

Oregano, scientifically known as Origanum vulgare, is a flavorful herb renowned for its culinary uses, aromatic properties, and potential health benefits.

Origins and Characteristics:

Aromatic Herb: Oregano is a perennial herb with a strong fragrance and a bold flavor, commonly associated with Mediterranean cuisine.

Global Cultivation: It's found in various regions worldwide and is a popular herb in many culinary traditions.

Culinary Uses

Flavorful Seasoning: Oregano is a staple herb in Italian, Mediterranean, and Mexican cuisines, adding depth to various dishes.

Pizza and Pasta: Widely used as a key ingredient in pizza, pasta sauces, and marinades.

Medicinal Applications:

Potential Antioxidant: Oregano contains compounds that have potential antioxidant properties.

Traditional Medicine: In some cultures, it's used for its potential digestive and respiratory health benefits.

Aromatic Significance:

Aromatherapy: Oregano's scent is used in aromatherapy for its invigorating and refreshing qualities.

Essential Oils: Oregano oil is extracted for its potential health benefits and aromatic uses.

Precautions:

Potency: Oregano can be potent, so moderate use is recommended in culinary and medicinal applications.

Oregano's rich flavor, aromatic properties, and potential health benefits have solidified its place as a beloved herb in culinary creations and traditional medicine. However, its potency calls for moderate use, especially in concentrated forms like essential oils, to avoid overwhelming flavors or potential adverse effects.

PASSIONFLOWER (PASSIFLORA SP.)

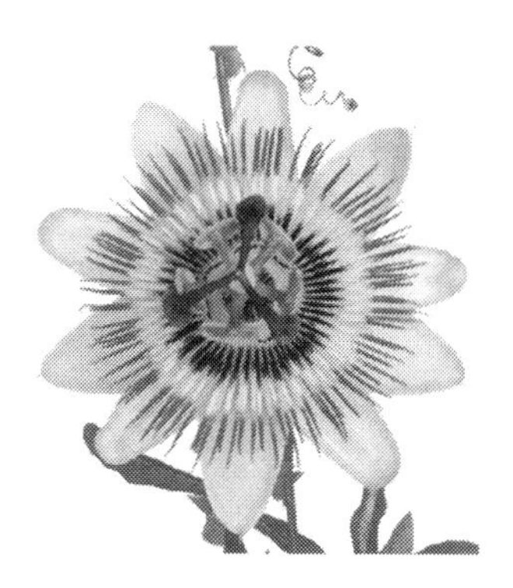

Passionflower, belonging to the Passiflora genus, is a stunning flowering plant admired for its unique appearance and potential medicinal applications.

Characteristics and Origins:

Exotic Flowers: Known for its vibrant and intricate flowers, which vary in colors and sizes, often symbolic due to their unique structure.

Global Distribution: Found in various regions, predominantly in tropical and subtropical climates.

Medicinal Uses:

Calming Effects: Passionflower is used for its potential to alleviate anxiety, aid in relaxation, and promote better sleep.

Traditional Medicine: It's employed in herbal medicine for its potential stress-reducing and calming properties.

Aromatic and Culinary Applications:

Aromatherapy: Its mild fragrance is sometimes used in aromatherapy for its calming effects.

Limited Culinary Use: In some regions, certain species of passionflower may be used in beverages or desserts.

Preparations and Supplements:

Herbal Teas: Passionflower is used in herbal teas or infusions to harness its potential calming effects.

Supplements: Extracts and capsules are available for individuals seeking its potential health benefits.

Precautions:

Pregnancy and Medication: Pregnant or nursing individuals and those taking medications should consult a healthcare professional before using passionflower.

Passionflower's captivating appearance and potential calming effects have made it a subject of interest in traditional medicine and wellness practices. However, it's essential to approach its use cautiously, particularly in the case of pregnancy, nursing, or medication, seeking guidance from a healthcare professional for safe and suitable usage.

PINE TREE (PINUS SP.)

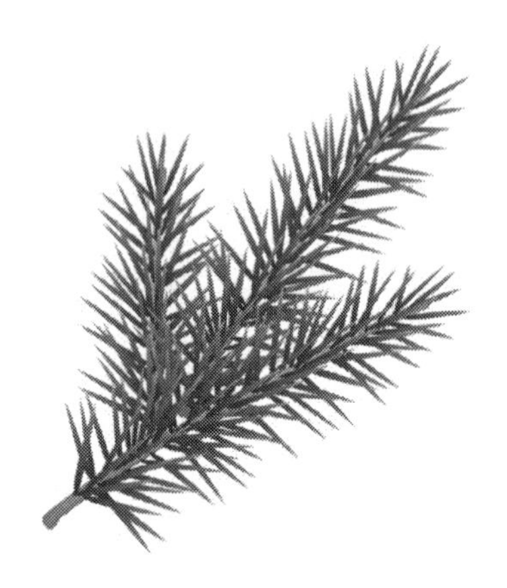

Pine trees, belonging to the Pinus genus, are a diverse group of evergreen conifers recognized for their longevity, distinct needles, and versatile uses.

Characteristics and Origins:

Evergreen Conifers: Pine trees retain their needles year-round, offering a constant green hue.

Global Distribution: Found across various continents, thriving in diverse climates from cold to temperate regions.

Practical Applications:

Lumber and Woodwork: Highly valued for their wood, used in construction, furniture, and paper production.

Resin and Turpentine: Pine resin is used for various products, including varnishes and turpentine.

Culinary and Aromatic Uses:

Pine Nuts: Pine trees produce edible pine nuts used in various cuisines and dishes.

Aromatherapy: Pine's fresh scent is utilized in aromatherapy for its potential calming effects.

Environmental and Landscaping Significance:

Ecosystem Contribution: Pine trees play a crucial role in ecosystems, providing habitats and stabilizing soil.

Landscaping and Ornamental Use: They're planted for their aesthetics and often used in landscaping.

Precautions:

Allergies: Some individuals may have sensitivities or allergies to pine pollen or resin.

Pine trees' multifaceted uses, from their wood and resin to culinary and aromatic applications, along with their environmental significance, make them an essential part of various industries and ecosystems. However, individual allergies or sensitivities to certain pine products should be taken into consideration when using or interacting with them.

PINEAPPLE WEED (MATRICARIA DISCOIDEA)

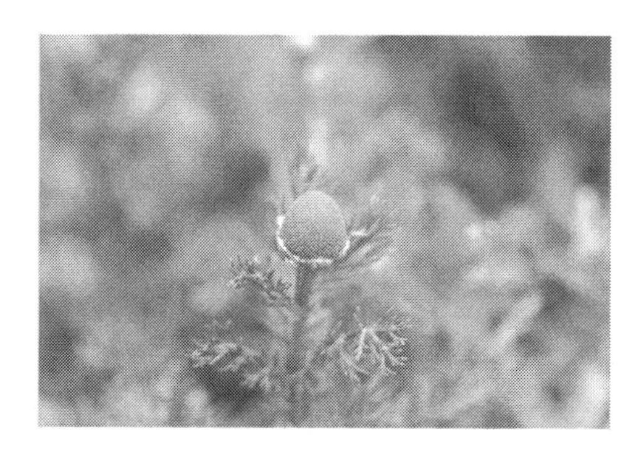

Pineapple weed, scientifically known as Matricaria discoidea, is a lesser-known herbaceous plant with small, daisy-like flowers and distinctive pineapple-like scent, valued for its diverse uses and aromatic qualities.

Characteristics and Origins:

Resemblance and Scent: Its flower heads resemble miniature daisies and emit a sweet, pineapple-like aroma when crushed.

Global Distribution: Found in various regions, especially in disturbed soils, along roadsides, and in open areas.

Culinary and Medicinal Uses:

Culinary Application: Used in herbal teas or infusions, or as a flavoring agent in culinary dishes due to its pleasant scent.

Traditional Medicine: Occasionally used in traditional herbal medicine for minor stomach discomfort.

Aromatic and Therapeutic Applications:

Aromatherapy: The pineapple-like scent is used for its potential calming and soothing effects in aromatherapy.

Relaxation and Stress Relief: It's believed to offer mild calming properties when inhaled.

Precautions:

Allergies: Some individuals may have sensitivities or allergies to certain plant species, including pineapple weed.

Pineapple weed's delightful pineapple scent, along with its potential culinary, aromatic, and mild medicinal applications, makes it an intriguing herb. However, as with any plant or herb, being mindful of potential allergies or sensitivities is important when using or interacting with pineapple weed.

PLANTAIN (PLANTAGO LANCEOLATA)

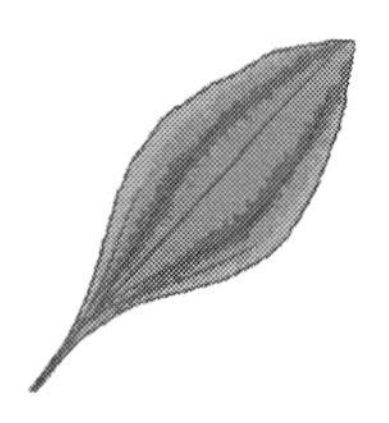

Plantain, scientifically known as Plantago lanceolata, is a common herbaceous plant recognized for its broad leaves and various traditional medicinal applications.

Characteristics and Origins:

Leaf Appearance: Plantain's leaves are broad, oval, and ribbed, often found close to the ground.

Global Distribution: Found in many regions, typically growing in lawns, gardens, and disturbed soils.

Medicinal Uses:

Wound Healing: Plantain is used topically to aid in healing minor cuts, insect bites, and skin irritations.

Respiratory Support: In traditional herbal medicine, it's used for potential mild respiratory discomfort.

Culinary and Nutritional Applications:

Limited Culinary Use: Young leaves are occasionally used in salads or cooked as a vegetable.

Nutritional Content: Rich in vitamins and minerals, it's valued for its nutritional profile.

Practical Uses:

Natural Remedy: It's a traditional remedy used in various cultures for its potential healing properties

Lawn and Garden Weed: Despite its beneficial properties, it's often considered a weed in lawns and gardens.

Precautions:

Allergic Reactions: Some individuals may have sensitivities or allergies to plantain.

Plantain's historical use in healing minor skin irritations and potential medicinal benefits make it a noteworthy herb. However, ensuring caution with potential allergies or sensitivities to plantain is essential when using it for medicinal purposes or handling it in natural remedies.

QUEEN ANNE'S LACE (DAUCUS CAROTA)

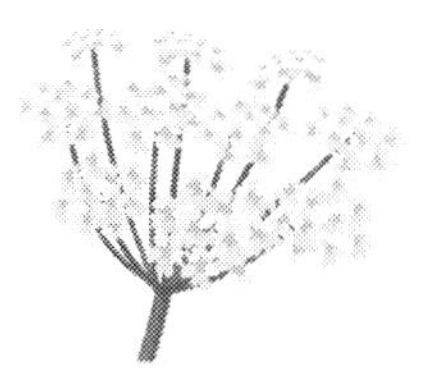

Queen Anne's lace, scientifically known as Daucus carota, is a flowering plant with delicate, lacy white flowers, recognized for its beauty and diverse applications.

Characteristics and Origins:

Flower Appearance: Its distinctive white flower clusters resemble lace, with a single purple floret at the center.

Global Distribution: Found in various regions, commonly along roadsides, meadows, and fields.

Culinary and Medicinal Uses:

Culinary Applications: Its roots are related to the domestic carrot and are used in some culinary traditions.

Traditional Medicine: In some cultures, it's used for potential medicinal purposes, although not as extensively as its domesticated carrot counterpart.

Aesthetic and Environmental Significance:

Ornamental Plant: Queen Anne's lace is admired for its delicate beauty and is sometimes used in floral arrangements.

Ecological Importance: It serves as a source of nectar for pollinators and supports biodiversity.

Precautions:

Identification: Caution is advised when foraging for wild plants, as Queen Anne's lace can resemble other plants, and misidentification may lead to consumption of toxic lookalikes.

Queen Anne's lace, with its delicate, lacy flowers and varied uses from culinary to ornamental, holds a unique place in various cultures and ecosystems. However, due to the potential risks of misidentification with toxic plants, it's important to exercise caution and proper knowledge when foraging or using wild plants for any purpose.

ROSE (ROSA SP.)

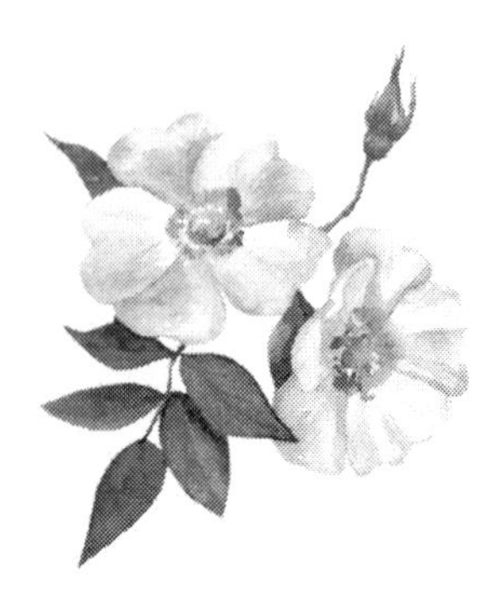

Roses, belonging to the Rosa genus, are beloved flowering plants appreciated for their beauty, fragrance, and diverse symbolic and practical uses.

Characteristics and Origins:

Flowering Plant: Roses are known for their beautiful, fragrant, and often thorny stems, producing various colored flowers.

Global Distribution: Found across the world, they're cultivated in different climates and soil conditions.

Symbolism and Cultural Significance:

Symbol of Love: Roses symbolize love, beauty, and passion, commonly used in romantic gestures.

Cultural Significance: They hold cultural importance in various traditions, ceremonies, and celebrations.

Ornamental and Aromatic Uses:

Gardening and Landscaping: Widely used in gardens and landscaping for their beauty and variety of colors and forms.

Aromatherapy: Rose oil is extracted and used in perfumery and aromatherapy for its calming and soothing properties.

Culinary Applications:

Culinary Decor: Rose petals are occasionally used as decorative elements in cuisine or infusions for flavoring.

Herbal Teas: They're used in herbal teas for their delicate fragrance and potential health benefits.

Precautions:

Thorns and Allergies: Thorns may cause skin irritation, and some individuals may have allergies to roses.

Roses' captivating beauty, aromatic essence, and multifaceted applications in culture, aesthetics, and even culinary uses have cemented their place as a timeless and cherished flower. However, it's important to be mindful of potential allergies or sensitivities when handling roses, especially regarding their thorns or fragrances.

ROSEMARY (ROSMARINUS OFFICINALIS)

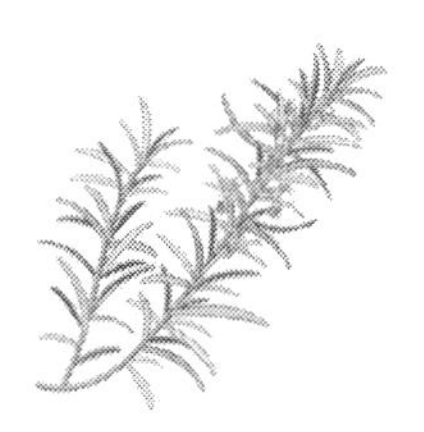

Rosemary, scientifically known as Rosmarinus officinalis, is an aromatic herb celebrated for its culinary, medicinal, and aromatic properties.

Characteristics and Origins:

Aromatic Herb: Rosemary features needle-like leaves, a robust aroma, and a woody appearance, commonly associated with Mediterranean cuisine.

Global Cultivation: Found in various regions globally, thriving in well-drained soil and sunny climates.

Culinary Uses:

Flavoring: Widely used in culinary applications, especially in Mediterranean dishes, to add a distinctive flavor.

Herbal Seasoning: It's employed in marinades, meats, stews, soups, and various dishes for its aromatic taste.

Medicinal and Aromatic Applications:

Traditional Medicine: Rosemary is used in traditional herbal medicine for its potential digestive and cognitive health benefits.

Aromatherapy: Its essential oil is utilized in aromatherapy for its potential invigorating and soothing effects.

Ornamental Significance:

Gardening: Planted for its ornamental value in gardens and landscapes due to its attractive appearance and fragrance.

Herbal Tea: Rosemary is used to prepare herbal teas, appreciated for its aroma and potential health benefits.

Precautions:

Moderate Use: While widely used in culinary and herbal preparations, excessive consumption may have adverse effects.

SAGE (SALVIA OFFICINALIS)

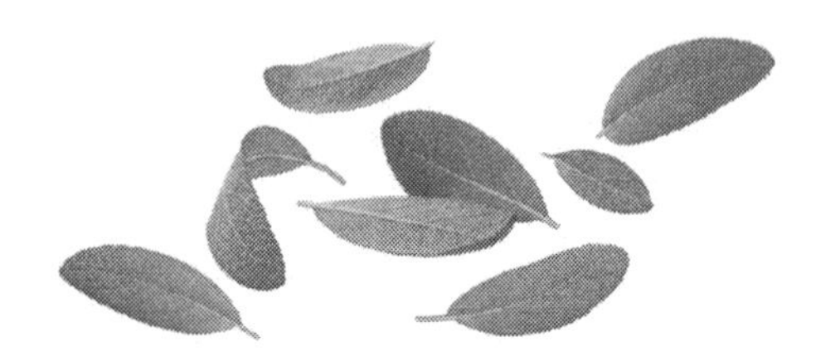

Rosemary's aromatic, culinary, and potential medicinal properties have solidified its status as a beloved herb. However, prudent use and consideration of individual sensitivities are recommended when incorporating rosemary into culinary dishes or utilizing it for its potential health benefits.

Sage, scientifically known as Salvia officinalis, is a revered herb famous for its culinary, medicinal, and aromatic properties.

Characteristics and Origins:

Aromatic Herb: Sage features soft, gray-green leaves, known for its strong aroma and slightly bitter taste.

Global Cultivation: Found in various regions worldwide, cultivated for its culinary and medicinal uses.

Culinary Uses:

Culinary Herb: Widely used in cooking, especially in Mediterranean cuisine, to flavor meats, sauces, stuffings, and various dishes.

Herbal Tea: Its leaves are used to prepare herbal teas, valued for their distinct taste and potential health benefits.

Medicinal and Aromatic Applications:

Traditional Medicine: Sage is used in traditional herbal medicine for its potential digestive and anti-inflammatory properties.

Aromatherapy: Its essential oil is used in aromatherapy for its potential calming and soothing effects.

Ornamental and Symbolic Significance:

Gardening: Planted for its ornamental value in gardens and landscapes due to its attractive appearance and fragrance.

Symbolism: Sage holds cultural significance in various traditions, symbolizing wisdom and purification.

Precautions:

Moderate Use: While widely used in culinary and herbal preparations, excessive consumption may have potential adverse effects.

Sage's versatile uses in cooking, herbal remedies, and aromatherapy, alongside its ornamental and symbolic value, make it a cherished and valuable herb. Nevertheless, mindful and moderate use is recommended to avoid potential adverse effects and fully enjoy its benefits.

SAINT JOHN'S WORT (HYPERICUM PERFORATUM)

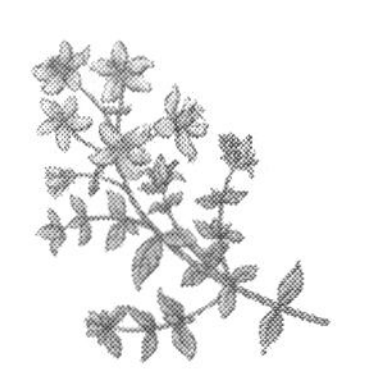

St. John's Wort, scientifically known as Hypericum perforatum, is an herb recognized for its historical use in herbal medicine and potential therapeutic properties.

Characteristics and Origins:

Herbaceous Plant: St. John's Wort has yellow, star-shaped flowers and perforated leaves, typically found in sunny areas.

Global Distribution: Found in various regions across the globe, commonly in meadows and fields.

Medicinal Uses:

Mood Support: Traditionally used for its potential to address mild mood imbalances and to support emotional well-being.

Topical Applications: Its oil is used for potential skin health benefits, like soothing minor skin irritations.

Herbal Preparations:

Infusions and Teas: Used in herbal teas or infusions, aiming to harness its potential calming effects.

Supplements: Available in various forms such as capsules or liquid extracts for those seeking its potential health benefits.

Precautions:

Interactions and Side Effects: St. John's Wort can interact with certain medications, and its use should be approached cautiously. Side effects may occur in some individuals.

St. John's Wort's historical use for mood support and potential therapeutic properties in traditional herbal medicine make it a subject of interest. However, its interactions with medications and potential side effects underscore the importance of consulting healthcare professionals before using it, especially for individuals taking medications or dealing with specific health conditions.

SEA BUCKTHORN (HIPPOPHAE RHAMNOIDES)

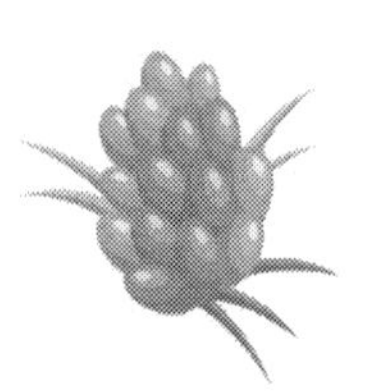

Sea buckthorn, scientifically known as Hippophae rhamnoides, is a remarkable fruit-bearing plant valued for its nutritional, medicinal, and cosmetic applications.

Characteristics and Origins:

Berry-Bearing Shrub: Sea buckthorn produces bright orange berries and is a deciduous shrub known for its resilience in harsh conditions.

Global Distribution: Found in various regions, especially in cold climates and sandy soils.

Nutritional Value:

Rich in Nutrients: Sea buckthorn berries are packed with vitamins, including C, E, and A, and are a source of omega fatty acids.

Culinary Uses: The berries are used in juices, jams, and various food products due to their nutritional content.

Medicinal Applications:

Traditional Medicine: Sea buckthorn is used for potential skin health benefits, immune support, and digestive health in traditional practices.

Supplements: Extracts and oils from the berries are used in supplements for their potential health properties.

Cosmetic and Skincare Use:

Cosmetic Products: Oil from the berries is used in skincare and cosmetics for its potential moisturizing and rejuvenating effects.

Hair Care: Its oil is utilized in hair care products for its potential nourishing properties.

Precautions:

Allergic Reactions: Some individuals may have sensitivities or allergies to sea buckthorn berries.

Sea buckthorn's extensive nutritional profile, medicinal potential, and cosmetic applications have made it a sought-after ingredient in various products. However, as with any natural substance, considering potential allergies or sensitivities is vital when using or consuming sea buckthorn products.

SKULLCAP (SCUTELLARIA SP.)

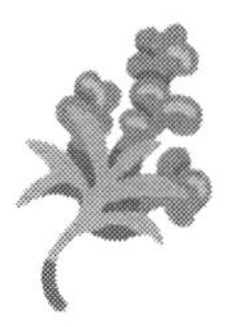

Skullcap, encompassing various species within the Scutellaria genus, is an herb admired for its potential medicinal uses and calming properties.

Characteristics and Origins:

Herbaceous Plant: Skullcap is a flowering herb known for its small, delicate flowers and diverse species within the Scutellaria genus.

Global Distribution: Found in different regions worldwide, often thriving in moist habitats.

Medicinal Uses:

Calming Effects: Skullcap is traditionally used for its potential to promote relaxation and calmness.

Traditional Herbal Medicine: It's utilized for potential stress relief and to support a calm mind.

Herbal Preparations:

Teas and Tinctures: Skullcap is used in herbal teas or tinctures, aiming to harness its potential calming effects.

Supplements: Available in various forms, including capsules and liquid extracts, for those seeking its potential health benefits.

Precautions:

Individual Reactions: Some individuals may experience side effects or interactions with certain medications, necessitating caution and, ideally, consultation with a healthcare professional before use.

Skullcap's potential calming properties and traditional use for relaxation have made it a subject of interest in herbal medicine. However, as with any herbal remedy, individual reactions, potential interactions, and suitable dosages should be carefully considered, particularly under the guidance of a healthcare professional.

SLIPPERY ELM (ULMUS RUBRA)

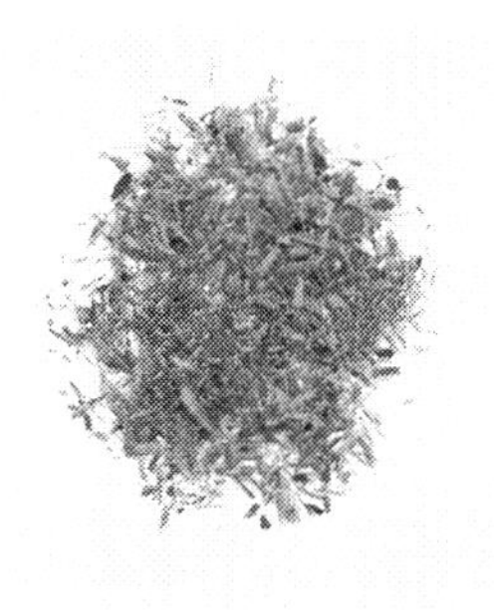

Slippery elm, scientifically known as Ulmus rubra, is a tree revered for its inner bark, historically used in traditional medicine for its potential health benefits.

Characteristics and Origins:

Deciduous Tree: Slippery elm is a tree known for its rough outer bark and mucilaginous inner bark.

Native to North America: Primarily found in North American forests and has been historically utilized by Indigenous peoples for its health properties.

Medicinal Applications:

Digestive Health: Slippery elm bark is traditionally used to soothe throat and gastrointestinal discomfort due to its mucilaginous properties.

Topical Use: Its inner bark has been applied topically to aid in minor skin irritations.

Preparations:

Herbal Teas: Ground inner bark is used to prepare herbal teas or infusions for its potential health benefits.

Lozenges and Supplements: Available in forms like lozenges or capsules for those seeking its potential health support.

Precautions:

Pregnancy and Medications: Pregnant individuals and those on medications should consult a healthcare professional before using slippery elm due to potential interactions or effects.

Slippery elm's historical use in addressing throat and gastrointestinal discomfort, along with potential skin benefits, has made it an integral part of traditional medicine. Nonetheless, considering potential interactions and proper usage, especially in specific health conditions or during pregnancy, is essential, warranting guidance from a healthcare professional.

STAGHORN SUMAC *(RHUS TYPHINA)*

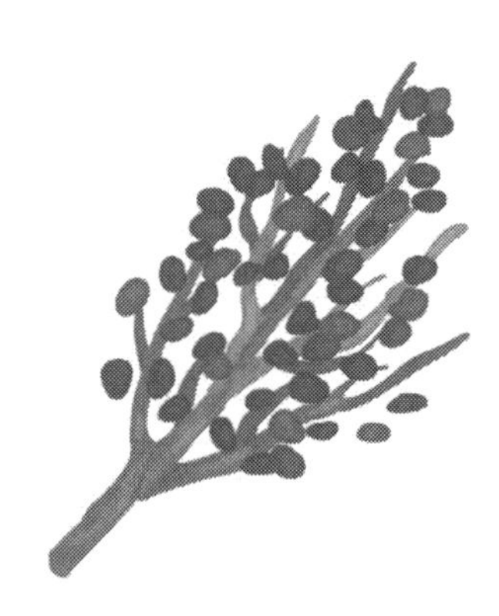

Staghorn sumac, scientifically known as Rhus typhina, is a deciduous shrub recognized for its unique red, hairy fruit clusters and diverse practical applications.

Characteristics and Origins

Shrub Appearance: Staghorn sumac features hairy, red fruit clusters resembling antlers, often seen in late summer and fall.

Global Distribution: Found in various regions, particularly in North America, in fields, roadsides, and open areas.

Culinary and Practical Uses:

Beverage Preparation: Its fruit clusters are used to make a tangy, lemonade-like beverage when properly prepared.

Landscape and Erosion Control: Planted for erosion control and as an ornamental shrub in landscaping.

Precautions:

Identification: While the fruit clusters are used to make a refreshing beverage, proper identification is crucial as certain sumac species can be toxic. It's important to differentiate between edible and toxic varieties.

Staghorn sumac's potential for making a refreshing beverage and its ornamental value in landscaping have made it a subject of interest. However, accurate identification is vital to ensure safe use for its intended purposes and to avoid potential contact with toxic sumac varieties.

TEA TREE (MELALEUCA ALTERNIFOLIA)

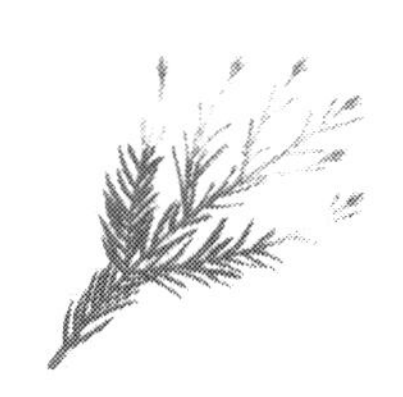

Tea tree, scientifically known as Melaleuca alternifolia, is a notable plant highly regarded for its essential oil, appreciated for its medicinal and cosmetic applications.

Characteristics and Origins:

Australian Native: Tea tree is indigenous to Australia, predominantly found in the eastern coastal regions.

Aromatic Leaves: It bears narrow, fragrant leaves that have been historically used for various purposes.

Medicinal and Cosmetic Applications:

Tea Tree Oil: The essential oil extracted from the leaves is famed for its potential antimicrobial and soothing properties.

Skincare: Its oil is used in skincare products for potential blemish control and skin soothing effects.

Health and Wellness:

Traditional Medicine: Tea tree oil has been used in traditional medicine for its potential antiseptic and healing properties.

Aromatherapy: Its oil is employed in aromatherapy for its potential calming and cleansing effects.

Precautions:

Skin Sensitivity: Some individuals may experience skin reactions, so patch testing is advisable before applying undiluted oil to the skin.

Tea tree oil's reputation for its antimicrobial and skincare properties has made it a popular ingredient in various products. Yet, due to potential skin sensitivities, it's recommended to dilute the oil and perform a patch test before using it topically.

THYME (THYMUS VULGARIS)

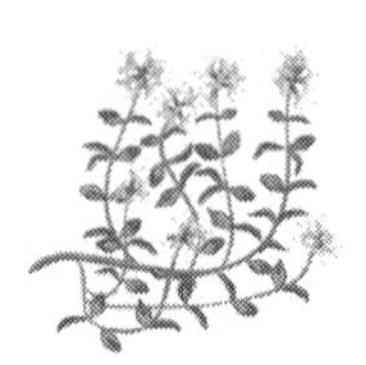

Thyme, scientifically known as Thymus vulgaris, is a popular herb recognized for its culinary uses, medicinal properties, and aromatic qualities.

Characteristics and Origins:

Aromatic Herb: Thyme features small, aromatic leaves on woody stems, known for its strong fragrance and flavorful taste.

Global Cultivation: Found in various regions worldwide, particularly in the Mediterranean.

Culinary Uses:

Culinary Herb: Widely used in cooking for its robust flavor, especially in Mediterranean and European cuisines.

Seasoning: Employed in a variety of dishes, including soups, stews, meats, and vegetable preparations for its aromatic taste.

Medicinal and Aromatic Applications:

Traditional Medicine: Thyme is used for potential respiratory health support and as an antiseptic in traditional herbal medicine.

Aromatherapy: Its essential oil is used in aromatherapy for its potential calming and cleansing effects.

Ornamental and Culinary Significance:

Gardening: Planted for its ornamental value in gardens and landscapes due to its attractive appearance and fragrance.

Herbal Teas: Thyme is used to prepare herbal teas, appreciated for its aroma and potential health benefits.

Precautions:

Moderate Use: While widely used in culinary and herbal preparations, excessive consumption may have potential adverse effects.

Thyme's rich flavor, aromatic properties, and potential health benefits have made it a staple in both culinary and traditional medicine practices. However, using it in moderation and being mindful of individual sensitivities is recommended to fully enjoy its benefits.

TULSI (OCIMUM TENUIFLORUM)

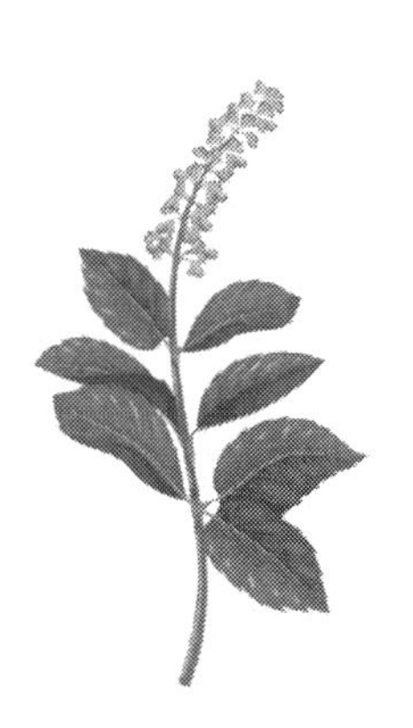

Tulsi, scientifically known as Ocimum tenuiflorum or Holy Basil, is a revered herb in Ayurvedic medicine, known for its medicinal properties and spiritual significance

Characteristics and Origins:

Sacred Herb: Tulsi is considered sacred in Hindu culture and is often cultivated around homes and temples.

Aromatic Leaves: It has fragrant, green leaves and is known for its strong aroma and taste.

Medicinal and Cultural Uses:

Ayurvedic Medicine: Tulsi is used in Ayurveda for potential immune support, respiratory health, and as an adaptogen to combat stress.

Cultural Significance: It holds religious and cultural significance in Hinduism and is revered for its spiritual and medicinal properties.

Herbal Preparations:

Herbal Teas: The leaves are used to prepare herbal teas or infusions, often consumed for potential health benefits.

Tinctures and Supplements: Available in various forms, including tinctures and supplements, for those seeking its potential health support.

Precautions:

Pregnancy and Medications: Pregnant individuals and those on medications should consult a healthcare professional before using Tulsi due to potential interactions or effects.

Tulsi's profound spiritual significance and potential health benefits have made it a cherished herb in both cultural and traditional medicinal practices. However, caution and guidance from healthcare professionals are advised, especially for pregnant individuals or those on medications, to ensure its safe and suitable usage.

TURMERIC (CURCUMA LONGA)

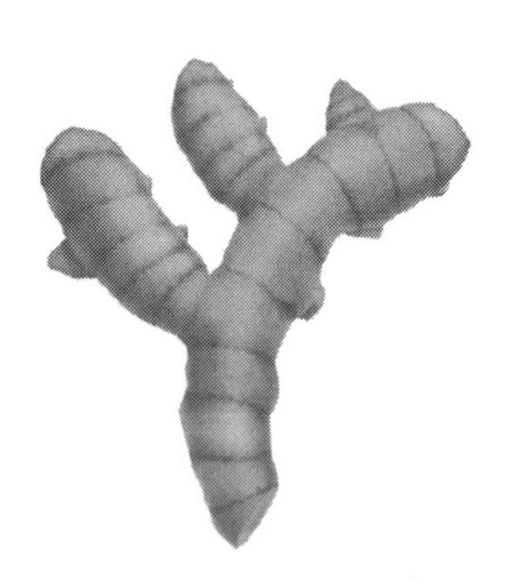

Turmeric, scientifically known as Curcuma longa, is a vibrant, golden-yellow spice celebrated for its culinary use, health benefits, and traditional medicinal properties.

Characteristics and Origins:

Vibrant Spice: Turmeric is a bright, golden-yellow spice derived from the rhizome of the Curcuma longa plant.

Cultivation: Primarily grown in India and Southeast Asia, it thrives in warm, humid climates.

Culinary and Nutritional Uses:

Flavorful Spice: Widely used in cooking, especially in Indian and Southeast Asian cuisines, imparting a warm, earthy flavor.

Nutritional Value: Known for its potential health benefits due to curcumin, its active compound with antioxidant and anti-inflammatory properties.

Medicinal Applications:

Traditional Medicine: Turmeric is utilized in traditional medicine for its potential anti-inflammatory and antioxidant effects.

Health Supplements: Available in various forms, including capsules, for those seeking its potential health support.

Precautions:

Staining and Allergies: It can stain surfaces and may cause allergies in some individuals.

Turmeric's versatility in cooking, potential health benefits, and traditional medicinal applications have made it a widely used and valued spice. However, being mindful of potential allergies and surface staining is recommended when using turmeric in various forms.

VALERIAN (VALERIANA OFFICINALIS)

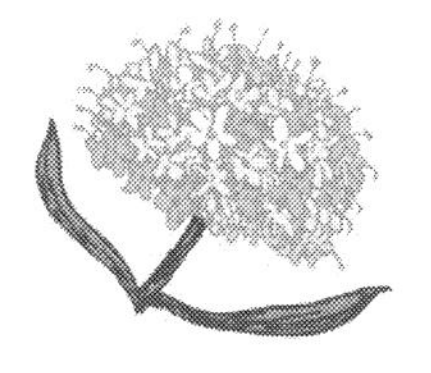

Valerian, scientifically known as Valeriana officinalis, is a herb esteemed for its potential calming effects and historical use in herbal medicine.

Characteristics and Origins:

Herbaceous Plant: Valerian is recognized for its sweetly scented pink or white flowers and fern-like foliage.

Global Distribution: Found in various regions, growing in temperate climates and damp conditions.

Medicinal Uses:

Calming Properties: Valerian is traditionally used for potential relaxation and to support sleep.

Herbal Medicine: Employed in traditional medicine for its calming effects and potential stress relief.

Herbal Preparations:

Teas and Infusions: Used in herbal teas or infusions, often consumed for its calming effects.

Supplements: Available in various forms like capsules or tinctures for those seeking its potential health benefits.

Precautions:

Drowsiness and Interactions: Valerian might cause drowsiness and can interact with certain medications, hence, consulting a healthcare professional is advisable.

Valerian's historical use for relaxation and its potential to support sleep have made it a popular choice in herbal medicine. However, considering its potential interactions with medications and effects on drowsiness, seeking guidance from a healthcare professional before use is recommended.

VERONICA (VERONICA OFFICINALIS)

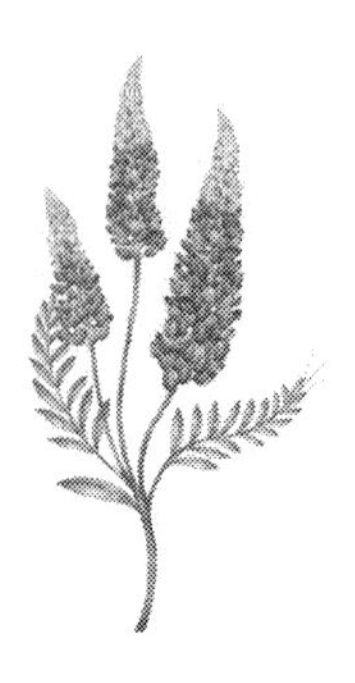

Veronica, specifically Veronica officinalis, is an herbaceous plant valued for its historical use in traditional medicine and potential health benefits.

Characteristics and Origins:

Herbaceous Herb: Veronica is recognized for its small, pale blue flowers and oval-shaped leaves.

Global Distribution: Found in various regions worldwide, often in grassy areas and open woods.

Medicinal Uses:

Traditional Medicine: Veronica has historical use in herbal remedies for potential digestive and respiratory support.

Herbal Teas: The leaves are used in herbal teas or infusions for potential health benefits.

Practical Applications:

Culinary Uses: While less common, some use Veronica leaves in salads or infusions

Ornamental Value: Appreciated for its delicate flowers, sometimes used in landscaping.

Precautions:

Individual Reactions: As with any herbal remedy, some individuals may experience allergies or adverse reactions.

Veronica's historical use in traditional medicine and potential health benefits have given it a place in herbal remedies. However, being cautious of individual reactions and sensitivities is important when using Veronica or any herbal remedy.

VIOLETS (VIOLA SP.)

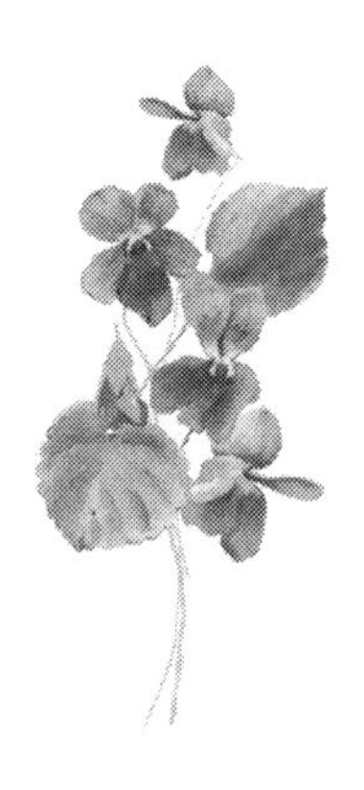

Violets, encompassing various species within the Viola genus, are delicate, colorful flowers admired for their ornamental value and occasional culinary use.

Characteristics and Origins:

Flowering Plants: Violets are characterized by heart-shaped leaves and colorful, fragrant flowers.

Global Diversity: Found in various regions worldwide, with a multitude of species and colors.

Culinary and Ornamental Uses:

Culinary Applications: Some species of violets are used in culinary creations, such as decorating desserts or infusing into beverages.

Gardening and Landscaping: Violets are planted for their ornamental value in gardens and landscapes.

Symbolism and Significance:

Symbol of Modesty: Violets are often associated with humility and modesty in various cultural contexts.

Botanical Interest: They hold a place of botanical interest due to their diversity and adaptability.

Precautions:

Species Variation: While some violets are edible and used in culinary practices, not all species are suitable for consumption. Careful identification is essential.

Violets' delicate beauty, symbolic significance, and occasional use in culinary applications have made them a charming addition to gardens and occasional culinary creations. However, due to variations in species and potential differences in edibility, careful identification is crucial before using them in culinary endeavors.

WATERCRESS (NASTURTIUM OFFICINALE)

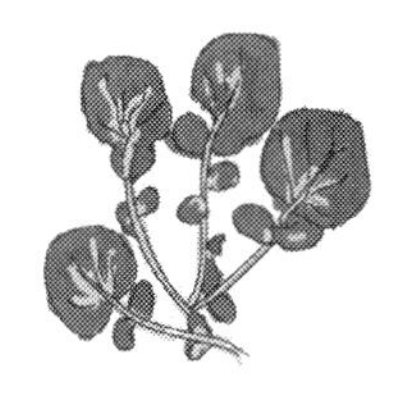

Watercress, scientifically known as Nasturtium officinale, is a leafy green plant renowned for its crisp, peppery flavor and potential health benefits.

Characteristics and Origins:

Aquatic Plant: Watercress thrives in shallow, slow-moving water bodies, known for its vibrant green, small, rounded leaves.

Global Cultivation: Found in various regions worldwide, particularly in clean, flowing water sources.

Culinary Uses:

Peppery Flavor: Often used in salads, sandwiches, and garnishes, providing a distinct, peppery taste.

Nutrient-Rich: Considered a nutrient-dense green, rich in vitamins and antioxidants.

Medicinal Applications:

Traditional Medicine: Watercress has been historically used for potential digestive health and as a source of vitamins and minerals.

Health Benefits: Known for its potential antioxidant and anti-inflammatory properties due to its nutrient content.

Precautions:

Water Source: Harvesting watercress from clean water sources is crucial to avoid potential contamination.

Watercress's crisp, peppery taste and nutrient richness make it a popular choice in culinary creations and as a potential source of health benefits. Yet, ensuring it's sourced from clean water environments is important to avoid potential health risks.

WILD LETTUCE (LACTUCA VIROSA)

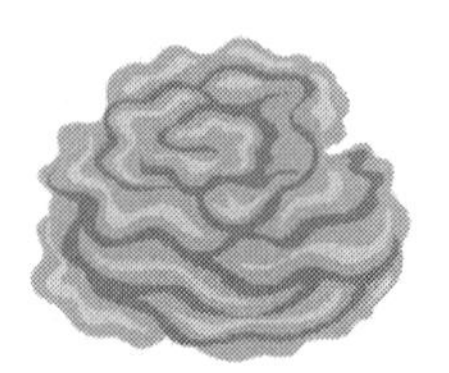

Wild Lettuce, scientifically known as Lactuca virosa, is an herb known for its potential sedative and mild pain-relieving properties.

Characteristics and Origins:

Leafy Plant: Wild Lettuce features leafy, serrated leaves and tall, leafy stems.

Global Distribution: Found in various regions, especially in Europe and parts of Asia.

Medicinal Applications:

Traditional Use: Wild Lettuce has a history of use for potential calming and sedative effects

Pain Relief: It's been utilized for mild pain relief due to its potential properties.

Herbal Preparations:

Tinctures and Extracts: The plant is used in tinctures or extracts for those seeking its potential health benefits.

Tea Infusions: Leaves can be brewed into teas, though caution is advised due to potential bitterness.

Precautions:

Dosage and Caution: Use of wild lettuce should be approached with care due to potential variations in potency and individual reactions.

Wild Lettuce's historical use for its potential sedative and mild pain-relieving properties has garnered attention. However, due to variations in potency and individual reactions, caution and guidance are recommended when considering its use for potential health benefits.

WILLOW (SALIX SP.)

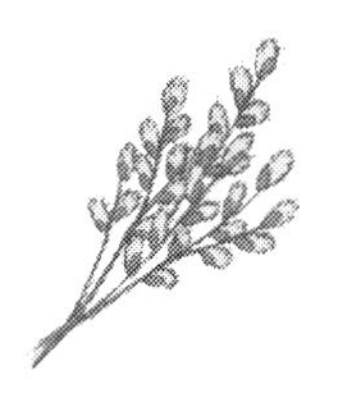

Willow, encompassing various species within the Salix genus, is a type of tree known for its flexible branches and potential medicinal properties.

Characteristics and Origins:

Tree Species: Willows are trees or shrubs with slender, flexible branches and narrow, elongated leaves.

Global Distribution: Found in various regions, commonly near water bodies, owing to their preference for moist conditions.

Medicinal Applications:

Traditional Medicine: The bark of willow trees contains salicin, a compound with potential pain-relieving properties.

Pain Relief: Historically used as a natural remedy for mild pain and discomfort.

Herbal Remedies:

Herbal Preparations: Willow bark has been used in teas, tinctures, or capsules for potential health benefits.

Caution: While considered natural, moderation and consulting a healthcare professional are advised due to potential side effects or interactions.

Precautions:

Consultation: Individuals should seek guidance before using willow bark for medicinal purposes, especially if on medications or dealing with health conditions.

Willow's historical use for its potential pain-relieving properties due to salicin content has made it a notable component in natural remedies. However, as with any herbal remedy, caution and expert guidance are recommended to avoid potential side effects or interactions, especially for individuals on medications or with health concerns.

WINTERGREEN (GAULTHERIA PROCUMBENS)

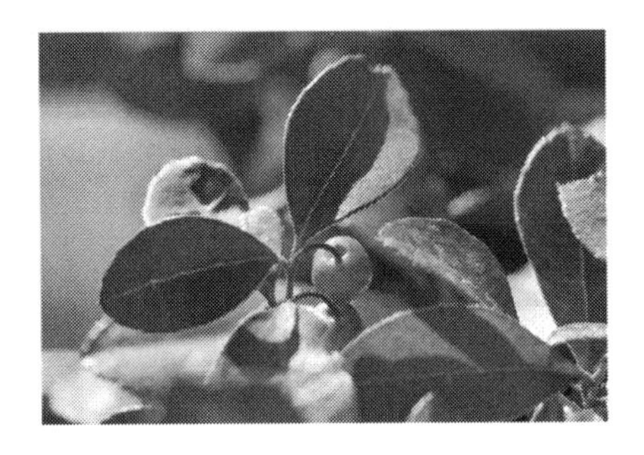

Wintergreen, scientifically known as Gaultheria procumbens, is a small, aromatic plant appreciated for its unique flavor and potential medicinal properties

Characteristics and Origins:

Aromatic Plant: Wintergreen features glossy, dark green leaves and produces red berries, known for its distinct, mint-like aroma.

Native to North America: Found in wooded areas in regions of North America.

Medicinal and Culinary Uses:

Minty Flavor: Wintergreen leaves possess a minty taste, often used to flavor food and beverages.Traditional Medicine: Historically used for its potential analgesic and anti-inflammatory properties.

Essential Oil:

Methyl Salicylate: The essential oil extracted from wintergreen contains methyl salicylate, akin to aspirin, giving it potential pain-relieving properties.

Topical Application: Often used in topical applications, diluted in carrier oils, for potential muscle or joint discomfort.

Precautions:

Caution in Usage: Wintergreen oil is potent and should be used in diluted forms. Direct application or excessive use may lead to potential side effects.

Wintergreen's distinctive flavor and the presence of methyl salicylate, which holds potential pain-relieving properties, have made it a component in both culinary uses and traditional remedies. However, due to its potency, dilution and caution in usage are strongly advised to avoid potential side effects.

WITCH HAZEL (HAMAMELIS VIRGINIANA)

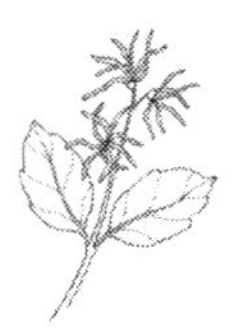

Witch hazel, scientifically known as Hamamelis virginiana, is a versatile shrub valued for its astringent properties and various applications in skincare and traditional medicine.

Characteristics and Origins:

Shrub Species: Witch hazel is a deciduous shrub with distinctive, fragrant yellow flowers that bloom in late fall.

Native to North America: Primarily found in North America and commonly grown for its beneficial properties.

Medicinal and Skincare Uses:

Astringent Properties: Witch hazel extract is known for its astringent properties, potentially tightening skin and reducing inflammation.

Skincare Tonic: Often used in skincare products as a natural toner or cleanser for its potential to soothe and cleanse the skin.

Traditional Medicine:

Topical Applications: Historically used topically for various skin conditions, minor irritations, and to soothe discomfort.

Anti-Inflammatory: Its extract is valued for potential anti-inflammatory effects, aiding in skin health.

Precautions:

Skin Sensitivity: While generally well-tolerated, some individuals may experience skin reactions. Patch testing before widespread use is recommended.

Witch hazel's astringent properties and historical use in skincare and traditional medicine have made it a popular ingredient in skincare products. However, individual skin sensitivities should be considered, warranting a patch test before extensive use.

YARROW (ACHILLEA MILLEFOLIUM)

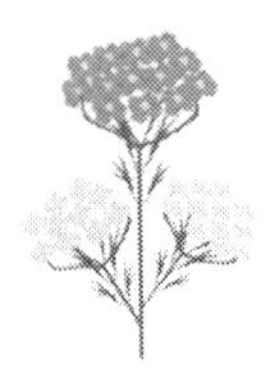

Yarrow, scientifically known as Achillea millefolium, is an herb revered for its diverse medicinal applications and ornamental value.

Characteristics and Origins:

Herbaceous Plant: Yarrow is recognized for its feathery, fern-like leaves and clusters of small, delicate flowers in various colors.

Global Distribution: Found in many regions worldwide, especially in meadows, pastures, and along roadsides.

Medicinal Uses:

Traditional Medicine: Yarrow has a history of use for potential wound healing and as a natural astringent.

Digestive Support: Utilized for potential digestive health benefits and as a mild diuretic.

Herbal Remedies:

Teas and Infusions: Leaves and flowers are used in herbal teas for their potential health benefits.

Topical Applications: Yarrow's leaves are used in poultices or as a topical treatment for potential skin healing.

Ornamental Value:

Gardening: Yarrow is planted in gardens for its attractive, colorful flowers and its ability to attract beneficial insects.

Dried Flowers: Its flowers are often used in dried flower arrangements for decorative purposes.

Precautions:

Pregnancy and Allergies: Pregnant individuals and those with known plant allergies should exercise caution when using yarrow.

Yarrow's versatile applications in traditional medicine, ornamental gardening, and potential health benefits have made it a valued herb. However, as with any herbal remedy, individuals should be cautious, especially during pregnancy or in the presence of known allergies.

YELLOW DOCK (RUMEX CRISPUS)

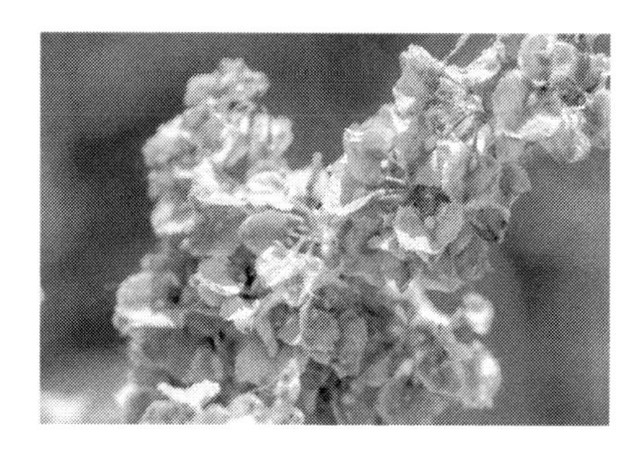

Yellow dock, scientifically known as Rumex crispus, is an herb recognized for its potential medicinal uses and nutritional content.

Characteristics and Origins:

Perennial Plant: Yellow dock is characterized by its tall, slender stems and distinctive, curly-edged leaves.

Global Distribution: Found in various regions worldwide, particularly in meadows and fields.

Medicinal Uses

Traditional Medicine: Yellow dock has been historically used for its potential as a mild laxative and for digestive support.

Nutritional Value: Its leaves are rich in vitamins and minerals, making them potentially beneficial in diets.

Herbal Remedies:Teas and Infusions: Leaves or roots are used in herbal teas or infusions for potential health benefits.

Digestive Support: Utilized for its potential to aid in digestion and support liver health.

Precautions:

Oxalates: Its leaves contain oxalates, and excessive consumption may affect individuals prone to kidney stones or oxalate-related issues.

Yellow dock's historical use as a mild laxative and its potential nutritional value have made it a part of traditional herbal remedies. However, moderation in consumption and consideration for individuals prone to oxalate-related concerns are advised.

BOOK 6: How to Grow, Harvest & Preserve for the Home Apothecary TO A FROM L

ALOE VERA

How to Grow, Harvest, and Preserve Aloe Vera for the Home Apothecary

Growing, harvesting, and preserving Aloe Vera involves specific steps:

Growing Aloe Vera:

Soil and Pot: Use well-draining soil, like a mix of sand and potting soil, in a pot with drainage holes to avoid waterlogging.

Temperature and Light: Aloe prefers moderate temperatures and indirect sunlight, so position it where it gets sun but avoid direct exposure during the hottest parts of the day.

Watering Technique: Water only when the soil is completely dry. The plant can tolerate some drought, so it's best to avoid excessive moisture.

Harvesting Aloe Vera:

Careful Selection: Choose the outermost, mature leaves as they contain the highest gel content.

Precise Cutting: Use a clean, sharp knife to cut the leaves close to the base of the plant, being careful not to harm the rest of the plant.

Preserving Aloe Vera:

Extraction and Cleansing: After cutting the leaves, cleanse the gel to remove any latex residues.

Optimal Storage: Store the gel in clean containers in the refrigerator for immediate use or in sealed bags in the freezer for long-term preservation.

Additional Tips:

Pruning Carefully: Remove dying or damaged leaves to encourage new growth.

Harvest Frequency: Avoid harvesting more than 1/3 of the leaves at a time to prevent excessive stress on the plant.

Adhering to these detailed guidelines will ensure proper cultivation, harvesting, and preservation of Aloe Vera, maintaining its valuable properties for your home apothecary.

ANGELICA

Growing Angelica (Angelica archangelica) can be a rewarding process. Here's a guide on how to cultivate this herb:

Planting Angelica:

Choose a Location: Select a spot with partial shade or full sun, depending on your climate. Angelica prefers moist, rich soil and cooler temperatures.

Soil Preparation: Ensure the soil is well-draining, fertile, and slightly acidic. Work in compost to enhance its richness.

Sowing Seeds: Sow seeds in early spring or late fall, about 18 inches apart and shallowly covered with soil.

Caring for Angelica:

Watering: Keep the soil consistently moist but not waterlogged. Mulch can help retain moisture.

Maintenance: Thin out seedlings to provide enough space for growth. Stake taller plants if they become top-heavy.

Fertilization: Consider adding a balanced fertilizer early in the growing season to promote healthy growth.

Harvesting Angelica:

Timing: Harvest the roots in the fall of the plant's second year. Leaves and stems can be harvested throughout the growing season.

Cutting: Use sharp scissors or shears to cut the stems and leaves, leaving enough for the plant's sustenance.

Preserving Angelica:

Drying: Dry leaves and stems by hanging them upside down in a dry, well-ventilated area. Roots can be air-dried or dehydrated.

Storage: Store dried leaves, stems, and roots in airtight containers away from light and moisture.

Tips:

Replantation: Angelica is a biennial, so allow some plants to go to seed to ensure reseeding.

Pests and Diseases: Monitor for pests and diseases, and address them promptly to maintain plant health.

Following these steps can help you successfully grow, harvest, and preserve Angelica, a versatile herb known for its culinary and medicinal uses.

ARNICA

Arnica, known for its medicinal properties, is a herbaceous plant used in various remedies. Here's an overview:

Characteristics:

Scientific Name: Arnica montana is the most common species used in herbal preparations.

Appearance: It typically bears bright yellow, daisy-like flowers.

Cultivation:Growing Conditions: Arnica prefers well-draining, slightly acidic soil in areas with partial shade.

Climate: Thrives in cooler climates, typically found in mountainous regions.

Medicinal Use:

Topical Applications: Arnica is popular for its potential to alleviate pain, reduce inflammation, and soothe bruises when applied topically.

Herbal Remedies: Often used in creams, ointments, or tinctures for its potential healing effects.

Harvesting and Preservation:

Harvesting: Flowers are usually collected at full bloom, while roots are typically gathered in the fall.

Drying: Flowers and roots are dried for preservation, ensuring they're kept in a well-ventilated area away from direct sunlight.

Precautions:

Toxicity: Arnica should not be ingested in its raw form as it can be toxic. External use is recommended.

Allergic Reactions: Some individuals might experience skin irritation or allergic reactions.

Arnica's potential healing properties, particularly in topical applications for pain relief and bruising, make it a valuable component in herbal remedies. However, precautions should be taken regarding its toxicity and possible allergic reactions. Consulting a healthcare professional before use is advisable.

ASH TREES

Ash trees, known for their elegance and sturdiness, are part of the Fraxinus genus. Here's an overview:

Characteristics:

Varieties: There are multiple species, including White Ash (Fraxinus americana) and Green Ash (Fraxinus pennsylvanica), among others.

Appearance: Typically tall with compound leaves and grayish bark.

Cultivation:

Growing Conditions: Ash trees prefer well-draining, loamy soil in full sun but can tolerate various soil types.

Climate: They are adaptable but commonly thrive in temperate regions.

Uses:

Ornamental Trees: Often planted for their decorative foliage and shape in landscapes.

Wood: Valued for their strong and elastic timber used in furniture making, tool handles, and sports equipment.

Threats:

Emerald Ash Borer: This invasive beetle species poses a significant threat to ash trees, causing widespread damage and often leading to tree loss.

Conservation Efforts:

Treatment: Various treatments aim to protect ash trees from Emerald Ash Borers, including insecticide applications and other control methods.

Research: Ongoing research focuses on breeding resistant ash trees and developing new methods to combat the beetle's impact.

Ash trees contribute significantly to landscaping and industries, but they face severe threats from pests like the Emerald Ash Borer. Efforts to protect and preserve these trees are ongoing to mitigate the damage caused by these invasive species.

ASHWAGANDHA

Ashwagandha, an herb with a prominent place in Ayurvedic medicine, offers numerous potential health benefits. Here's an overview:

Characteristics:

Scientific Name: Withania somnifera, also known as Indian ginseng or winter cherry.

Appearance: It's a small shrub with yellow flowers and red fruit, primarily found in India, the Middle East, and parts of Africa.

Medicinal Use:

Adaptogen: Known for its potential to help the body manage stress and anxiety.

Anti-Inflammatory: It may aid in reducing inflammation and boosting the immune system.

Energy and Vitality: Often used to enhance energy levels and support overall vitality.

Preparation and Use:

Roots: The roots are typically dried and ground to create powders or extracts for consumption.

Supplements: Available in various forms such as capsules, powders, or liquid extracts for easy consumption.

Cautions and Considerations:

Pregnancy: Pregnant individuals should avoid using ashwagandha due to its potential effects on hormonal regulation.

Interactions: It may interact with certain medications, so consulting a healthcare professional before use is advisable.

Research and Popularity:

Scientific Interest: Ongoing research explores its potential in various health areas, including stress management and cognitive health.

Global Usage: Its popularity has grown worldwide, largely due to its perceived adaptogenic and overall health-supporting properties.

Ashwagandha's potential as an adaptogen and its use in managing stress and overall well-being have led to its increased global usage and scientific interest. However, individuals should exercise caution, especially during pregnancy or when taking medications, and seek advice from a healthcare professional before use.

ASTRAGALUS

Astragalus, scientifically known as Astragalus propinquus, is a perennial herb native to Northern and Eastern China, Mongolia, and Korea. It has a long history of use in traditional Chinese medicine and is known for its potential health benefits. Here's an overview of Astragalus:

Characteristics:

Scientific Name:** Astragalus propinquus.

Appearance:** Astragalus is a leguminous plant with small yellow flowers. The root is the part most commonly used for its medicinal properties.

Medicinal Use:

Immune System Support:** Astragalus is well-regarded for its potential to boost the immune system and help the body fight off infections.

Anti-Inflammatory:** It may have anti-inflammatory properties and is used to address various inflammatory conditions.Adaptogen:** Astragalus is considered an adaptogen, which means it may help the body adapt to stress and maintain balance.

Preparation and Use:

Root:** The dried root is commonly used to make teas, tinctures, and extracts.

Supplements:** Astragalus is also available in various supplement forms, including capsules and powders.

Cautions and Considerations:

Astragalus is generally considered safe when used as directed, but it may interact with certain medications, so consult a healthcare professional before use.

It's advisable to use Astragalus under the guidance of a healthcare practitioner, especially if you have specific health concerns or are taking other medications.

Research and Popularity:

Astragalus has gained popularity for its immune-boosting potential, especially in traditional Chinese medicine.

While more research is needed to fully understand its benefits, it's widely used and recognized for its potential health-promoting properties.

Astragalus is primarily known for its immune-supporting capabilities and its use as an adaptogen to help the body manage stress. It has a long history of use in traditional Chinese medicine and is increasingly gaining recognition in the Western world. As with any herbal remedy, it's important to use Astragalus responsibly and seek guidance from a healthcare professional if you have any concerns.

BALSAM POPLAR

Balsam poplar, scientifically known as Populus balsamifera, is a species of poplar tree native to North America. Here's an overview of the Balsam Poplar:

Characteristics:

Scientific Name: Populus balsamifera.Habitat:

Balsam poplars are typically found in wetlands, riparian zones, and moist forests in North America.

Appearance:

These trees are tall and can reach heights of up to 25 meters. They're recognizable by their green, ovate leaves and resinous buds that exude a balsamic scent.

Medicinal Use:

Historical Uses:Traditionally, various parts of the Balsam Poplar tree have been used by indigenous peoples for medicinal purposes.

Balsam: The resin obtained from the buds was historically used in salves or ointments for skin irritations or as an inhalant.

Preparation and Use:

Balsam: The resinous substance obtained from the buds has been used traditionally in various topical applications. However, contemporary medicinal use isn't as widespread.

Cautions and Considerations:

While Balsam Poplar has historical usage in traditional medicine, contemporary medicinal practices or consumption of parts of the tree may require further evaluation or guidance from healthcare professionals.

It's important to note that traditional uses may not have been scientifically validated, and using any part of the tree for medicinal purposes should be approached with caution.

Balsam Poplar, like many plants in traditional medicine, has a history of use among indigenous communities, particularly for its balsamic resin. However, its contemporary medicinal use or efficacy may require more scientific validation. Always exercise caution and seek guidance from healthcare professionals before using any plant for medicinal purposes.

BARBERRY

Barberry, or Berberis, is a beautiful shrub with colorful flowers and fruits. Here's how to cultivate it and make the most of its properties!

How to Grow Barberry

Berberis is resilient and suitable for various climates.

Optimal Location

Plant Barberry in a sunny or partially shaded spot. It prefers well-draining soil and can tolerate dry conditions.

Planting

Plant Barberry seedlings in the spring or fall. Ensure you dig a hole large enough to accommodate the roots.

Maintenance

It requires minimal maintenance once established. Prune it to maintain the desired shape and remove dead or damaged branches.

How to Harvest Barberry Berries

Barberry berries are edible and rich in antioxidants. To harvest them, wait until they reach maturity and take on a vibrant color. Carefully cut the berry clusters.

Extraction of Barberry Juice

Barberry berries can be used to extract a juice rich in health benefits. Gently crush them and strain the juice through a fine cloth to remove the seeds.

Preservation of Barberry Juice

Store the juice in sterilized glass bottles. You can freeze it to extend its shelf life or use it fresh within a few days.

Uses of Barberry Juice

Barberry juice is used in cooking to flavor dishes, prepare beverages, or as a dietary supplement for its health benefits.

Berberis is a versatile plant with much to offer, from its decorative features to its culinary and health benefits!

BAY LAUREL

Bay Laurel, or Laurus nobilis, is a fantastic plant with both culinary and ornamental value. Here's an in-depth guide on growing, harvesting, and utilizing this wonderful herb!

How to Cultivate Bay Laurel

Bay Laurel thrives in various climates and is relatively low-maintenance.

Optimal Location

Plant your Bay Laurel in a sunny spot with well-draining soil. It can tolerate both full sun and partial shade.

Planting

When planting, ensure the soil is rich and well-drained. Consider using a potting mix if you're growing it in a container.

Maintenance

Bay Laurel doesn't demand much attention once established. Pruning can help shape the plant and encourage denser growth.

Harvesting Bay Laurel Leaves

The leaves are best harvested fresh. Pick the mature, dark green leaves. They are flavorful and ideal for culinary uses.

Extracting Bay Laurel Essential Oil

Bay Laurel leaves can be used to produce essential oil. Dry the leaves and steam-distill them to extract the aromatic oil, which has various applications, from aromatherapy to natural remedies.

Storing Bay Laurel Leaves and Oil

Store the dried leaves in airtight containers in a cool, dark place. As for the essential oil, store it in dark glass bottles away from direct sunlight to preserve its potency.

Uses of Bay Laurel

The leaves are an essential ingredient in many cuisines, imparting a unique flavor to soups, stews, and sauces. The essential oil is also utilized in aromatherapy for its calming and cleansing properties.

Bay Laurel is a wonderful addition to any garden, offering both practical and sensory delights!

BEE BALM

Bee Balm, also known as Monarda, is a vibrant and fragrant herb that's a favorite among gardeners and pollinators alike. Let's dive into how to cultivate, harvest, and use this remarkable plant!

How to Grow Bee Balm

Bee Balm is a hardy plant that thrives in diverse conditions.

Optimal Conditions

Plant Bee Balm in well-draining soil under full sun to partial shade. It enjoys slightly acidic soil but is adaptable to different pH levels.

Planting

Sow seeds or plant seedlings in early spring. Space them about 18 inches apart, as they can spread.

Maintenance

Keep the soil consistently moist, especially during dry spells. Regular deadheading can encourage more blooms.

Harvesting Bee Balm

Harvest the flowers when they're in full bloom for the best flavor and potency. The leaves can be picked at any time during the growing season.

Extracting Bee Balm Essential Oil

The leaves of Bee Balm can be distilled to extract an essential oil. This oil possesses a pleasant fragrance and can be used for various purposes, from aromatherapy to homemade skincare products.

Storing Bee Balm

Dry the leaves in a cool, dark place and store them in airtight containers. The essential oil should be kept in dark glass bottles away from direct light to maintain its quality.

Uses of Bee Balm

Apart from its ornamental value, Bee Balm has several uses. The leaves make a delightful tea with a hint of citrus and mint, while the flowers attract bees, butterflies, and hummingbirds to your garden.

Bee Balm is not just a beautiful addition to your garden; it's a multi-functional herb that adds both visual and practical charm to your outdoor space!

BEECH TREE

The Beech tree, a majestic and resilient species, holds both ornamental and ecological significance. Here's a detailed exploration on cultivating, utilizing, and appreciating this remarkable tree.

How to Cultivate a Beech Tree

Beech trees are hardy, but proper care is essential for their growth.

Optimal Conditions

They prefer well-drained soil and a sunny to partially shaded environment. Beech trees are adaptable but thrive in slightly acidic soil.

Planting

Transplanting a young beech tree is ideal. Choose a spot where it has space to grow to its full size.

Maintenance

Regular watering, especially during dry spells, is necessary to establish the tree. Pruning, if required, should be minimal.

Harvesting Beech Nuts

Beech trees produce small, triangular nuts encased in spiky husks. Harvest the nuts when they fall to the ground, then remove the husks and dry the nuts for consumption.

Uses of Beech Wood

Beech wood is valuable and used in various applications, from furniture making to flooring and even in culinary tools due to its non-porous nature.

Ecological Importance

Beech trees support biodiversity, providing shelter and food for various wildlife. Their dense canopy also aids in oxygen production and soil stability.

Appreciating Beech Trees

Beech trees stand out in landscapes, especially during autumn when their leaves turn a beautiful golden color, adding visual appeal to any environment.

The Beech tree is not only a stunning addition to nature's palette but also an essential contributor to ecosystems and a source of various practical and aesthetic utilities.

BELLADONNA

Belladonna, scientifically known as Atropa belladonna, is a captivating yet highly toxic plant. Here's a comprehensive guide on its cultivation, properties, and precautions.

How to Cultivate Belladonna

Note: Growing Belladonna is not recommended for most gardeners due to its extreme toxicity.

Optimal Conditions

Belladonna prefers partial shade and well-drained, alkaline soil. However, it's crucial to emphasize that this plant is toxic and should be handled with care.

Planting

If you still wish to proceed, sow Belladonna seeds in early spring. Ensure you wear protective gear and keep it out of reach of children and pets.

Maintenance

Maintenance is minimal due to its toxic nature. Handle the plant with extreme caution and avoid ingestion or contact with the skin.

Harvesting Belladonna

Caution: Harvesting Belladonna is extremely dangerous due to its toxic compounds. It's strongly advised against for anyone without professional knowledge.

Uses of Belladonna

Belladonna contains alkaloids like atropine and scopolamine, which are potent toxins. Historically, it has been used in minute quantities for medicinal purposes, but it should only be handled by experts.

Precautions

Belladonna is one of the most toxic plants in the world. Ingestion or even skin contact can lead to severe poisoning. Do not attempt to cultivate or use it without proper expertise.

Due to its extreme toxicity, Belladonna is not recommended for general cultivation or use. It should be approached with the utmost caution and only by individuals with the necessary knowledge and expertise in handling toxic plants.

The Betula species, commonly known as Birch trees, are graceful and versatile trees that can enhance your landscape. Here's a guide on how to cultivate, appreciate, and utilize these beautiful trees.

BIRCH TREES

How to Cultivate Birch Trees (Betula sp.)

Birch trees are relatively low-maintenance and can thrive in various conditions.

Optimal Conditions

Plant Birch trees in well-draining soil with exposure to full sun or partial shade. They prefer slightly acidic soil but are adaptable to different pH levels.

Planting

Transplant young Birch trees into your garden, ensuring they have sufficient space to grow to their full size.

Maintenance

Regular watering during the establishment phase is essential. Pruning, if necessary, should be done with care to maintain the tree's natural form.

Harvesting Birch Bark

Birch trees have a distinctive bark that can be harvested for various uses. It's best to collect the bark from fallen branches rather than harming the living tree.

Uses of Birch Bark

Birch bark has been traditionally used for crafting, including making canoes, baskets, and shelters. It's also employed in modern crafts for its rustic appeal.

Appreciating Birch Trees

Birch trees are known for their striking white bark and delicate foliage. They add elegance to any landscape, and their leaves turn a lovely golden color in the fall.

Birch trees are a captivating addition to your garden or landscape, providing both aesthetic beauty and practical uses through their distinctive bark.

BLACK COHOSH

Black Cohosh, scientifically known as Actaea racemosa, is a herbaceous perennial with both medicinal and ornamental properties. Here's a comprehensive guide on cultivating, harvesting, and utilizing Black Cohosh.

How to Cultivate Black Cohosh

Black Cohosh requires specific conditions to thrive.

Optimal Conditions

Plant in partially shaded areas with rich, moist, well-drained soil. The plant benefits from sheltered spots and requires consistent moisture.

Planting

Plant the rhizomes or seeds in early spring. Ensure they are placed at the right depth and spacing for optimal growth.

Maintenance

Regular watering is essential, especially during dry spells. Mulching can help retain moisture and regulate the soil temperature.

Harvesting Black Cohosh

Harvest the roots in late summer or early fall when the plant reaches maturity. Use caution and harvest responsibly to ensure the plant's sustainability.

Uses of Black Cohosh

Black Cohosh has a history of use in traditional medicine, primarily for women's health. Its roots are utilized in various forms, such as tinctures, teas, or capsules, to alleviate menopausal symptoms.

Precautions

While Black Cohosh has been used for medicinal purposes, it's important to consult a healthcare professional before using it, especially for prolonged or extensive treatments.

Black Cohosh is a plant with notable medicinal value, particularly in addressing women's health concerns. When used responsibly and with proper guidance, it can offer relief from specific conditions.

BLACK EYED SUSAN

How to Cultivate Black-Eyed Susan (Rudbeckia Hirta)

Planting Black-Eyed Susan:

Ideal Conditions: These vibrant flowers thrive in various conditions.

Soil & Sun: They prefer well-draining soil and bask in full sun to partial shade.

Planting Method: Sow seeds or plant seedlings during early spring. Allow around 18 inches of space between plants to accommodate their spreading nature.

Maintenance:

Watering: Ensure consistent moisture, especially during dry spells.

Pruning: Regular deadheading can stimulate prolonged flowering.

Harvesting Black-Eyed Susan

Flowering Stage:

Harvest the flowers at their peak bloom for the best appearance and use.

Using Black-Eyed Susan

Visual Appeal:

These flowers are not only charming but also attract butterflies and bees, adding natural beauty and biodiversity to your garden.

Landscaping Uses:

Ideal for borders, containers, or wild gardens due to their bright and striking appearance.

Overall, Black-Eyed Susan is not just a garden favorite for its appearance, but also for its ability to attract pollinators and enhance the landscape's visual appeal.

BLACK WALNUT

Growing Black Walnut (Juglans Nigra)

Planting Black Walnut:

Ideal Conditions: Black walnuts prefer deep, fertile, well-drained soil with plenty of sunlight.

Planting Time: Optimal planting time is in the early spring or late fall.

Spacing: Ensure enough space between trees to accommodate their eventual size.

Maintenance:

Watering: Maintain consistent moisture, especially during the tree's initial growth.

Pruning: Regularly trim dead or diseased branches.

Harvesting Black Walnuts

Maturation:

Harvest the nuts when the husks split, revealing the dark, hard shells inside.

Processing Black Walnuts

Drying and Storage:

After harvesting, dry the nuts thoroughly in a well-ventilated area to prevent molding.

Store the nuts in a cool, dry place in airtight containers to maintain their quality.

Using Black Walnuts

Culinary Uses:

Black walnuts have a robust, distinct flavor and are often used in baking or as a topping for various dishes.

They can also be ground into flour or used in salads for a unique taste.

Wood Utilization:

The wood of black walnut trees is highly valued for furniture and woodworking due to its durability and attractive color.

Black Walnut trees are not only a source of flavorful nuts but also provide valuable wood, making them a dual-purpose addition to your landscape.

BLESSED THISTLE

Cultivating Blessed Thistle (Cnicus Benedictus)

Planting Blessed Thistle:

Soil Preference: Plant in well-draining, loamy soil with good sunlight exposure.

Planting Time: Sow seeds in late spring after the last frost.

Spacing: Allow adequate space between plants to accommodate their growth.

Care and Maintenance:

Watering: Keep the soil consistently moist but not waterlogged.

Pruning: Regular deadheading can encourage continuous blooming.

Harvesting Blessed Thistle

Harvesting Flowers and Leaves:

Gather the flowering tops when the flowers are in full bloom.

Leaves can be harvested throughout the growing season.

Drying and Storing:

Dry the harvested parts in a well-ventilated, dark area to preserve their quality.

Store the dried thistle in airtight containers away from direct light and moisture.

Utilizing Blessed Thistle

Medicinal Uses:

Blessed thistle is known for its traditional medicinal uses, often brewed into teas or tinctures for digestive issues or as a general tonic.

It's advisable to consult a healthcare professional before using it for medicinal purposes.

Blessed thistle is not only visually striking in the garden but also holds historical significance for its medicinal properties.

BLUE VERVAIN

Cultivating Blue Vervain (Verbena Hastata)

Planting Blue Vervain:

Soil Preference: Plant in moist, well-drained soil in full sun to partial shade.

Planting Time: Sow seeds in early spring or late fall.

Spacing: Allow adequate space between plants to support growth.

Care and Maintenance:

Watering: Keep the soil consistently moist, especially during dry periods.

Pruning: Regular deadheading encourages continuous blooming.

Harvesting Blue Vervain

Harvesting Flowers and Leaves:

Collect the flowering tops when they reach their peak bloom.

Leaves can be harvested throughout the growing season.

Drying and Storing:

Dry the harvested parts in a cool, dark, and well-ventilated area.

Store the dried vervain in airtight containers, away from direct light and moisture.

Utilizing Blue Vervain

Medicinal and Herbal Uses:

Blue Vervain has a history of use in traditional herbal medicine for various purposes, including relaxation and immune support.

It's recommended to seek advice from a healthcare professional before using it for medicinal purposes.

With its medicinal potential and graceful appearance, Blue Vervain is a delightful addition to any garden.

BORAGE

Growing Borage (Borago Officinalis)

Planting Borage:

Soil and Sun: Thrives in well-draining soil with full sun.

Sowing Seeds: Directly sow seeds into the ground as they don't transplant well due to their deep taproot.

Maintenance and Care:

Watering: Keep the soil consistently moist, but avoid waterlogged conditions.

Thinning Out: Thin seedlings to ensure proper spacing for healthy growth.

Weeding: Regularly remove weeds around the plant to avoid competition for nutrients.

Harvesting Borage

Harvesting Flowers and Leaves:

Flowers: Harvest when fully bloomed for culinary or decorative purposes.

Leaves: Pick young leaves for culinary use throughout the growing season.

Preserving Borage:

Drying Flowers and Leaves: Dry in a cool, dry place, ensuring good air circulation.

Storage: Store dried leaves and flowers in airtight containers, away from direct sunlight.

Using Borage

Culinary Applications:

Borage is prized for its edible flowers and leaves, often used in salads, garnishes, or to flavor drinks.

Medicinal Uses:

Historically, borage has been used in herbal remedies, particularly for its potential anti-inflammatory properties.

Borage is not just a culinary delight but also a beneficial addition to any garden, attracting pollinators and serving multiple purposes!

BURDOCK

Cultivating Burdock (Arctium Lappa)

Planting Burdock:

Soil and Sun: Requires well-drained, loamy soil and partial shade to full sun.

Sowing Seeds: Plant seeds in early spring or late autumn. They should be sown directly into the ground.

Maintenance and Care:

Thinning: Thin seedlings to about 2 feet apart for optimal growth.

Watering: Keep the soil consistently moist but not waterlogged.

Mulching: Mulch around the plants to retain moisture and suppress weeds.

Harvesting Burdock

Harvesting Roots and Leaves:

Roots: Dig up mature roots in their first year during autumn or early spring.

Leaves: Gather leaves before the plant starts flowering for culinary purposes.

Preserving Burdock:

Root Storage: Clean and dry roots, store in a cool, dark place in airtight containers.

Drying Leaves: Dry leaves in a shaded, well-ventilated area and store them in airtight containers.

Using Burdock

Culinary Applications:

The root is a common ingredient in Asian cuisine, used in stir-fries, soups, and stews.

Young leaves can be cooked similarly to spinach or used in salads.

Medicinal Uses:

Burdock has a history in herbal medicine, known for its potential detoxifying properties and as a blood purifier.

Burdock's culinary versatility and potential health benefits make it a valuable addition to both your garden and kitchen!

CALENDULA

Growing Calendula (Calendula Officinalis)

Cultivation:

Soil and Sun: Thrives in well-drained soil and full sun.

Sowing Seeds: Plant seeds directly in the garden after the last frost or start indoors and transplant. Space them about 12 inches apart.

Care and Maintenance:

Watering: Keep the soil consistently moist, especially during dry spells.

Deadheading: Regularly remove spent flowers to encourage continuous blooming.

Fertilizing: Minimal fertilization needed; too much can reduce flower production.

Harvesting Calendula

Harvesting Blooms:

Timing: Pick flowers in the morning when they're fully open for the highest concentration of beneficial compounds.

Drying: Dry the blooms by hanging them upside down in a dark, well-ventilated area.

Preservation:

Storing Dried Flowers: Once completely dry, store in airtight containers in a cool, dark place for later use.

Utilizing Calendula

Culinary and Medicinal Applications:

Teas and Infusions: Create teas or infusions with the dried flowers for a soothing beverage.

Skincare Products: The petals can be infused into oils or added to homemade lotions and salves for their skin-soothing properties.

Calendula's vibrant blooms and diverse uses make it a wonderful addition to any garden, offering not just beauty but also practical applications in health and skincare!

CALIFORNIA POPPY

Growing California Poppy (Eschscholzia californica)

Cultivation:

Soil and Sun: Prefers well-drained soil and full sun.

Sowing Seeds: Plant seeds directly in the garden in the fall for early spring blooms. Scatter the seeds lightly and press them gently into the soil.

Utilizing California Poppy

Ornamental and Medicinal Uses

Ornamental: These vibrant flowers make stunning garden additions, especially in arid or dry regions.

Medicinal Purposes: California Poppy has been traditionally used for its sedative and calming properties. However, it's crucial to seek guidance from a healthcare professional before using it for medicinal purposes.

Care and Maintenance:

Watering: Requires little water once established; avoid overwatering.

Thinning: Thin the seedlings to ensure proper spacing, usually 6-12 inches apart.

Minimal Maintenance: California Poppies are relatively low-maintenance.

Harvesting California Poppy

Blooms:

Timing: Pick flowers in the morning when they're open for the best color and potency.

Preservation:

Drying: Allow harvested blooms to air dry in a cool, dark area. Store in airtight containers once dry for later use.

California Poppy's striking appearance and potential medicinal properties make it a captivating addition to gardens while holding historical significance in traditional medicine!

CAYENNE

Cultivating Cayenne (Capsicum annuum)

Growing Conditions:

Warmth and Sunlight: Thrives in warm temperatures and full sunlight.

Soil Preference: Well-draining soil rich in organic matter.

Planting:

Seeds or Transplants: Start seeds indoors about 8-10 weeks before the last frost or directly sow them in warm soil.

Spacing: When transplanting, space the plants about 18-24 inches apart.

Care:

Watering: Keep the soil consistently moist but not waterlogged. Mulching can help retain moisture.

Fertilizing: Apply a balanced fertilizer once the plants start flowering.

Harvesting Cayenne

Fruit Harvest

Timing: Harvest peppers when they reach the desired size and color. For cayenne, this is typically when they turn red and mature.

Drying Cayenne Peppers:

Air Drying: String the peppers and hang them in a well-ventilated, warm area until they are thoroughly dried.

Alternative Drying Methods: Dehydrators or low-heat ovens can also be used to dry the peppers.

Utilizing Cayenne

Culinary Uses:

Spice: Ground cayenne peppers add heat and flavor to various dishes, from salsas to soups and sauces.

Homemade Pepper Flakes: Crush dried cayenne peppers to make your own red pepper flakes.

Cayenne, with its spicy heat, is not just a culinary delight but also adds a fiery punch to numerous dishes, bringing both flavor and heat to the table!

CHICKWEED

Cultivating Chickweed (Stellaria media)

Growing Chickweed:

Growing Conditions: Grows best in cool, moist environments.

Soil Type: Thrives in rich, well-draining soil.

Planting:

Sowing Seeds: Directly sow seeds in early spring or fall.

Spacing: Allow about 6 inches between plants.

Maintenance:

Watering: Keep the soil consistently moist, especially during dry spells.

Trimming: Regularly trim the plant to encourage bushier growth.

Harvesting Chickweed

Storage:

Fresh Use: Chickweed is best used fresh. If storing, keep it in a plastic bag in the refrigerator for a short period.

Utilizing Chickweed

Culinary Uses:

Salads and Soups: Add fresh chickweed to salads or use it as a garnish. It can also be used in soups.

Tea: Infuse the leaves for a mild, earthy tea.

Chickweed, with its delicate taste and versatility, can be a delightful addition to salads, soups, and even as a refreshing tea!

RED CLOVER

Cultivating Red Clover (Trifolium pratense)

Growing Red Clover:

Environmental Preferences: Flourishes in temperate climates.

Soil Type: Thrives in well-draining, loamy soil.

Planting:

Sowing Seeds: Plant seeds in early spring or late summer.

Harvest Time:

Leaves and Stems: Harvest young, tender leaves and stems.

Depth: Sow seeds shallowly, around ¼ inch deep.

Spacing: Maintain spacing of about 6-8 inches between plants.

Maintenance:

Watering: Ensure consistent moisture in the soil, particularly during dry spells.

Mulching: Apply mulch to retain moisture and inhibit weed growth.

Harvesting Red Clover

Harvest Time:

Blooming Phase: Harvest when the plant is in full bloom.

Cutting: Trim the flowers along with the upper stems.

Storage:

Drying: Dry the harvested blooms and store them in a cool, dry place.

Utilizing Red Clover

Culinary Uses:

Tea: Brew dried red clover flowers for a floral, herbal tea.

Cosmetic and Medicinal Applications:

Herbal Remedies: Red clover is often used in herbal remedies and tinctures.

Skincare: Its flowers can be used in skincare preparations for their soothing properties.

Red clover's blossoms are not only visually appealing but also serve as a delightful addition to teas and herbal remedies, contributing to both taste and well-being.

COMFREY

Cultivating Comfrey (Symphytum officinale)

Growing Comfrey:

Environmental Preferences: Flourishes in most soils, tolerating shade but prefers full sun to partial shade.

Soil Type: Adaptable to various soil types.

Planting:

Propagation: Can be grown from seeds or root cuttings.

Depth: Plant root cuttings about 2-3 inches deep.

Maintenance:

Watering: Requires moderate watering, especially during dry periods.

Pruning: Regular pruning can promote leaf growth.

Harvesting Comfrey

Harvest Time:

Timing: Harvest young leaves before flowering for optimal potency.

Storage:

Drying: Dry leaves in a cool, dark place for future use.

Utilizing Comfrey

Garden Aid:

Mulch or Compost: The large leaves make great mulch or can be composted.

Medicinal and Topical Uses:

Poultices: Leaves can be used to create poultices for minor skin irritations.

Traditional Medicine: Often used in traditional herbal medicine.

Comfrey, with its rapid growth and multi-purpose use in both gardening and traditional medicine, can be a valuable addition to any garden or herbal remedy collection.

CORNFLOWER

Growing Cornflower (Centaurea cyanus

Cultivation:

Ideal Conditions: Thrives in well-draining soil and prefers full sun.

Sowing: Directly sow seeds into the ground in early spring or fall.

Care:

Watering: Moderate watering requirements, particularly during dry spells.

Thinning: Thin seedlings to ensure proper spacing for healthy growth.

Harvesting:

Blooms: Harvest when the flowers are in full bloom for the best color and potency.

Preservation:

Drying: Dry the flowers in a dark, well-ventilated space for storage.

Utilization:

Ornamental Beauty: Known for its striking blue hue, it's often used in floral arrangements.

Culinary Uses: Petals are edible and used as a decorative element in salads or teas.

Cornflowers not only add a vivid touch to gardens but also offer a unique culinary contribution, making them a versatile and visually stunning choice for both aesthetics and practical applications.

CHAMOMILE

Growing Chamomile (Matricaria recutita and Anthemis nobilis)

Cultivation:

Optimal Conditions: Prefers well-draining soil and full sun to partial shade.

Sowing: Plant seeds in early spring or fall directly into the ground.

Maintenance:

Watering: Keep the soil consistently moist, especially when establishing the plants.

Thinning: Thin seedlings for proper spacing.

Harvesting:

Flowers: Harvest flowers in the morning once they're fully open for the highest oil content and flavor.

Preservation:

Drying: Dry flowers in a cool, dark place to retain their beneficial properties.

Utilization:

Culinary Uses: Infuse fresh or dried flowers for a soothing herbal tea with calming properties.

Medicinal Applications: Chamomile is renowned for its calming and sleep-inducing effects. It's also used in skincare for its anti-inflammatory properties.

Chamomile, with its serene fragrance and versatile uses, is a delightful addition to any garden, offering both practical and therapeutic benefits.

CRAMP BARK

Cultivating Cramp Bark (Viburnum opulus)

Growing Conditions:

Soil: Thrives in moist, well-draining soil.

Sunlight: Prefers partial shade to full sun.

Hardiness: Adaptable and resilient in various climates.

Planting:

Time: Plant in the spring or fall.

Spacing: Ensure appropriate spacing, roughly 5 to 10 feet apart, as it can grow quite large.

Care and Maintenance:

Watering: Keep the soil consistently moist, especially during dry spells.

Pruning: Regular pruning can help maintain a healthy shape and size.

Harvesting:

Bark: Harvest the bark during the dormant season for its medicinal properties.

Uses:

Medicinal Purposes: Cramp Bark is known for its muscle-relaxing and anti-spasmodic properties, commonly used for menstrual cramps and muscle tension.

Preparation: It's often used in tinctures, teas, or capsules for consumption.

Storage:

Drying: Dry the harvested bark for future use, storing it in a cool, dark place.

Cramp Bark, with its therapeutic qualities, serves as a valuable addition to any herb garden, offering natural remedies for various conditions.

CRANBERRY

Cultivating Cranberry (Vaccinium macrocarpon)

Growing Conditions:

Soil: Cranberries thrive in acidic, sandy peat or loamy soils with good drainage.

Sunlight: They require full sun exposure.

Hardiness: Cranberries are hardy in USDA zones 2 to 7.

Planting:

Time: Plant in the spring or early fall.

Spacing: Plant cranberries in rows with about 2 to 4 feet between plants.

Care and Maintenance:

Watering: Maintain consistently moist soil. Cranberries benefit from irrigation.

Mulching: Apply a layer of acidic mulch to conserve moisture and suppress weeds.

Pruning: Prune to remove dead or damaged vines

Harvesting:

Timing: Cranberries are typically ready for harvest in the fall, from late September to early November.

Collection: Harvest by either dry or wet picking methods. Wet picking involves flooding the bog and using mechanical harvesters to collect the floating berries.

Uses:

Culinary: Cranberries are widely used in dishes like cranberry sauce, cranberry juice, and baked goods.

Health Benefits: They are rich in antioxidants and have various health benefits, including supporting urinary tract health.

Storage:

Fresh Berries: Store fresh cranberries in the refrigerator for up to a month.

Freezing: Cranberries can be frozen for longer-term storage.

Cranberries are not only a delightful addition to holiday meals but also a nutritious fruit with a range of culinary and health applications. Cultivating them in your garden can provide a fresh, homegrown source of these vibrant berries.

DANDELIONS

Growing Dandelions (Taraxacum officinale)

Cultivation:

Soil: Dandelions are adaptable but prefer well-drained, loamy soil.

Sunlight: They thrive in full sun but tolerate partial shade.

Hardiness: These resilient plants grow in various climates.

Propagation:

Seeds: Scatter seeds in early spring or fall, lightly covering them with soil.

Division: Dandelions also propagate through division, replanting the root crowns.

Maintenance:

Watering: These plants are drought-tolerant but benefit from occasional watering during dry spells.

Pruning: Regularly deadhead to prevent seeding and promote continuous blooming.

Harvesting:

Leaves: Harvest leaves while young and tender, typically before the plant flowers for the best flavor.

Roots: Dig up roots in the fall for medicinal uses or as a coffee substitute.

Utilization:

Culinary: Dandelion leaves are edible and used in salads, sautés, and teas. The flowers can be used for making wine or syrups.

Medicinal: Dandelion has a long history in herbal medicine, particularly for liver health and digestion.

Coffee Substitute: Roasted dandelion roots can be ground and brewed as a caffeine-free coffee alternative.

Storage:

Leaves: Keep freshly harvested leaves in the refrigerator for a few days. They wilt quickly.

Roots: Dry the roots thoroughly before storing in a cool, dry place.

Note: When harvesting dandelions, ensure they are sourced from areas free of pesticides or other contaminants.

Dandelions are much more than pesky lawn invaders; they're versatile, nutritious, and offer a range of culinary and medicinal uses, making them a valuable addition to any garden.

ELECAMPANE

Cultivating Elecampane (Inula helenium)

Growing Conditions:

Soil: Elecampane thrives in well-drained, loamy soil. It prefers a slightly acidic to neutral pH.

Sunlight: Plant in a location that receives full sun to partial shade.

Hardiness: It's a hardy perennial that can withstand various climates.

Planting:

Seeds: Sow seeds in early spring or late fall, lightly covering them with soil.

Space: Leave ample space, as these plants can grow quite large.

Care:

Watering: Keep the soil consistently moist, especially during the plant's initial growth period.

Mulching: Apply mulch to help retain moisture and regulate soil temperature.

Harvesting:

Roots: Dig up roots in the plant's second or third year during late fall or early spring. Wash and dry them thoroughly.

Leaves and Flowers: Harvest leaves and flowers during the plant's blooming period for medicinal uses.

Utilization:

Medicinal: Elecampane has been traditionally used to support respiratory health and alleviate coughs. The roots are the primary medicinal part and can be used in teas or tinctures.

Culinary: The young leaves can be used in salads, and the flowers can be added for a touch of color and flavor.

Storage:

Roots: Once dried completely, store the roots in airtight containers in a cool, dry place.

Leaves and Flowers: Dry these parts separately and store them in airtight containers away from direct sunlight.

Caution: If planning to use Elecampane for medicinal purposes, it's advisable to consult with a healthcare professional due to its potency.

Elecampane's vibrant flowers, along with its diverse medicinal properties, make it a valuable addition to any herb garden, providing both aesthetic beauty and potential health benefits.

EDELBERRY

Growing Elderberry (Sambucus nigra)

Cultivation

Location: Elderberries prefer well-drained soil and full sun. They tolerate various soil types but thrive in loamy, fertile soil.

Planting: Choose either potted plants or cuttings. Plant in early spring.

Spacing: Plant them 5 to 6 feet apart due to their eventual size.

Care:

Watering: Elderberries need consistent moisture, especially during dry periods. Mulch around the plants to retain moisture and regulate temperature.

Pruning: Regular pruning is essential to encourage growth and maintain shape. Remove dead or damaged wood.

Harvesting:

Berries: Harvest the berries when they are fully ripe, usually late summer to early fall. They should be dark and plump.

Flowers: The flowers can also be harvested for teas or infusions in late spring.

Utilization:

Culinary: Elderberries are commonly used in jams, pies, and syrups. The flowers are used in teas and cordials.

Medicinal: They're celebrated for their immune-boosting properties and are often used in syrups and tinctures for cold and flu relief.

Storage:

Berries: Consume fresh or dry them thoroughly for longer shelf life. Store in airtight containers in a cool, dark place.

Flowers: Dry the flowers completely and store them in airtight containers away from light.

Note: Be cautious with elderberry consumption as the raw berries and other parts contain cyanide-inducing glycosides. Proper preparation, like cooking or drying, neutralizes this substance.

Elderberries are not only a delightful addition to your culinary endeavors but also hold traditional medicinal value, making them a versatile and valuable plant in any garden.

EUCALYPTUS

Growing Eucalyptus (Eucalyptus sp.)

Cultivation:

Climate: Eucalyptus thrives in warm climates and well-drained soil. They prefer full sun.

Planting: Plant from seeds or seedlings in spring or early summer. Ensure frost has passed.

Care:

Watering: Eucalyptus trees are drought-tolerant once established, but regular watering is crucial during their initial growth period.

Pruning: Prune for shape and to remove damaged or crossing branches.

Harvesting:

Leaves: Harvest leaves for various uses when the plant is mature. Select healthy, mature leaves from different parts of the tree.

Utilization:

Aromatherapy: Eucalyptus oil, extracted from the leaves, is used in aromatherapy due to its refreshing scent and potential health benefits.

Medicinal: The oil is also used for respiratory conditions and as an antiseptic.

Storage:

Leaves: Dry the leaves thoroughly, and store them in airtight containers away from light and moisture. If extracting oil, store it in dark glass bottles.

Note: Eucalyptus oil can be toxic if ingested. Always use it according to recommended guidelines and keep it away from children and pets.

Eucalyptus, with its aromatic leaves and valuable oil, can be a wonderful addition to your garden.

It not only adds visual appeal but also offers various practical and health-related benefits.

EVENING PRIMROSE

Cultivating Evening Primrose (Oenothera biennis)

Growing Conditions

Soil and Sun: Evening primrose thrives in well-draining soil and prefers full sun but can tolerate partial shade.

Planting: Sow seeds directly in the garden in early spring or late summer. Thin seedlings to about 12 inches apart.

Care:

Watering: Maintain consistent moisture, especially during dry periods.

Pruning: Remove spent blooms to encourage more flowering and prevent self-seeding if not desired.

Harvesting:

Seeds: Collect seeds from the mature flower heads when they turn brown and dry.

Leaves: Young leaves are edible and can be harvested throughout the growing season.

Utilization:

Culinary: Evening primrose seeds are edible and nutritious. They can be used in salads or ground into a meal.

Medicinal: Evening primrose oil, extracted from the seeds, is known for its potential health benefits, particularly for skin and women's health.

Storage:

Seeds: Store seeds in a cool, dry place in airtight containers. Ensure they are completely dry before storing.

Leaves: Use fresh or dry for later use, storing them in a cool, dark place in sealed containers.

Note: Evening primrose oil is widely used in supplements. However, it's advisable to consult a healthcare professional before use, especially if you have existing medical conditions or are taking medications.

Evening primrose, with its delicate blooms and versatile seeds, not only beautifies your garden but also offers nutritional and potential medicinal value.

FEVERFEW

Cultivating Feverfew (Tanacetum parthenium)

Cultivation:

Growing Conditions: Feverfew thrives in well-draining soil and prefers full sun but can tolerate partial shade.

Planting: Sow seeds in early spring or plant seedlings in well-prepared soil, spaced about 12 inches apart.

Care:

Watering: Maintain consistent moisture in the soil. Avoid overwatering, as feverfew prefers slightly drier conditions.

Pruning: Regular deadheading can prolong blooming and prevent self-seeding.

Harvesting:

Leaves and Flowers: Harvest leaves and flowers when they are in full bloom for the best potency.

Utilization:

Medicinal: Feverfew is renowned for its potential medicinal properties, particularly for migraines and other health issues. The leaves and flowers are often used in teas or tinctures.

Culinary: In some cultures, feverfew leaves are used sparingly in salads or as a garnish. However, it's crucial to be cautious due to its bitter taste.

Storage:

Drying: Dry the leaves and flowers in a cool, dark place and store them in sealed containers.

Fresh Use: Feverfew can be used fresh, but for long-term use, dried forms are more convenient.

Caution: Feverfew, while known for its potential benefits, can cause adverse effects in some individuals. Always consult a healthcare professional before using it medicinally, especially if you have existing health conditions or are on medication.

Feverfew's delicate, daisy-like blooms not only add charm to your garden but may also offer potential health benefits when utilized properly. Always approach its usage with caution and seek guidance if intending to use it for medicinal purposes.

FLAXSEED

Growing Flaxseed (Linum usitatissimum)

Cultivation:

Soil and Sun: Flaxseed thrives in well-draining soil with a neutral pH level. It prefers full sun.

Planting: Sow seeds directly in the garden or containers in early spring or early fall. Ensure the seeds are covered lightly with soil.

Care:

Watering: Flaxseed requires consistent moisture, especially during germination and flowering.

Thinning: Once seedlings appear, thin them to ensure proper spacing, typically 4-6 inches apart.

Harvesting:

Seeds: Harvest flaxseeds when the seed capsules turn brown and begin to split. Remove the seed capsules and allow them to dry further before extraction.

Utilization:

Culinary: Flaxseeds are highly nutritious and can be used in various dishes, from baked goods to smoothies, offering a boost of omega-3 fatty acids and fiber.

Medicinal: Flaxseeds are known for their potential health benefits, aiding in digestive health and potentially reducing the risk of heart disease.

Storage:

Seeds: Store flaxseeds in airtight containers in a cool, dark place to maintain their nutritional properties.

Caution: When consuming flaxseeds, it's crucial to drink plenty of water as they can absorb liquids and might cause digestive issues if not consumed with enough fluid.

Flaxseeds not only provide nutritional value but also add a charming touch to gardens. Their dual functionality, both in the kitchen and potentially in supporting health, makes them a valuable addition to any gardening endeavor.

FLOXGLOVE

Cultivating Foxglove (Digitalis lanata)

Growth Conditions:

Soil and Sun: Foxglove flourishes in fertile, well-draining soil, thriving in partial shade to full sun.

Planting: Sow seeds in early spring or late summer. Ensure the seeds are lightly covered with soil for successful germination.

Maintenance:

Watering: Keep the soil consistently moist, especially during dry spells, without waterlogging the plant.

Thinning: Once seedlings sprout, thin them to ensure proper spacing, typically 18-24 inches apart.

Care:

Pruning: Regularly deadhead spent flowers to encourage prolonged blooming and prevent self-seeding, as the plant can be invasive.

Mulching: Applying mulch around the base helps retain moisture and keeps the roots cool

Harvesting:

Seeds: Harvest ripe seeds when the seed pods dry and turn brown. Collect and store them for future planting.

Caution: Foxglove contains digitalis, a compound used in heart medications. However, it is highly toxic if ingested. Care should be taken when handling the plant, especially around pets and children.

Aesthetic and Utility:

Foxglove adds a vertical elegance to gardens with its tall spires of tubular flowers in various shades.

Though primarily ornamental, foxglove's compounds have historical medicinal uses. However, the toxicity necessitates extreme caution and professional guidance before any use.

Foxglove's beauty and historical significance make it a captivating addition to any garden, requiring attentive care due to its toxic nature.

GARLIC

Cultivating Garlic (Allium sativum

Planting Garlic:

Season: Plant cloves in the fall for a summer harvest or in early spring for a smaller, but still viable, late summer harvest.

Soil: Plant in well-draining, fertile soil with good organic content.

Plant Care:

Planting Depth: Place individual cloves root-side down, around 2 inches deep, with about 4-6 inches of space between them.

Mulching: Apply mulch to regulate soil temperature and retain moisture.

Maintenance:

Watering: Ensure consistent soil moisture, especially during the early growth stages.

Fertilizing: Provide a nitrogen-rich fertilizer during the growing season.

Harvesting:

Timing: Harvest when the lower leaves begin to yellow and wilt, typically mid-summer for fall-planted garlic.

Curing: Dry harvested bulbs in a well-ventilated area for a few weeks to enhance flavor and storage potential.

Uses

Culinary: Garlic is a versatile ingredient in various cuisines, adding depth and flavor to dishes.

Medicinal: Historically, it has been used for its purported health benefits, including potential antimicrobial and antioxidant properties.

Garlic is not only a flavorful addition to numerous dishes but also a relatively low-maintenance plant that rewards growers with its distinct aroma and taste, along with potential health benefits.

GINGER

Cultivating Ginger (Zingiber officinale)

Growing Ginger:

Starting: Begin with a ginger root purchased from a store, ensuring it's plump with well-developed growth buds, called eyes.

Soil: Plant in a well-draining, fertile potting mix or in the ground in a warm, partially shaded area

Planting Process:

Preparation: Soak the ginger root overnight to encourage sprouting.

Planting Depth: Place the ginger root with the eyes facing up in soil, covering it lightly with around an inch of soil.

Container Size: Use a wide, shallow container to accommodate the roots' spreading growth.

Maintenance:

Watering: Keep the soil consistently moist, but not waterlogged.

Temperature: Maintain a warm, humid environment, avoiding temperatures below 50°F (10°C).

Care and Growth:

Mulching: Apply mulch to retain moisture and suppress weed growth.

Fertilizing: Feed the plant with a balanced fertilizer regularly during the growing season.

Harvesting:

Timing: Ginger can be harvested after 8-10 months once the plant matures. You can unearth and harvest the rhizomes or harvest a portion, allowing the rest to continue growing.

Uses:

Culinary: Fresh ginger root is widely used in various cuisines, adding a unique, spicy flavor to dishes.

Medicinal: It's renowned for potential health benefits, including aiding digestion and having anti-inflammatory properties.

Growing ginger at home can be a rewarding experience, providing a fresh supply of this versatile spice for culinary uses and potentially for health benefits.

GINKGO

Cultivating Ginkgo (Ginkgo biloba

Growing Ginkgo:

Planting: Ginkgo trees are typically grown from seeds or nursery-purchased saplings.

Soil: Plant in well-draining, loamy soil that's slightly acidic

Planting Process

Seed Planting: If growing from seeds, plant them in spring or fall.

Saplings: When using nursery saplings, transplant them carefully, ensuring they are well-watered and planted at the same depth they were in the nursery container.

Maintenance:

Watering: Keep the soil consistently moist, especially during the tree's initial growth phase.

Sunlight: Ginkgo trees thrive in full sun but can tolerate partial shade

Care and Growth:

Pruning: Shape the tree when it's young and later only for maintenance or to remove dead branches.

Fertilizing: Use a balanced fertilizer in the early spring to support growth.

Harvesting

Seed Collection: Ginkgo trees produce seeds within fleshy fruit. Harvest and remove the fruit, then let the seeds dry for a few days before planting.

Uses:

Ornamental: Ginkgo trees are prized for their unique fan-shaped leaves, turning a brilliant yellow in the fall.

Medicinal: The leaves have been used in traditional medicine and herbal remedies, although it's essential to seek guidance from a healthcare professional before using them.

Ginkgo trees not only offer aesthetic appeal in landscapes but also hold historical and potential medicinal significance, making them a valuable addition to gardens and environments.

GINSENG

Growing Ginseng (Panax sp.

Cultivation:

Shade-loving Plant: Ginseng thrives in shaded, wooded areas with well-draining, loamy soil.

Site Selection: Choose a spot with about 70-80% shade, such as under deciduous trees, where it's protected from direct sunlight.

Planting Process:

Preparation: Clear the area of debris and weeds, ensuring the soil is loose and rich.

Sowing: Plant seeds in the fall or early spring, around 1 inch deep.

Maintenance:

Moisture: Keep the soil consistently moist but not waterlogged.

Mulching: Apply a natural mulch to help retain moisture and control weeds.

Care and Growth:

Patience: Ginseng takes several years to mature. It grows slowly, and its seeds can take up to 18 months to germinate.

Weeding: Regularly weed the area to prevent competition for resources.

Harvesting:

Maturity: Ginseng is typically harvested after about 4-6 years when the roots have matured.

Harvesting Roots: Carefully dig up the roots, being cautious not to damage them.

Uses:

Medicinal: The roots of ginseng are widely used in herbal medicine and are believed to have various health benefits. Consult with an expert before using it for medicinal purposes.

Ginseng cultivation demands patience and dedication, but the potential health benefits and its cultural significance make it a valuable addition to a shaded garden or wooded area.

GOLDENSEAL

Growing Goldenseal (Hydrastis canadensis)

Cultivation

Shade-Loving Plant: Goldenseal thrives in shady, well-drained, and loamy soil, preferably in woodland conditions.

Planting Process:

Site Selection: Choose a location with around 70-80% shade, mimicking a woodland environment.

Soil Preparation: Loosen the soil and ensure good drainage.

Planting Goldenseal:

Rhizomes: Plant the rhizomes in early spring, burying them about an inch deep in the soil.

Spacing: Keep about 6 to 12 inches between each rhizome.

Maintenance:

Moisture: Keep the soil consistently moist without waterlogging.

Mulching: Apply a natural mulch to maintain moisture and prevent weed growth.

Care and Growth:

Patience: Goldenseal takes several years to mature. It's a slow grower and might not be ready for harvesting until it's around 4-6 years old.

Harvesting:

Maturity: Goldenseal roots are usually ready for harvesting after 4-6 years. Harvest by carefully digging up the rhizomes.

Uses:

Medicinal Properties: Goldenseal has been traditionally used for its medicinal properties, primarily in natural remedies. Its roots are believed to contain compounds with various health benefits.

Goldenseal cultivation requires patience due to its slow growth, but the potential health benefits and its role in traditional medicine make it a sought-after herb.

GROUND IVY

Growing Ground Ivy (Glechoma hederacea)

Cultivation:

Adaptability: Ground Ivy is a low-growing perennial that thrives in shaded areas, though it can adapt to varying light conditions.

Soil Preference: It grows well in moist, well-drained soil and can tolerate a range of soil types

Planting Process:

Location: Select a spot that receives some shade, as direct sunlight might scorch the leaves.

Soil Preparation: Ensure the soil is well-drained and has adequate moisture.

Planting Ground Ivy

Propagation: It can be propagated through seeds or division of existing plants.

Spacing: Plant seedlings or divisions approximately 12 inches apart to allow for spreading

Maintenance:

Watering: Keep the soil consistently moist, especially during dry spells.

Weeding: Regularly weed to prevent competition for nutrients.

Care and Growth:

Vigilance: Ground Ivy tends to spread rapidly, so monitor its growth to prevent it from overtaking other plants.

Harvesting:

Leaves: Harvest the leaves as needed throughout the growing season. They can be used fresh or dried for various purposes.

Uses:

Culinary and Medicinal Uses: Ground Ivy has been utilized for its culinary potential, often used in salads or herbal teas. Medicinally, it's been used for its potential health benefits, but usage should be moderated.

Ground Ivy can be a beneficial addition to your garden, offering both culinary and potential medicinal uses. However, its rapid spreading nature requires attentive management to prevent it from becoming invasive.

HAWTHORN

Cultivating Hawthorn (Crataegus sp.

Growing Conditions:

Climate: Hawthorn thrives in temperate climates.

Soil Preference: It prefers well-draining, loamy soil and can tolerate various soil types.

Exposure: It grows best in full sun to partial shade.

Planting Process:

Seed Planting: Sow seeds in a prepared bed in the fall for natural stratification, or in the spring after cold stratification.

Seedlings: Plant seedlings in well-prepared soil, ensuring they're adequately spaced for growth.

Maintenance:

Watering: Keep the soil consistently moist, especially during dry periods.

Pruning: Regular pruning helps shape the tree and promotes healthy growth.

Growth and Care:

Vigilance: Monitor for pests or diseases, addressing any issues promptly.

Harvesting

Berries: Harvest the berries in the late summer or fall when they're ripe and have a deep red color.

Uses:

Culinary and Medicinal: Hawthorn berries are commonly used in herbal preparations for their potential health benefits. They can be made into teas, tinctures, or extracts.

Ornamental: Hawthorn trees also have ornamental value with their beautiful blooms and can be used in landscaping.

Hawthorn's berries are particularly esteemed for their medicinal properties, but as with any herbal use, it's recommended to seek advice before consuming or using for medicinal purposes.

HERB ROBERT

Cultivating Herb Robert (Geranium robertianum)

Growing Conditions:

Habitat: Herb Robert is an adaptable and hardy plant that thrives in various environments.

Soil Preference: It prefers well-draining, moderately fertile soil

Planting Process:

Seed Planting: Sow seeds directly into the ground in spring or fall.

Spacing: Plant them about 6-12 inches apart to allow for their spreading nature.

Maintenance:

Watering: Keep the soil consistently moist, especially during dry spells, but avoid waterlogging.

Pruning: Regularly deadhead spent flowers to encourage continuous blooming.

Growth and Care:

Vigilance: Herb Robert is generally low-maintenance and resistant to pests and diseases.

Harvesting:

Leaves and Flowers: Harvest leaves and flowers as needed throughout the growing season. They're best used fresh.

Uses:

Medicinal: Herb Robert has been used in traditional medicine for various purposes due to its reported antibacterial and astringent properties. It's commonly made into teas or tinctures.

Companion Plant: Its pungent scent is believed to repel certain pests, making it a beneficial companion plant in gardens.

Herb Robert is a versatile herb, known for its potential health benefits. As always, consult with a healthcare professional before using it for medicinal purposes.

HOREHOUND

Cultivating Horehound (Marrubium vulgare)

Growing Conditions:

Hardiness: Horehound is a tough, perennial herb that thrives in various climates and soil types.

Soil Preference: Well-draining soil is preferable, but it can adapt to different soil conditions.

Planting Process:

Seeds or Transplants: It can be grown from seeds or transplanted from root divisions in the spring.

Spacing: Plant individual horehound plants about 18-24 inches apart.

Maintenance:

Watering: It's relatively drought-tolerant once established, but regular watering in the early stages aids growth.

Pruning: Regularly trim back the plant to encourage new growth and prevent it from becoming leggy.

Growth and Care:

Pest and Disease: Horehound is relatively resistant to most pests and diseases.

Harvesting:

Leaves and Flowers: Harvest the leaves and flowers just before the plant blooms for the highest concentration of essential oils and active compounds.

Uses:

Medicinal: Horehound has been used in traditional medicine for respiratory ailments, coughs, and sore throats. It can be brewed into teas, lozenges, or cough syrups.

Flavoring: It's also utilized as a flavoring agent in candies and herbal liqueurs due to its slightly bitter taste.

Horehound is a robust herb with historical significance in traditional medicine and culinary applications. Always seek professional advice before using it for medicinal purposes.

HORSE CHESTNUT

Cultivating Horse Chestnut (Aesculus hippocastanum)

Growing Conditions:

Climate: Flourishes in temperate regions with well-distributed rainfall.

Soil Type: Thrives in fertile, well-drained soil.

Planting Process

Seeds: Plant fresh seeds in the fall or spring. Sow them 2-4 inches deep.

Maintenance:

Watering: Requires regular watering, especially in the early growth stages.

Pruning: Trim to shape the tree or remove damaged branches in late winter.

Growth and Care:

Pest and Disease: Susceptible to leaf-mining insects and certain diseases, but proper care can mitigate these issues.

Harvesting:

Seeds: Collect the seeds from the spiky husks in autumn. They need proper processing before they're safe for use due to their toxic nature.

Uses:

Traditional Medicine: Historically used in herbal medicine for certain conditions, but ingestion of raw seeds can be toxic.

Ornamental: Often planted for its decorative value, admired for its large, showy flowers in spring and interesting fruits in autumn.

The Horse Chestnut tree offers ornamental beauty and historical medicinal significance, but caution is necessary due to the toxic nature of its seeds. Always consult with experts before using it for any medicinal purposes.

HOLLYHOCK

Cultivating Hollyhock (Alcea rosea)

Growing Conditions:

Climate: Thrives in temperate climates with moderate summers and mild winters.

Soil: Well-draining, fertile soil with a slightly acidic to neutral pH.

Planting Process:

Seeds: Start seeds indoors or sow directly in the garden. Ensure a sunny location.

Spacing: Plant the seeds or seedlings about 18-24 inches apart.

Maintenance:

Watering: Regular watering, particularly during dry spells, to establish strong root systems.

Support: As they grow tall, stake or provide support to prevent them from toppling over.

Growth and Care:

Pruning: Deadhead spent flowers to encourage new blooms and prevent self-seeding.

Pest and Disease: Watch for rust, a common disease among hollyhocks. Proper air circulation can help prevent it.

Harvesting:

Seeds: Collect seeds from spent blooms for propagation in the next season.

Uses:

Ornamental: Adds a vertical dimension to gardens, available in various colors, and attracts pollinators.

Historical and Medicinal: In the past, used for medicinal purposes, although caution is advised as certain parts may be toxic.

Hollyhocks are stunning additions to gardens, boasting vibrant blooms and attracting pollinators. Their historical medicinal use requires careful consideration and consultation before any application.

HOPHORNBEAM TREE

Cultivating Hophornbeam Tree (Ostrya virginiana)

Growing Conditions:

Climate: Adaptable to various climates, but typically thrives in temperate regions.

Soil: Well-draining soil, tolerates various soil types, including rocky or sandy soils.

Planting Process:

Seeds or Seedlings: Plant seeds or young trees in the desired location in spring or fall.

Depth: Ensure proper planting depth, similar to the nursery container.

Maintenance:

Watering: Regular watering during the tree's establishment phase, especially in dry conditions.

Mulching: Apply a layer of mulch around the base to retain moisture and regulate soil temperature.

Pruning: Minimal pruning required; mainly remove dead or damaged branches.

Growth and Care:

Growth Rate: Relatively slow-growing but steady.

Pest and Disease: Generally resistant to many pests and diseases, making it a low-maintenance tree.

Harvesting:

Hophornbeam trees are not typically harvested for consumable products.

Uses:

Landscape: Valued for its attractive bark and unique branching pattern, often used in landscaping.

Wildlife: Provides nesting sites for birds and habitats for various wildlife.

Wood: The wood is dense and hard, suitable for woodworking.

The Hophornbeam tree, with its low-maintenance characteristics and distinct appearance, serves as a valuable addition to landscapes, benefiting wildlife and offering durable wood for various applications.

HORSETAIL

Growing Horsetail (Equisetum arvense

Cultivation:

Environment: Horsetail, a perennial, thrives in moist environments and can adapt to various soil types.

Light: Prefers partial to full sunlight.

Planting:

Rhizomes or Division: Plant rhizomes or divided plants in spring or fall in a location with ample moisture.

Spacing: If planting multiple, space them about 18 inches apart to accommodate their spread.

Maintenance:

Watering: Keep the soil consistently moist but not waterlogged.

Containment: Consider planting in containers to manage its spreading nature in garden settings.

Pruning: Trim or cut back any invasive growth to maintain control.

Growth and Care:

Growth Rate: Horsetail grows vigorously and may become invasive if not contained.

Propagation: Easily spreads via rhizomes, so keep an eye on its growth and spread.

Disease and Pest Resistance: Generally resilient to pests and diseases.

Harvesting:

Aerial Parts: Harvest young shoots for culinary or medicinal purposes before they become too mature and tough.

Uses:

Medicinal: Horsetail has historical use in traditional medicine for its potential diuretic and antioxidant properties.

Garden Ornament: It can be used ornamentally in gardens for its unique appearance.

Pond Plant: Suitable for water gardens or damp areas due to its affinity for moisture.

Horsetail, while visually intriguing and historically used in various applications, requires vigilant containment due to its invasive nature. When managed properly, it can be a unique addition to a garden or utilized for its potential medicinal properties.

JASMINE

Cultivating Jasmine (Jasminum officinale)

Growing Environment

Climate: Jasmine thrives in warm and temperate climates, preferring temperatures above freezing.

Sunlight: Requires full sun to partial shade.

Planting:

Soil: Well-draining, fertile soil is ideal for jasmine.

Container vs. Ground: It can be grown in containers or directly in the ground.

Maintenance:

Watering: Keep the soil consistently moist but not waterlogged, especially during the growing season.

Fertilization: Feed with a balanced fertilizer during the growing season to encourage flowering.

Pruning: Regularly prune to shape and control its growth.

Growth and Care:

Support: Provide trellises or support for climbing varieties.

Propagation: Can be propagated from seeds, cuttings, or layering.

Disease and Pest Control: Watch for pests like aphids and caterpillars, and treat promptly if noticed.

Harvesting:

Flowers: Harvest the blossoms as they open for various uses.

Uses:

Aromatherapy: Jasmine flowers are highly fragrant and are often used in essential oils and perfumes.

Tea: The blossoms can be used for making fragrant teas.

Ornamental: Adds a beautiful, fragrant touch to gardens and outdoor spaces.

Jasmine, prized for its aromatic blossoms, can be a lovely addition to a garden and provides various practical uses, from aromatherapy to tea-making. With proper care and attention, it can thrive and reward you with its delightful fragrance.

JEWELWEED

Cultivating Jewelweed (Impatiens capensis)

Growing Conditions:

Habitat: Jewelweed thrives in moist, shady conditions and is often found near water sources like streams or in damp woodland areas.

Sunlight: Prefers partial to full shade.

Planting:

Soil: Well-draining, moist, fertile soil is ideal.

Sowing Seeds: Plant seeds directly in the soil in early spring or late fall.

Maintenance:

Watering: Ensure consistent moisture, especially in drier conditions.

Spacing: Thin seedlings to about 18 inches apart for proper growth.

Mulching: Applying a layer of organic mulch can help retain moisture and regulate soil temperature.

Growth and Care:

Invasive Tendency: Monitor its spread as jewelweed can grow rapidly and might become invasive.

Pruning: Regularly trim to control growth and encourage bushier plants.

Division: Divide clumps every few years to manage growth and rejuvenate the plant.

Uses:

Medicinal Properties: Jewelweed is traditionally used as a natural remedy for skin irritations like poison ivy rashes.

Attracting Wildlife: The nectar-rich flowers attract hummingbirds and certain insects.

Ornamental: Its unique, spurred flowers add visual interest to shaded garden areas.

Harvesting:

Leaves: Collect the leaves for making topical treatments like poultices or salves.

Jewelweed, with its vibrant, unique flowers and medicinal properties, can be a beneficial addition to a shade garden, especially for its potential in aiding skin irritations. However, given its rapid growth, it's essential to manage its spread in cultivated areas.

JOE PYE WEED

Cultivating Joe Pye Weed (Eutrochium sp.)

Growing Conditions:

Sunlight: Thrives in full sun to partial shade.

Soil: Prefers moist, well-draining soil but can adapt to various soil types.

Planting:

Seed Sowing: Plant seeds directly into the soil in the fall or early spring.

Spacing: Allow enough space between plants to accommodate their mature size.

Maintenance:

Watering: Keep the soil consistently moist, especially during dry periods.

Mulching: Apply a layer of mulch to retain moisture and regulate soil temperature.

Growth and Care:

Pruning: Deadhead spent flowers to encourage prolonged blooming.

Support: Taller varieties might benefit from staking to prevent flopping.

Uses:

Attracting Wildlife: The flowers attract butterflies and bees, adding to the garden's biodiversity.

Aesthetic Value: With its tall, striking blooms, it's an excellent addition to cottage-style gardens and naturalized areas.

Medicinal Qualities: Some varieties have traditional medicinal uses.

Harvesting:

Seeds: Collect seeds for propagation or sharing with other gardeners.

Pruning: Trimming spent flowers can encourage further blooming.

Joe Pye Weed, with its attractive, feathery blooms, serves both aesthetic and ecological purposes in a garden setting. Its adaptability to various conditions makes it a versatile addition for those looking to attract pollinators and introduce native plants into their landscape.

LADY SLIPPER ORCHIDS

Cultivating Lady Slipper Orchids (Cypripedium parviflorum

Growing Conditions:

Shade Preference: Flourishes in shaded or partially shaded areas.

Soil: Requires well-draining, organic-rich soil, typically found in woodland environments.

Planting:

Transplanting: Best to obtain nursery-grown plants as they're sensitive to disturbance in the wild.

Location: Plant in areas mimicking their natural habitat, such as woodland gardens.

Maintenance:

Watering: Requires consistent moisture, especially during the growing season.

Mulching: Apply a layer of mulch to retain moisture and insulate roots.

Growth and Care:

Protection: Protect from direct sunlight and strong winds.

Fertilization: Generally not necessary; they derive nutrients from the organic matter in the soil.

Uses

Ornamental Value: Coveted for their unique, slipper-shaped blooms, adding elegance to shaded gardens.

Conservation: Some varieties are protected and should not be collected from the wild.

Harvesting:

Reproduction: Propagation is often done through division by experts to avoid damaging wild populations.

Cypripedium parviflorum, or Lady Slipper Orchids, present an alluring and delicate addition to shaded garden spaces. As these orchids are often found in woodland settings, replicating their natural environment is crucial for their successful growth and blooming. Given their vulnerable status, it's essential to exercise care when obtaining these plants to preserve their natural populations.

LAVENDER

Cultivating Lavender (Lavandula angustifolia)

Growing Conditions:

Sunlight: Lavender thrives in full sunlight, at least 6 to 8 hours daily.

Well-Draining Soil: Requires soil with excellent drainage to prevent root rot.

Planting:

Timing: Best planted in the spring or fall.

Spacing: Allow ample space between plants for good air circulation.

Container Planting: Suitable for containers with proper drainage holes.

Maintenance

Watering: Requires regular watering until established, then moderate watering.

Pruning: Trim spent blooms to encourage growth and shape the plant.

Fertilization: Minimal feeding, avoid nitrogen-rich fertilizers.

Growth and Care:

Winter Protection: In colder climates, protect from harsh winter conditions.

Mulching: Apply a thin layer of mulch to retain moisture.

Uses:

Aromatherapy: Harvest and dry the flowers for aromatic sachets or oils.

Culinary: The flowers can be used in cooking, especially in desserts or teas.

Medicinal: Lavender is known for its calming properties, often used in herbal remedies.

Harvesting:

Timing: Harvest just before the flowers are fully open for the most potent fragrance and oil content.

Drying: Bundle and hang in a dry, airy place away from direct sunlight for drying.

Lavender, with its soothing fragrance and multiple uses, not only adds aesthetic appeal to gardens but also serves culinary, medicinal, and aromatic purposes. Its success relies on well-draining soil, ample sunlight, and appropriate care, ensuring a bountiful harvest of aromatic blooms.

LEMONS

Cultivating Lemons (Citrus limon)

Growing Conditions:

Climate: Thrives in subtropical to tropical climates.

Sunlight: Requires full sun exposure for optimal fruiting.

Planting:

Location: Choose a well-drained, sunny spot for planting.

Soil: Loamy, well-draining soil with a slightly acidic to neutral pH.

Care and Maintenance:

Watering: Regular watering, ensuring the soil is moist but not waterlogged.

Fertilization: Use citrus-specific fertilizers during the growing season.

Pruning: Prune to shape and remove dead branches.

Protection and Care:

Cold Protection: Shield from frost or cold weather in non-tropical regions.

Pest Control: Regularly check for pests and treat as necessary.

Harvesting:

Timing: Harvest when the fruits have developed their full color and give slightly to gentle pressure.

Twisting Method: Twist the lemon gently to detach it from the tree.

Uses:

Culinary: Lemons are versatile and used in numerous dishes, beverages, and desserts.

Health Benefits: High in vitamin C and antioxidants, aiding in immune health.

Aromatherapy: Lemon essential oil is used for its refreshing and uplifting scent.

Note: In regions with colder climates, consider potted lemon trees that can be brought indoors during chilly seasons to protect them from frost. With proper care, lemon trees can provide an abundant harvest, bringing a zesty touch to various culinary delights and aromatherapy.

LEMONGRASS

Growing Lemongrass (Cymbopogon flexuosus)

Cultivation:

Climate: Lemongrass thrives in warm, tropical regions.

Sunlight: Prefers full sun for optimal growth.

Planting:

Soil: Well-draining soil with organic matter.

Propagation: Usually planted via stalk divisions.

Care and Maintenance:

Watering: Regular, consistent watering without waterlogging the soil.

Fertilization: Occasional feeding with a balanced fertilizer.

Pruning: Trim dead leaves to encourage new growth.

Protection:

Cold Protection: In cooler climates, plant in pots to move indoors during colder seasons

Harvesting:

Timing: Harvest when the stalks are about half an inch thick.

Cutting Method: Snip the stalks close to the ground.

Uses:

Culinary: Adds a unique, citrusy flavor to various dishes, especially in Southeast Asian cuisine.

Medicinal: Known for its calming properties and as a remedy for digestive issues.

Aromatherapy: Lemongrass essential oil is used in aromatherapy for its invigorating scent.

Note: Lemongrass is versatile and offers both culinary and medicinal benefits, making it a valuable addition to gardens or as a potted plant, especially in regions with warm climates.

LEMON BALM

Growing Lemon Balm (Melissa officinalis)

Cultivation

Climate: Grows well in temperate climates.

Sunlight: Prefers full sun but tolerates partial shade.

Planting:

Soil: Well-draining soil enriched with organic matter.

Propagation: Seeds, cuttings, or plant divisions.

Care and Maintenance

Watering: Keep the soil consistently moist but not waterlogged.

Pruning: Regular trimming to encourage bushy growth.

Fertilization: Occasional feeding with balanced fertilizer.

Protection:

Pests: Susceptible to aphids and spider mites; watch for infestations.

Diseases: Prone to powdery mildew in humid conditions

Harvesting

Timing: Leaves are best harvested just before flowering for optimal flavor.

Cutting Method: Trim the leaves, leaving some for the plant to continue growing.

Uses:

Culinary: Leaves add a lemony flavor to teas, salads, and various dishes.

Medicinal: Often used to ease stress, anxiety, and aid in sleep.

Aromatherapy: Essential oils derived from lemon balm are used in aromatherapy for their calming properties.

Note: Lemon balm is a versatile herb, offering both culinary and medicinal benefits. It's relatively low-maintenance and can be a delightful addition to any herb garden.

LICORICE ROOT

Cultivating Licorice Root (Glycyrrhiza glabra)

Growing Conditions:

Climate: Thrives in warm, Mediterranean-like climates.

Soil: Well-draining, loamy soil with a slightly acidic to neutral pH.

Sunlight: Requires full sun for optimal growth.

Planting:

Propagation: Usually grown from root divisions or seedlings.

Spacing: Plant individual root divisions at least 2 to 3 feet apart.

Care and Maintenance:

Watering: Regular, deep watering, especially during dry periods.

Mulching: Apply mulch to retain soil moisture and regulate temperature.

Fertilization: Not usually necessary; mature plants benefit from occasional organic fertilizers.

Protection:

Pests: Vulnerable to aphids and root-knot nematodes. Employ organic pest control methods.

Diseases: Keep an eye out for root rot and fungal issues. Ensure proper drainage to prevent waterlogging.

Harvesting:

Timing: Roots are typically harvested in the fall, after three to four years of growth.

Method: Carefully dig up the roots, ensuring minimal damage.

Uses:

Medicinal: Licorice root is prized for its various medicinal properties, including soothing sore throats, aiding digestion, and supporting adrenal function.

Culinary: It's used as a flavoring agent in candies, herbal teas, and some traditional cuisines.

Cosmetic: Extracts from licorice root are used in some skincare products for their skin-soothing properties.

Note: Licorice root cultivation can be a long-term endeavor, as it takes several years for the roots to mature enough for harvesting. However, the health benefits and its culinary uses make it a valuable addition to any herb garden.

LINDEN

Cultivating Linden (Tilia sp.)

Growing Conditions:

Climate: Thrives in temperate climates.

Soil: Prefers loamy, well-draining soil with a slightly acidic to neutral pH.

Sunlight: Grows best in full sun to partial shade.

Planting:

Propagation: Typically from seeds, although some species can be grown from cuttings.

Spacing: Plant saplings at least 15 to 20 feet apart.

Care and Maintenance:

Watering: Requires moderate and consistent watering.

Mulching: Apply mulch to maintain soil moisture and deter weed growth.

Fertilization: Generally doesn't require additional fertilizers

Protection:

Pests: Vulnerable to aphids and caterpillars. Employ natural pest control methods.

Diseases: Watch for issues like leaf spot or powdery mildew. Adequate air circulation can prevent fungal problems.

Pruning:

Regular pruning helps shape the tree and removes dead or damaged branches.

Harvesting:

Not typically harvested for consumption but for ornamental or potentially medicinal purposes.

Flowers can be collected when in bloom for teas or infusions.

Uses:

Medicinal: Linden flowers are often used in herbal teas and infusions, believed to have calming and mild sedative effects.

Ornamental: Planted for its attractive foliage and fragrant flowers, enhancing gardens and landscapes.

Cultural Uses: Linden trees hold cultural significance in some societies, often symbolizing strength and tranquility.

Note: Linden trees are revered for their beauty and cultural importance. The fragrant and soothing properties of their flowers make them a popular choice for both gardeners and those seeking natural remedies.

LOTUS

Growing Lotus (Nelumbo nucifera)

Cultivation:

Climate: Ideal in warm, tropical regions but can thrive in temperate climates.

Water: Grows in water; best in calm, shallow ponds or containers.

Soil: Requires rich, loamy soil or mud with good organic content.

Sunlight: Full sun exposure is preferred.

Planting:

Seeds: Plant the seeds in spring when the water temperature is consistently above 70°F.

Depth: Submerge seeds in shallow water (4-6 inches) in containers or ponds.

Maintenance:

Watering: Ensure the water level is consistent and does not dry out.

Fertilization: Occasional application of aquatic plant fertilizer during the growing season.

Care:

Protection: Protect young plants from strong winds.

Pests: Watch for pests like aphids or red spider mites.

Harvesting:

Flowers: Typically not harvested but appreciated for their ornamental beauty.

Seeds: Pods can be collected for propagation or culinary use.

Uses

Ornamental: Lotus flowers are celebrated for their elegance and cultural significance.

Culinary: Lotus seeds and rhizomes are used in various Asian cuisines, often in soups, stir-fries, or desserts.

Medicinal: Some traditional medicine systems use various parts of the lotus plant for their supposed health benefits.

Note: Lotus plants are not just visually stunning but also hold cultural, culinary, and even potential medicinal significance, making them a fascinating addition to both gardens and various cultural practices.

BOOK 7: How to Grow, Harvest & Preserve for the Home Apothecary TO M FROM Z

MAPLE TREES

Growing Maple Trees (Acer species)

Cultivation:

Climate: Various species thrive in different climates. Some prefer cooler temperate climates, while others tolerate warmer regions.

Soil: Well-draining soil with good moisture retention, slightly acidic to neutral pH.

Sunlight: Most prefer full sun, but some varieties can tolerate partial shade.

Planting:

Time: Best planted in early spring or fall.

Depth: Plant the root ball slightly higher than the soil level.

Spacing: Allow enough space for the tree's mature canopy.

Maintenance:

Watering: Regular watering for young trees; established trees are often drought-tolerant.

Mulching: Mulch around the base to retain moisture and suppress weeds.

Pruning: Minimal pruning when young to shape and remove dead or diseased branches.

Care:

Protection: Protect young trees from strong winds and extreme weather conditions.

Pests and Diseases: Keep an eye out for common pests like aphids, scale insects, and diseases like powdery mildew or verticillium wilt.

Harvesting:

Sap: Some maple species yield sap that can be harvested in late winter or early spring for making maple syrup.

Uses:

Ornamental: Maple trees are popular for their stunning foliage and vibrant colors during the fall.

Wood: Some species provide high-quality timber for furniture and flooring.

Maple Syrup: Certain maple species produce sap that can be boiled down to make the beloved maple syrup.

Note: Maple trees are not just a beautiful addition to landscapes; they offer various practical uses, from providing shade to yielding maple syrup, making them a valuable and multi-purpose tree in many settings.

MARSHMALLOW

Cultivating Marshmallow (Althaea officinalis)

Planting Marshmallow:

Location: Choose a sunny or partially shaded spot with well-draining soil.

Soil: Thrives in moist, fertile soil, slightly acidic to neutral pH.

Sowing: Sow seeds indoors in early spring or directly in the garden once the frost has passed.

Maintenance:

Watering: Keep the soil consistently moist, especially during dry spells.

Mulching: Apply organic mulch to retain moisture and control weeds.

Fertilization: Apply organic compost to enrich the soil.

Pruning:

Cutting Back: Prune the plants in early spring to encourage new growth.

Deadheading: Remove spent flowers to encourage continuous blooming.

Harvesting Marshmallow:

Roots: Harvest the roots in the fall of the second year. Wash and dry them for later use.

Leaves and Flowers: Collect leaves and flowers during the growing season for immediate use.

Uses of Marshmallow:

Medicinal: Known for its medicinal properties, the roots are used in teas and tinctures for respiratory and digestive issues.

Culinary: The leaves can be used in salads, and the flowers can make a sweet addition to desserts.

Cosmetic: The mucilage from the roots is used in various skincare products for its soothing properties.

Note: Marshmallow is a versatile plant with various uses, making it a valuable addition to gardens for both its practical and ornamental benefits.

MILK THISTLE

Cultivating Milk Thistle (Silybum marianum)

Planting Milk Thistle:

Location: Plant in a sunny area with well-draining soil.

Sowing: Directly sow seeds in early spring or fall. Thin seedlings to prevent overcrowding.

Maintenance:

Watering: Provide consistent moisture, but ensure the soil doesn't become waterlogged.

Weeding: Regularly remove weeds to reduce competition for nutrients.

Mulching: Apply organic mulch to retain moisture and regulate soil temperature.

Pruning:

Deadheading: Remove spent flowers to prevent self-seeding and encourage continuous blooming.

Harvesting Milk Thistle:

Seeds: Harvest seeds when the flower heads turn brown. Dry them thoroughly before storage or use.

Leaves: Gather leaves throughout the growing season for immediate consumption or drying.

Uses of Milk Thistle:

Medicinal: Well-regarded for its liver-supporting properties. Seeds are used in teas or tinctures.

Culinary: Young leaves can be used in salads or cooked like spinach. The roasted seeds can be ground and added to dishes.

Cosmetic: Extracts from the seeds are used in certain skincare products for their beneficial properties.

Note: Milk Thistle is not just visually striking but also offers a range of practical applications, making it a versatile addition to gardens.

MINT

Cultivating Mint (Mentha sp.

Growing Conditions:

Soil: Plant in well-draining, moist soil with a slightly acidic to neutral pH.

Sunlight: Prefers partial shade to full sun, depending on the variety.

Planting:

From Cuttings: Easily propagated from cuttings or root divisions. Ensure each division has roots and stems for successful transplantation.

Spacing: Plant in separate containers or space at least 18 inches apart in the garden to prevent overcrowding.

Maintenance

Watering: Keep the soil consistently moist but not waterlogged.

Mulching: Apply mulch to retain moisture and inhibit weed growth.

Pruning: Regularly trim to encourage bushier growth and prevent legginess.

Harvesting Mint:

Leaves: Harvest leaves at any time during the growing season. The flavor is best before flowering, so early morning harvesting is ideal.

Stems: Cut the stems just above a leaf node to encourage new growth.

Uses of Mint:

Culinary: Adds a refreshing flavor to beverages, salads, sauces, and desserts. Can also be dried or frozen for later use.

Medicinal: Known for its digestive properties. It can be brewed into a tea or used in aromatherapy.

Repellent: Its strong scent deters pests; consider planting it near other vulnerable plants.

Note: Mint is a versatile herb with various uses, from flavoring culinary delights to promoting wellness and naturally repelling pests in the garden.

MOTHERWORT

Cultivating Motherwort (Leonurus cardiaca)

Growing Conditions:

Soil: Thrives in well-draining soil, tolerating a wide pH range.

Sunlight: Flourishes in full sun to partial shade.

Planting:

Seeds: Sow seeds directly in the garden or start indoors and transplant when the seedlings are robust.

Spacing: Provide ample space, around 18 to 24 inches between plants, as it can grow quite expansively.

Maintenance:

Watering: Keep the soil consistently moist but not waterlogged, especially during dry spells.

Pruning: Regularly deadhead spent flowers to encourage continuous blooming and prevent self-seeding.

Harvesting Motherwort:

Flowering Tops: Harvest when the plant is in full bloom, usually in the summer. Collect the upper part of the stem with flowers for medicinal use.

Leaves: Can be harvested throughout the growing season, but they're best before the plant flowers.

Uses of Motherwort:

Medicinal: Traditionally used to support heart health, ease menstrual discomfort, and reduce anxiety. Can be brewed as tea or used in tinctures.

In the Garden: Attracts beneficial insects and pollinators to the garden, supporting a healthy ecosystem.

Caution: Consult with a healthcare professional before using for medicinal purposes as it may interact with certain medications or conditions.

Note: Motherwort is not only a lovely addition to a garden but also holds a history of medicinal uses, making it a multi-functional and beneficial herb when used properly.

MUGWORT

Cultivating Mugwort (Artemisia vulgaris)

Growing Conditions:

Soil: Thrives in well-draining, moderately fertile soil.

Sunlight: Prefers full sun but can tolerate partial shade.

Planting:

Seeds: Sow seeds directly into the soil after the last frost, or start indoors and transplant seedlings.

Spacing: Provide ample space, around 18 to 24 inches between plants, as it can spread vigorously

Maintenance:

Watering: Regular watering, especially during dry periods, but avoid waterlogging.

Pruning: Trim back to prevent overgrowth and encourage bushiness.

Harvesting Mugwort:

Leaves: Best harvested before flowering for culinary or medicinal purposes. Gather young leaves in the morning for the best flavor.

Uses of Mugwort:

Medicinal: Often used in traditional medicine for its potential digestive, diuretic, and anti-inflammatory properties. It's also believed to aid in menstrual issues.

Culinary: Leaves can be used sparingly in salads or cooked as a flavoring herb in various dishes.

Caution: Mugwort can cause allergic reactions in some individuals and should be avoided during pregnancy and breastfeeding.

Note: Mugwort, while a versatile herb, requires caution in its use due to potential allergic reactions and its effects on specific health conditions. Always consult a healthcare professional before using it medicinally.

MULLEIN

Cultivating Mullein (Verbascum thapsus)

Growing Conditions:

Soil: Prefers well-draining, even rocky soil, but adapts to various soil types.

Sunlight: Thrives in full sun.

Planting:

Seeds: Sow seeds in early spring or late fall directly into the soil.

Spacing: Space plants about 2 feet apart.

Maintenance:

Watering: Mullein is drought-tolerant but benefits from watering during dry spells.

Pruning: Deadhead spent flowers to encourage continuous blooming and prevent self-seeding.

Harvesting Mullein:

Leaves and Flowers: Harvest leaves in the first year, and in the second year, the tall flowering stalks can be harvested for various uses.

Uses of Mullein:

Medicinal: Leaves and flowers are commonly used in herbal remedies for respiratory conditions. They can be brewed into tea or used in tinctures.

Culinary: The leaves are occasionally used as a mild flavoring in salads.

Crafts: The tall, dried flower stalks have been used historically as torches.

Note: Mullein has a long history in herbal medicine but should be used cautiously and preferably under the guidance of a healthcare professional due to its effects and potential interactions with certain medications. Always consult a healthcare provider before using it medicinally.

NETTLE

Cultivating Stinging Nettle (Urtica dioica)

Growing Conditions:

Soil: Nettles thrive in moist, nitrogen-rich soil.

Sunlight: Prefers partial shade but tolerates full sun.

Planting:

Seeds: Directly sow seeds in early spring or fall.

Spacing: Plant them about 18 inches apart.

Maintenance:

Watering: Keep the soil consistently moist.

Pruning: Regular harvesting encourages new growth. Use gloves when handling to avoid stings.

Harvesting Nettle:

Leaves: Harvest the leaves before flowering for culinary or medicinal use.

Roots: The roots can be harvested in the fall.

Uses of Stinging Nettle:

Culinary: The young leaves can be cooked and eaten like spinach, added to soups, or brewed into tea.

Medicinal: Often used in herbal medicine for various purposes, including as a diuretic or for joint pain relief.

Fiber: Historically, the plant has been used for making textiles.

Note: The stinging nettle's stings are caused by tiny hairs that can cause skin irritation. Always handle with care and consider wearing gloves. Also, consult with a healthcare professional before using it medicinally.

OREGANO

Cultivating Oregano (Origanum vulgare)

Growing Conditions:

Soil: Well-draining soil is ideal.

Sunlight: Full sun is preferred for optimum growth.

Planting:

Seeds: Start seeds indoors 6-10 weeks before the last frost or sow directly in the garden.

Spacing: Plant seedlings 8-10 inches apart.

Maintenance:

Watering: Allow the soil to dry out between waterings. Overwatering can cause root rot.

Pruning: Regularly trim to encourage bushier growth and prevent it from becoming too leggy.

Harvesting Oregano:

Leaves: Gather leaves once the plant is established and before it flowers for the best flavor.

Drying: Air-dry or use a dehydrator to preserve oregano for later use.

Uses of Oregano:

Culinary: A staple herb in Mediterranean cuisine, it flavors various dishes, from sauces and pizzas to salads.

Medicinal: Oregano contains antioxidants and has potential antibacterial properties. It's used in traditional medicine for various ailments.

Note: Oregano is a hardy herb but can be invasive, so consider planting it in a container to control its spread. It attracts beneficial insects and pollinators to your garden.

PASSIONFLOWER

Cultivating Passionflower (Passiflora sp.)

Growing Conditions:

Climate: Thrives in subtropical and tropical regions.

Soil: Well-draining, fertile soil with a slightly acidic pH.

Sunlight: Full sun for at least six hours a day.

Planting:

Seeds or Cuttings: Start from seeds or cuttings in spring after the last frost.

Spacing: Provide ample space, as these vines can spread vigorously.

Maintenance:

Watering: Regular watering is essential, especially during dry spells.

Support: As a climbing vine, it requires a trellis or structure to climb and spread.

Harvesting Passionflower:

Flowers and Fruit: Harvest the ripe fruits and flowers when they're mature and at their peak.

Uses of Passionflower:

Medicinal: Often used in traditional medicine to aid sleep and reduce anxiety. It's also believed to have calming properties.

Ornamental: Apart from its medicinal use, its unique flowers make it a beautiful addition to any garden.

Note: Some species produce edible fruits known as passionfruit, loved for their unique taste and used in various culinary dishes. Certain varieties of passionflower can be invasive, so keep an eye on their growth to prevent overtake.

PINE TREES

Cultivating Pine Trees (Pinus sp.)

Growing Conditions:

Climate: Pine trees thrive in diverse climates, from temperate to subtropical regions.

Soil: Well-draining, slightly acidic soil is preferred.

Sunlight: Full sun exposure is ideal for most species.

Planting:

Seedlings or Seeds: Plant seedlings or seeds in late winter or early spring for best results.

Spacing: Allow plenty of space between trees to accommodate their mature size.

Maintenance:

Watering: Young trees need consistent watering until established; mature trees are generally drought-tolerant.

Pruning: Minimal pruning for shaping or removing dead branches.

Harvesting Pine:

Needles and Cones: Collect fresh pine needles and cones for various uses.

Uses of Pine:

Wood: Valued for its timber used in construction, furniture, and paper production.

Resin: Pine resin is utilized in making varnishes, adhesives, and other industrial applications.

Aesthetic Value: Ornamental pine trees add beauty to landscapes and are popular choices for Christmas trees.

Note: Some species produce edible pine nuts that are a popular culinary ingredient, prized for their rich flavor and nutritional value. Additionally, pine needle tea is known for its health benefits and pleasant aroma.

PINEAPPLEWEED

Cultivating Pineapple Weed (Matricaria discoidea)

Growing Pineapple Weed:

Pineapple weed, resembling chamomile, is easy to cultivate and offers various practical and aromatic uses.

Growing Conditions:

Soil: Thrives in well-drained, poor soils, often found in disturbed areas.

Sunlight: Grows best in full sun but can tolerate partial shade.

Planting:

Seeds: Directly sow seeds in the desired area in early spring or fall.

Spacing: Thin seedlings to about 6 inches apart to allow for proper growth.

Maintenance:

Watering: Tolerant of drought conditions but benefits from moderate watering.

Weeding: Remove competing weeds to allow pineapple weed to flourish.

Harvesting Pineapple Weed:

Collect flowers when in bloom for various uses.

Uses of Pineapple Weed:

Herbal Tea: Its flowers make a pleasant, chamomile-like tea, offering relaxation and digestive benefits.

Aromatic Potpourri: Dried flowers can be used in sachets or potpourri for their sweet scent.

Natural Pest Repellent: Its aroma can deter insects, making it useful in natural pest control.

Note: Pineapple weed is considered a common wild plant and is often used for its calming properties and delightful aroma, making it a unique addition to a garden or herbal collection.

PLANTAIN

Cultivating Plantain (Plantago lanceolata

Growing Plantain:

Plantain, known for its various medicinal properties, is a hardy herb commonly found in many regions. Cultivating it in your garden offers access to its healing benefits.

Growing Conditions:

Soil: Adaptable to various soil types but thrives in well-draining soil.

Sunlight: Grows well in full sun to partial shade.

Planting

Seeds: Plant seeds directly in the garden in early spring or early fall.

Spacing: Allow about 6 inches between plants to ensure adequate space for growth.

Maintenance:

Watering: Regular, moderate watering without over-saturating the soil.

Weeding: Ensure minimal competition from weeds for better growth.

Harvesting Plantain:

Gather leaves when they are young and tender for medicinal uses.

Uses of Plantain:

Medicinal Purposes: Leaves are used in poultices or salves for wound healing and insect bites.

Internal Use: Leaves can be dried and used for teas or infusions for various health benefits.

Skin Care: Useful in skincare products due to its soothing and healing properties.

Note: Plantain is a versatile and beneficial herb often used in traditional medicine, offering a range of applications from healing wounds to promoting internal wellness.

QUEEN ANNE'S LACE

Growing Queen Anne's Lace (Daucus carota)

Cultivating Queen Anne's Lace:

Queen Anne's Lace, with its delicate and intricate flowers, is a stunning addition to any garden. Here's a guide to grow and care for this lovely herb.

Optimal Growing Conditions:

Soil: Well-draining soil, although it can tolerate various soil types.

Sunlight: Full sun to partial shade.

Planting:

Seeds: Sow seeds directly in the ground in early spring or late fall.

Spacing: Allow ample space for the plants, as they tend to spread out

Maintenance:

Watering: Moderate watering, ensuring the soil remains moist but not waterlogged.

Weeding: Regularly remove competing weeds to aid in the plant's growth.

Harvesting Queen Anne's Lace:

Gather flowers when in full bloom. Be cautious, as this plant closely resembles wild carrots, and harvesting must be done carefully.

Uses of Queen Anne's Lace:

Ornamental Value: Adds beauty to gardens and attracts beneficial insects.

Caution: This plant closely resembles the wild carrot, so proper identification is crucial before use. The root is edible, but it must be correctly identified to avoid confusion with poisonous plants.

Note: Queen Anne's Lace, with its lacy, white flowers, brings a delicate charm to gardens. However, it's essential to be cautious when harvesting, as proper identification is key to avoiding any risks associated with mistaken identity.

ROSES

Cultivating Roses (Rosa sp.)

Growing Roses:

Roses are timeless beauties and cultivating them can be a delightful endeavor. Here's a guide to grow and care for these classic flowers.

Optimal Growing Conditions:

Soil: Well-draining, fertile soil.

Sunlight: Full sun is ideal, at least six hours of direct sunlight.

Planting:

Time: Plant bare-root roses in early spring, but container roses can be planted at any time during the growing season.

Depth: Ensure the bud union (the swollen area where the canes meet the rootstock) is just above the soil level.

Maintenance:

Watering: Regular and consistent watering, especially during dry periods.

Pruning: Regular pruning, usually in early spring, to encourage new growth and maintain shape.

Fertilizing: Feed with rose-specific fertilizer to promote healthy growth and abundant blooms.

Pest and Disease Control:

Prevention: Keep an eye out for common rose pests like aphids or diseases like powdery mildew. Regular inspections and appropriate treatments can help manage these issues.

Harvesting Roses:

Collect blooms when they're fully open for the best fragrance and appearance.

If gathering petals for culinary or decorative purposes, ensure they're from unsprayed, organically grown roses.

Uses of Roses:

Ornamental Value: Adds classic beauty to gardens and landscapes.

Culinary: Edible petals can be used in various dishes or to make fragrant teas and jams.

Aromatherapy: Rose petals are often used for their soothing aroma in potpourri or essential oils.

Note: Roses are versatile and cherished for their beauty and diverse uses, from ornamental value to culinary and aromatherapy applications. Regular care and attention are key to ensuring a flourishing rose garden.

ROSEMARY

Cultivating Rosemary (Rosmarinus officinalis)

Growing Rosemary:Rosemary is a fragrant and versatile herb that's a wonderful addition to any garden. Here's how to cultivate, care for, and utilize this aromatic herb.

Optimal Growing Conditions:

Soil: Well-draining soil is essential; sandy or loamy soil works well.

Sunlight: Full sun, at least six hours of direct sunlight.

Planting:

Propagation: Typically grown from cuttings rather than seeds.

Spacing: Plant in an area where it has space to spread, usually about 2 to 3 feet apart.

Maintenance:

Watering: Rosemary prefers slightly dry conditions, so be cautious not to overwater. Allow the soil to dry out between waterings.

Pruning: Regular pruning encourages bushy growth and helps maintain its shape.

Pest and Disease Control:

Rosemary is relatively resistant to pests and diseases, especially when grown in well-draining soil and with adequate air circulation.

Harvesting Rosemary:

Snip off sprigs as needed, but avoid harvesting more than one-third of the plant at a time to ensure continued growth.

Uses of Rosemary:

Culinary: Widely used in Mediterranean cuisine, especially with roasted meats, stews, and vegetables.

Aromatherapy: Rosemary's fragrance is known for its calming and invigorating properties, often used in essential oils and herbal baths.

Medicinal: It's believed to have various health benefits, including improving digestion and boosting memory.

Note: Rosemary is a hardy and versatile herb that not only adds flavor to dishes but also offers aromatic and potential health benefits. Its resilience makes it an excellent choice for both gardeners and culinary enthusiasts.

SAGE

Cultivating Sage (Salvia officinalis)

Growing Sage:

Sage is a beautiful herb renowned for its aromatic leaves and various uses. Let's explore how to cultivate, care for, and utilize this remarkable herb.

Optimal Growing Conditions:

Soil: Well-draining soil, slightly alkaline, with good aeration.

Sunlight: Full sun, at least six hours of direct sunlight.

Planting:

Propagation: Can be grown from seeds or cuttings.

Spacing: Plant sage about 24 inches apart to allow for its growth.

Maintenance:

Watering: Sage prefers drier conditions, so be cautious not to overwater. Water deeply but infrequently.

Pruning: Regularly trim to maintain shape and encourage new growth.

Pest and Disease Control:

Sage is relatively resistant to pests and diseases due to its aromatic oils, but watch for issues in overly moist conditions.

Harvesting Sage:

Harvest leaves as needed; for the most flavor, pick before flowering. Dry them in a well-ventilated area for later use.

Uses of Sage:

Culinary: A versatile herb used in various cuisines, especially with poultry, pork, and in stuffing.

Medicinal: Sage is believed to have medicinal properties, aiding digestion and potentially having antibacterial properties.

Aromatherapy: Its fragrant leaves are often used in essential oils and herbal remedies.

Note: Sage is a resilient and flavorful herb that not only enhances culinary dishes but also offers potential health benefits. Its adaptability and various uses make it a valuable addition to any herb garden.

SAINT JOHN'S WORT

Cultivating Saint John's Wort (Hypericum perforatum

Growing Saint John's Wort:

Saint John's Wort, known for its bright yellow flowers and potential medicinal properties, is a versatile herb to cultivate.

Optimal Growing Conditions:

Soil: Well-draining soil, preferably slightly alkaline.

Sunlight: Thrives in full sun, though it can tolerate partial shade.

Planting:

Propagation: Can be grown from seeds, cuttings, or divisions.

Spacing: Plant about 18 inches apart, as it tends to spread.

Maintenance:

Watering: Ensure regular watering, especially during dry spells.

Pruning: Trimming back after flowering can promote new growth.

Pest and Disease Control:

Relatively resistant to pests and diseases, but watch for root rot in overly wet conditions.

Harvesting Saint John's Wort:

Collect the flowers when in full bloom. Dry them in a well-ventilated area for medicinal use.

Uses of Saint John's Wort

Medicinal: Believed to have antidepressant and anti-inflammatory properties, often used in herbal remedies for mental health.

Topical Applications: Oil extracted from the flowers is used in various skin treatments.

Herbal Tea: The dried flowers can be used to prepare a soothing herbal tea.

Note: Saint John's Wort is a resilient herb with multiple uses, from potential medicinal benefits to ornamental beauty. Its ease of cultivation and diverse applications make it a valuable addition to any herb garden.

SEA BUCKTHORN

Cultivating Sea Buckthorn (Hippophae rhamnoides)

Growing Sea Buckthorn:

Sea Buckthorn, known for its nutritional berries and hardy nature, can be a great addition to a garden.

Optimal Growing Conditions:

Soil: Well-draining, sandy, or loamy soil with good aeration.

Sunlight: Requires full sun exposure for optimal growth.

Planting:

Sowing: Best planted in the early spring or late fall.

Spacing: Allow ample space, as the plant tends to grow large. Space them about 5 to 10 feet apart.

Maintenance:

Watering: Regular watering during the first year to establish roots, then minimal maintenance.

Pruning: Prune to shape and remove dead or damaged branches.

Pest and Disease Control:

Generally resistant to pests and diseases but watch for root rot in excessively wet conditions.

Harvesting Sea Buckthorn:

Berries are best harvested when fully ripe, usually in late summer or early fall. They're quite acidic but highly nutritious.

Uses of Sea Buckthorn:

Nutritional Value: The berries are rich in vitamins, especially Vitamin C, and have various health benefits.

Culinary Uses: Berries can be used to make juices, jams, or incorporated into baked goods.

Cosmetic and Medicinal: The oil extracted from the berries is used in skincare products and has medicinal applications due to its high nutritional content.

Note: Sea Buckthorn, with its resilience and nutritional value, is a wonderful addition to any garden, offering both practical uses and visual appeal.

Growing Skullcap (Scutellaria sp.)

Cultivation of Skullcap:

Skullcap, a herbaceous perennial, is valued for its medicinal properties and can be a rewarding addition to a garden.

Ideal Growing Conditions:

Soil: Well-draining soil with good moisture retention.

Sunlight: Prefers partial shade to full sun.

Planting:

Sowing Seeds: Plant seeds in early spring or autumn.

Spacing: Allow ample space between plants, approximately 12 to 18 inches apart.

Maintenance:

Watering: Keep the soil consistently moist, but avoid waterlogging.

Pruning: Regularly trim to promote bushy growth and remove spent flowers.

Pest and Disease Control:

Relatively resistant to pests and diseases but keep an eye out for mildew in humid conditions.

Harvesting Skullcap:

Harvest the aerial parts (leaves and flowers) when in full bloom for the best potency.

Uses of Skullcap:

Medicinal Applications: It's known for its calming and relaxing properties, often used in herbal medicine.

Herbal Tea: The leaves can be dried and brewed into a soothing tea.

Note: Skullcap is a versatile herb that not only adds charm to a garden but also offers herbal remedies for relaxation and well-being.

SLIPPERY ELM

Cultivating Slippery Elm (Ulmus rubra)

Growing Conditions:

Climate: Slippery Elm thrives in various climates and soil types.

Soil: Prefers well-draining, moist, and fertile soil.

Sunlight: Grows best in full sun but can tolerate partial shade.

Planting:

Time: Plant in early spring or late fall.

Depth: Sow seeds about 1/8 inch deep in the soil.

Spacing: Allow ample space between saplings to accommodate their growth.

Care:

Watering: Keep the soil consistently moist, especially during dry spells.

Pruning: Minimal pruning required; remove dead or damaged branches.

Pests and Diseases:

Generally robust, but watch for common elm pests like leaf beetles and caterpillars.

Harvesting Slippery Elm:

Bark can be collected from mature trees. Harvesting the bark should be done carefully to avod harming the tree.The inner bark is traditionally used for its mucilaginous properties.

Utilization of Slippery Elm:

Medicinal Uses: The inner bark is commonly used in herbal remedies for various ailments, especially for soothing sore throats and digestive issues.

Cosmetic Uses: Extracts from the bark are used in some skincare products for their soothing properties.

Note: Slippery Elm, with its medicinal properties and adaptability to various environments, is a valuable addition to any garden, providing both practical and medicinal benefits.

STAGHOM SUMAC

Cultivating Staghorn Sumac (Rhus typhina)

Growing Conditions:

Climate: Adaptable and can thrive in various climates.

Soil: Tolerant of different soil types, but well-draining soil is preferable.

Sunlight: Grows well in full sun to partial shade.

Planting:

Time: Best planted in the spring or fall.

Depth: Plant seeds just below the soil surface.

Spacing: Allow ample room between saplings to accommodate their growth.

Care:

Watering: Staghorn Sumac is relatively drought-tolerant once established, but regular watering aids growth.

Pruning: Minimal pruning is necessary; trim dead branches for a tidy appearance.

Pests and Diseases:

Generally hardy with few issues; watch for pests like aphids and scale insects.

Harvesting Staghorn Sumac:

Berries can be harvested in late summer through fall. They can be dried for various uses.

Utilization of Staghorn Sumac:

Culinary Uses: Berries are commonly used to make sumac spice, imparting a tangy, lemony flavor to dishes.

Medicinal Uses: Some traditional medicine practices use sumac for its potential health benefits.

Aesthetic Value: Staghorn Sumac's red, cone-like fruit clusters add visual interest to landscapes, especially in the fall.

Note: Staghorn Sumac, with its hardiness and versatile uses, is an excellent choice for both culinary purposes and landscape aesthetics.

TEA TREE

Cultivating Tea Tree (Melaleuca alternifolia)

Growing Conditions:

Climate: Prefers warm, temperate climates.

Soil: Well-draining, slightly acidic soil is optimal.

Sunlight: Requires full sun for proper growth.

Planting:

Propagation: Usually through seeds or cuttings.

Depth: Plant seeds or saplings in shallow holes, not too deep.

Spacing: Provide adequate space for mature growth.

Care:

Watering: Regular watering is crucial, especially in the early stages. Once established, it becomes somewhat drought-tolerant.

Pruning: Trim dead or diseased branches to encourage healthy growth

Pests and Diseases:

Generally resistant to pests and diseases; watch for scale or mites.

Harvesting Tea Tree:

Leaves and branches can be harvested throughout the year, but essential oil extraction is typically done when the oil content is highest.

Utilization of Tea Tree

Essential Oil: Valued for its potent antibacterial and antifungal properties, widely used in aromatherapy and skincare products.

Medicinal Uses: Tea tree oil is known for its antimicrobial and anti-inflammatory properties and is used in various treatments.

Aesthetic Value: Tea Tree's slender leaves and occasional white flowers make it a visually appealing addition to gardens.

Note: Tea Tree is a valuable plant with a myriad of applications, especially prized for its essential oil's diverse benefits in health and skincare. Its cultivation demands attention to watering and ensuring adequate sunlight for optimal growth.

TULSI

Growing Tulsi (Ocimum tenuiflorum)

Cultivation:

Climate: Thrives in warm, tropical climates; can be grown indoors in cooler areas.

Soil: Well-draining soil with good fertility.

Sunlight: Requires plenty of sunlight.

Planting:

Seeds or Cuttings: Propagate from seeds or cuttings.

Depth: Plant seeds or cuttings at a shallow depth.

Care:

Watering: Keep the soil consistently moist but not waterlogged.

Pruning: Regularly pinch off the flowers to encourage leaf growth.

Pests and Diseases: Generally resistant but can be susceptible to aphids and fungal issues in damp conditions.

Harvesting Tulsi:

Harvest leaves once the plant reaches a mature height. Pinch off individual leaves or small stems.

Uses of Tulsi

Culinary: Leaves are used in teas or as flavoring in dishes.

Medicinal: Renowned in Ayurvedic medicine for its diverse medicinal properties, aiding in respiratory issues, stress relief, and more.

Spiritual: Considered sacred in Hindu culture and often used in religious rituals.

Note: Tulsi is a revered plant in many cultures for its medicinal and spiritual significance. Easy to cultivate, it requires sunlight, well-draining soil, and consistent moisture, making it a valuable addition to both gardens and spiritual spaces.

TURMERIC

Cultivating Turmeric (Curcuma longa)

Growing Conditions:

Climate: Thrives in warm, humid climates but can also be grown indoors in containers.

Soil: Well-draining soil rich in organic matter.

Sunlight: Prefers partial to full sunlight.

Planting Turmeric:

Rhizomes: Plant fresh turmeric rhizomes (similar to ginger roots) in the soil with the buds facing upwards.

Depth: Plant the rhizomes about 2 inches deep.

Care:

Watering: Keep the soil consistently moist but not waterlogged.

Temperature: Protect from cold temperatures, as turmeric prefers warmth.

Fertilization: Periodically supplement with organic fertilizers.

Harvesting Turmeric:

Harvest when the leaves start to dry out, typically after 8-10 months. Gently unearth the rhizomes using a garden fork.

Uses of Turmeric:

Culinary: Widely used as a spice in various cuisines, known for its vibrant color and earthy flavor.

Medicinal: Celebrated for its anti-inflammatory and antioxidant properties; commonly used in traditional medicine for various health benefits.

Note: Turmeric is not just a spice; it's a versatile plant with both culinary and medicinal value. Growing it involves patience as it takes several months to mature, but the beautiful foliage and the rewarding harvest of rhizomes make it a fascinating addition to any garden.

VALERIAN

Cultivating Valerian (Valeriana officinalis)

Growing Conditions:

Soil: Prefers well-draining, loamy soil with rich organic matter.

Sunlight: Partial shade to full sun.

Moisture: Keep the soil consistently moist, but avoid waterlogging.

Planting Valerian:

Seeds: Sow seeds directly in the garden or in containers during early spring or fall.

Depth: Plant seeds about 1/8 inch deep in the soil.

Spacing: Space seeds or seedlings about 12-18 inches apart.

Care:

Watering: Regularly water to maintain consistent moisture, especially during dry periods.

Mulching: Apply mulch to retain moisture and control weeds.

Fertilization: Use organic fertilizers sparingly.

Harvesting Valerian:

Roots: Harvest the roots in the plant's second or third year during autumn. The roots are the valuable part for their medicinal properties.

Uses of Valerian:

Medicinal: Valerian root is renowned for its calming properties and is used to make teas, tinctures, or capsules to promote relaxation and sleep.

Note: Valerian is prized for its medicinal properties, particularly its role in promoting relaxation and sleep. The roots are the main focus for harvesting, and while the plant may take a couple of years to mature, the wait is worth it for its potent qualities.

VERONICA

Growing Veronica (Veronica officinalis)

Cultivation:

Soil: Thrives in well-draining, slightly acidic to neutral soil.

Sunlight: Prefers full sun but can tolerate partial shade.

Watering: Regular watering to keep the soil consistently moist.

Planting Veronica:

Seeds: Sow seeds in the desired location in early spring or fall.

Depth: Plant seeds about 1/8 inch deep in the soil.

Spacing: Space seeds or seedlings about 12-18 inches apart.

Care:

Maintenance: Trim or deadhead spent flowers to encourage continuous blooming.

Fertilization: Use a balanced fertilizer during the growing season.

Harvesting Veronica:

Leaves and Flowers: Leaves and flowers can be harvested during the growing season for various uses, such as teas or herbal preparations.

Uses of Veronica:

Medicinal: Traditionally used in herbal medicine for respiratory issues, it's known for its expectorant properties.

Ornamental: Its beautiful blooms make it a charming addition to gardens and landscapes.

Note: Veronica, commonly known as Speedwell, is not only an attractive garden plant but also holds significance in herbal medicine, particularly for its benefits in respiratory health. Harvesting leaves and flowers for medicinal uses can be done during the plant's growing season, offering multiple applications for health and aesthetics.

VIOLETS

Growing Violets (Viola sp.)

Cultivation:

Soil: Violets prefer well-draining, slightly acidic soil rich in organic matter.

Sunlight: Partial shade to full shade. They thrive under trees or in areas with dappled sunlight.

Watering: Regular, moderate watering to keep the soil consistently moist.

Planting Violets:

Seeds: Plant seeds in a prepared bed or potting soil, barely covering them with a thin layer of soil.

Spacing: If planting multiple violet plants, space them about 6-12 inches apart.

Care:

Mulching: A layer of mulch around the plants can help retain moisture and suppress weeds.

Fertilization: Use a balanced, water-soluble fertilizer to support healthy growth.

Harvesting Violets:

Flowers and Leaves: Both flowers and leaves are edible and can be harvested during the growing season for culinary uses.

Uses of Violets:

Culinary: Their delicate flowers and leaves are often used in salads, desserts, or as garnishes.

Medicinal: Violets have been historically used in herbal medicine for their potential anti-inflammatory and healing properties.

Ornamental: Apart from their practical uses, violets add vibrant color to gardens and landscapes.

Note: Violets are versatile plants known for their culinary and ornamental value. Their delicate flowers and leaves offer a touch of elegance in both cooking and aesthetics. Additionally, they possess potential medicinal properties, making them a multi-faceted addition to gardens.

WATERCRESS

Growing Watercress (Nasturtium officinale)

Cultivation:

Water Requirements: Watercress thrives in wet environments. It grows best in shallow, slow-moving water or in consistently moist soil.

Soil: Opt for loamy, fertile soil with good drainage if planting watercress in a garden bed.

Planting Watercress:

In Water: If planting in water, consider a container or a shallow area of a pond or stream where water is slow-moving and consistently moist.

In Soil: For planting in soil, prepare a moist bed with good drainage and sow the seeds about 6 inches apart.

Care:

Watering: Ensure a consistent water supply, keeping the soil or water around the plant consistently moist.

Sunlight: Watercress prefers partial shade to full sun. In hotter climates, partial shade is ideal to prevent scorching.

Harvesting Watercress:

Leaves: Harvest the leaves once they've reached a desirable size, usually within 6 to 8 weeks after planting.

Uses of Watercress:

Culinary: Watercress adds a peppery, fresh taste to salads, sandwiches, and various dishes.

Nutritional: It's rich in vitamins and minerals, making it a nutritious addition to meals.

Medicinal: Traditionally, watercress has been used in herbal medicine for various health benefits.

Note: Watercress is a versatile and nutritious plant, commonly used in culinary dishes for its peppery flavor. It thrives in consistently moist conditions and can be grown both in water or in a well-prepared garden bed. With its rich nutritional profile, it's a fantastic addition to a home garden for both taste and health.

WILD LETTUCE

Cultivating Wild Lettuce (Lactuca virosa

Growing Environment:

Soil Preference: Wild lettuce thrives in rich, well-draining soil. Loamy soil with good fertility is ideal.

Sunlight: It prefers full sun but can tolerate partial shade.

Planting Wild Lettuce:

Sowing Seeds: Plant seeds directly into the soil after the last frost. Sow seeds thinly and cover lightly with soil.

Spacing: Maintain a spacing of around 8 to 12 inches between plants.

Care:

Watering: Keep the soil consistently moist, but not waterlogged. Regular watering, especially during dry spells, is beneficial.

Weeding: Remove competing weeds to allow the wild lettuce to flourish.

Harvesting:

Leaves: Harvest the leaves when they are young and tender, typically before the plant flowers. This is when they are most flavorful.

Utilization of Wild Lettuce:

Culinary Use: While not as common as cultivated lettuces, the leaves of wild lettuce are edible and can be used in salads or as a cooked green.

Medicinal Applications: Traditionally, wild lettuce has been used for its potential sedative and pain-relieving properties.

Note: Wild lettuce is an interesting addition to a garden, appreciated for its potential medicinal properties and sometimes for culinary uses. Proper care in terms of watering and weeding can result in a healthy and vibrant plant that can offer both utility and aesthetic appeal.

WILLOW TREES

Growing Willow Trees (Salix sp.)

Cultivating Willow:

Soil: Willows thrive in moist, well-drained soil. They are quite adaptive and can tolerate a variety of soil types.

Sunlight: Full sun is preferable, although some species can handle partial shade.

Planting Willow:

Propagation: Willows can be started from seeds or cuttings. Cuttings often root easily.

Spacing: Provide adequate space between trees, as willows tend to grow quickly and can spread wide.

Care:

Watering: Ensure consistent moisture, especially during the initial growth stages. Established trees are generally drought-tolerant.

Pruning: Prune to maintain shape and remove dead or damaged branches.

Harvesting Willow:

While not typically harvested in a traditional sense, branches or stems might be collected for craftwork or to create rooting hormone solutions.

Utilization of Willow:

Ornamental Value: Willows are often planted for their aesthetic appeal, particularly their gracefully drooping branches.

Medicinal Uses: Some traditional medicine uses willow bark for its salicin content, which is similar to aspirin.

Note: Willows are beautiful and versatile trees. Their adaptability to various soil conditions and relatively fast growth make them a popular choice in landscaping and gardening. Additionally, their potential medicinal properties and craft uses add to their overall appeal.

WINTEERGREEN

How to Grow Wintergreen (Gaultheria procumbens)

Wintergreen Cultivation:

Ideal Environment: Wintergreen prefers acidic, well-draining soil and partial to full shade. It's often found in forest settings with moist, cool conditions.

Soil Type: Sandy or loamy soils with high acidity suit wintergreen best.

Planting Wintergreen:

Propagation: Wintergreen can be propagated from seeds or cuttings. Plant in early spring for optimal growth.

Spacing: Provide about 6 to 12 inches between each plant.

Wintergreen Maintenance:

Watering: Keep the soil consistently moist but not waterlogged. Mulching can help retain moisture.

Pruning: Minimal pruning is needed. Remove dead or damaged leaves or stems.

Harvesting Wintergreen:

Leaves and Berries: Leaves can be harvested throughout the growing season. The berries, containing wintergreen oil, can be harvested when ripe for culinary or medicinal purposes.

Extracting Wintergreen Oil:

Wintergreen oil is obtained from the leaves and berries and is used in various applications such as flavorings, aromatherapy, and topical pain relief.

Storing Wintergreen:

Dry the leaves and store in airtight containers away from direct sunlight. Wintergreen oil should be stored in dark glass bottles.

Utilization of Wintergreen:

Medicinal Use: Wintergreen is known for its oil, which contains methyl salicylate, similar to aspirin, and is often used topically for pain relief.

Culinary Applications: The leaves or oil can be used for flavoring in food or beverages.

Note: Wintergreen, with its aromatic leaves and beneficial oil, serves both culinary and medicinal purposes. Its preference for acidic soil and shade makes it an excellent addition to gardens or natural wooded areas. Proper care and harvesting ensure its sustainability for various uses.

WITCH HAZEL

How to Grow Witch Hazel (Hamamelis virginiana)

Witch Hazel Cultivation:

Ideal Environment: Witch hazel thrives in well-draining, slightly acidic to neutral soil and partial shade. It's a hardy shrub that tolerates various soil types and can withstand cold temperatures.

Planting Witch Hazel:

Time of Planting: Plant young witch hazel shrubs in the early spring or fall.

Spacing: Leave about 6 to 10 feet between each shrub for proper growth.

Witch Hazel Maintenance:

Watering: Regular but not excessive watering is essential, especially during dry periods.

Mulching: Applying a layer of mulch helps retain moisture and keeps the roots cool.

Pruning and Shaping:

Pruning can be minimal and primarily for shaping. Remove dead or diseased branches to encourage healthy growth.

Harvesting Witch Hazel:

Witch hazel leaves, bark, and twigs are harvested to create extracts used in medicinal applications.

Extracting Witch Hazel Extract:

The bark and leaves are used to create witch hazel extract, which is known for its astringent and anti-inflammatory properties, often used in skincare and medicinal products.

Storing Witch Hazel Extract:

Preserve the extract in airtight containers and store it in a cool, dry place away from direct sunlight to maintain its potency.

Utilization of Witch Hazel:

Medicinal Use: Witch hazel extract is employed for its skin-soothing properties, aiding in conditions such as minor irritations, bruises, and insect bites.

Cosmetic Applications: It's a common ingredient in skincare products like toners and cleansers due to its astringent and cleansing qualities.

Note: Witch hazel is a versatile shrub known for its medicinal and cosmetic benefits. Its ease of maintenance and adaptability to various conditions make it a valuable addition to gardens, providing both practical uses and ornamental value. Proper care and harvesting ensure its usefulness in various applications.

YARROW

How to Cultivate Yarrow (Achillea millefolium)

Growing Yarrow:

Preferred Conditions: Yarrow thrives in well-draining soil and full sun but can tolerate various soil types. It's a hardy perennial that can withstand drought conditions.

Planting Yarrow:

Timing: Plant yarrow seeds or transplants in the early spring or fall.

Spacing: Plant yarrow 1 to 2 feet apart, as it can spread rapidly.

Maintenance:

Watering: Yarrow is drought-resistant but benefits from occasional watering during dry spells.

Pruning: Regular deadheading can encourage prolonged blooming and prevent self-seeding.

Harvesting Yarrow:

Flowers: Harvest yarrow flowers when they are in full bloom for their highest medicinal potency.

Leaves: Leaves can be collected at any point during the growing season for various uses.

Using Yarrow:

Medicinal Properties: Yarrow has long been utilized for its medicinal properties, especially in traditional herbal medicine. It's known for its anti-inflammatory and antiseptic qualities.

Tea: The leaves and flowers make a pleasant tea when dried and brewed.

Storing Yarrow:

Drying: Dry the harvested yarrow in a well-ventilated, shaded area.

Storage: Once dried, store yarrow in airtight containers in a cool, dark place to preserve its potency.

Note: Yarrow is a versatile and beneficial herb, not only as an ornamental plant in gardens but also for its numerous medicinal applications. Proper cultivation, harvesting, and storage are

Weeding: Regular weeding prevents competition for nutrients.

Harvesting Yellow Dock:

Roots: Harvest the roots in the fall for their medicinal use.

Leaves: Leaves can be harvested throughout the growing season.

Using Yellow Dock:

essential to harness its full potential for herbal remedies and teas.

YELLOW DOCK

How to Cultivate Yellow Dock (Rumex crispus)

Growing Yellow Dock:

Preferred Conditions: Yellow Dock is a perennial that thrives in moist, well-drained soil and full sun to partial shade. It’s highly adaptable and can grow in various soil types.

Planting Yellow Dock:

Timing: Plant seeds or transplants in early spring or fall.

Spacing: Provide ample space as Yellow Dock can spread; about 18-24 inches apart is recommended.

Maintenance:

Watering: Ensure the soil stays consistently moist, especially during dry periods.

Medicinal Purposes: The roots are valued for their various medicinal properties and are often used in herbal remedies.

Edible Leaves: Young leaves can be consumed, but older leaves may have a strong taste.

Storing Yellow Dock:

Roots: After harvesting, wash and dry the roots thoroughly. Store them in a cool, dry place to maintain their potency.

Note: Yellow Dock is a versatile herb, appreciated for its medicinal qualities. Proper cultivation, careful harvesting, and appropriate storage ensure the best utilization of its benefits.

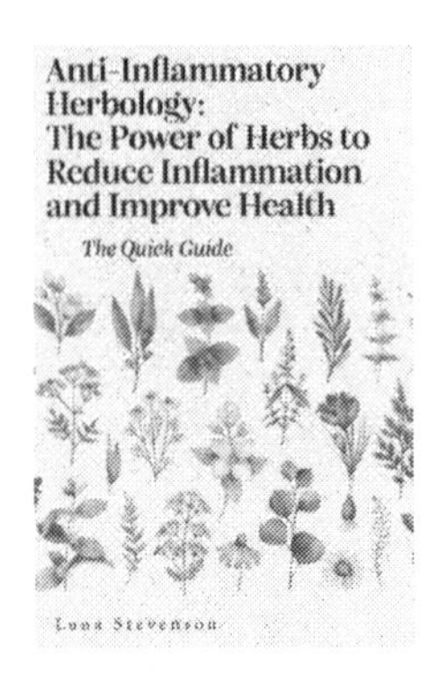

Dear reader, thank you so much for delving into 'The Herb Bible.' Your support means the world to me! I hope this book has sparked your interest in the fascinating world of herbs and natural wellness.

Your feedback is valuable, so I invite you to share your experience through a review. As a token of gratitude, you can download the 'Guide to Anti-Inflammatory Herbs' for free.

It's a special gift for you, a way to further explore the benefits of herbs. Thank you again for choosing this book and being a part of this incredible journey into the world of herbs!

Dear reader, thank you so much for delving into 'The Herb Bible.' Your support means the world to me! I hope this book has sparked your interest in the fascinating world of herbs and natural wellness.

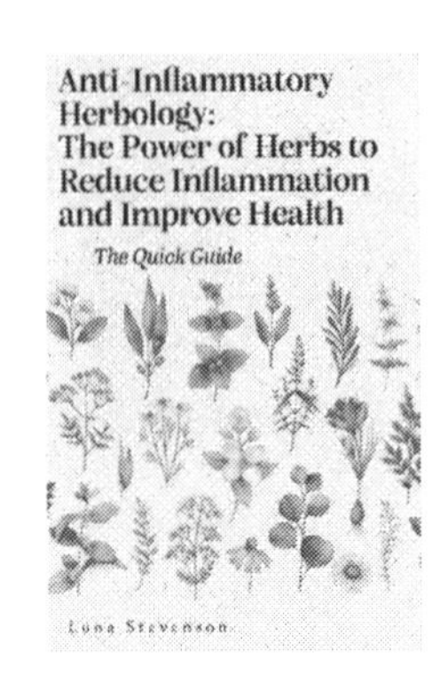

Your feedback is valuable, so I invite you to share your experience through a review. As a token of gratitude, you can download the 'Guide to Anti-Inflammatory Herbs' for free.

It's a special gift for you, a way to further explore the benefits of herbs. Thank you again for choosing this book and being a part of this incredible journey into the world of herbs!

BOOK 8: HOMEOPATHIC HERB FLOWER TERAPY,AROMA THERAPY

Chapter 1:
Flower Therapy

Flower therapy, also known as flower essence therapy or flower remedies, is a complementary and alternative medicine practice that makes use of the positive emotional and mental effects associated with flower energy. The theory holds that flowers' vibrational characteristics have a beneficial effect on our mental and physical wellbeing.

In the 1930s, British physician and homeopath Dr. Edward Bach originated the idea of flower therapy. Dr. Bach created a collection of floral essences now often referred to as the Bach Flower Remedies. In his view, a person's emotional and mental states are often to fault for their physical health problems. He thought that correcting these irrational emotions would help the body repair itself.

There are 38 unique flower essences that make up the Bach Flower Remedies, each of which is meant to treat a distinct mood, trait, or condition. To create the essences, flowers are infused in water, which records the flowers' energy signature. These essences can be ingested sublingually, applied topically, or diluted in water and consumed orally.

The right flower essences are chosen after some sort of consultation or introspective procedure. To restore equilibrium, the practitioner or individual first determines the nature of the emotional or mental disturbance and then selects the appropriate floral essences. Rock Rose or Mimulus essence, for instance, would be advised to a fearful or anxious person, whereas Star of Bethlehem or Sweet Chestnut essence might help a grieving or sorrowful person.

It is thought that the essences help restore emotional balance by subtly altering the person's electromagnetic field. Flower therapy is a sort of alternative medicine that is safe for people of all ages, including kids and pets. It is frequently employed in tandem with standard medical care and psychotherapy as a complimentary therapy.

It's crucial to remember that flower therapy and flower essences aren't meant to detect, treat, or cure any medical or psychological issue. Instead, they strive to encourage a sense of harmony and balance in one's emotional life. If you're thinking about trying flower therapy, it's best to go to an expert who can help you choose and apply flower essences that are tailored to your specific situation.

Chapter 2: Homeopathic Remedies

Alternative medicine like homeopathy dates to the 18th century. A chemical that generates symptoms in a healthy person can be used to treat comparable symptoms in a sick person; this is the core principle of homeopathy, also known as "like cures like."

Natural components like plants, minerals, or animal products are often used in homeopathic medicines, which are then diluted in water or alcohol. Repeatedly diluting and shaking the original chemical is termed potentization, and it is done to increase the healing benefits while decreasing the potentially hazardous effects.

Homeopathic medicines are extremely diluted, often to the point where there is no detectable amount of the original chemical left in the end product. Homeopaths think that the "energetic imprint" of the original substance is preserved in the water or alcohol, which then triggers the body's natural healing processes.

Acute and chronic ailments, as well as mental health problems, are all treated using homeopathy. However, there is few and contradictory research to back up homeopathy's claims of success. Despite a large body of high-quality research, homeopathic treatments have not been shown to outperform a placebo.

Homeopathy should be used with carefully, and certainly not in place of conventional medical care. It's best to talk to a doctor about any health issues you may be having so they can recommend the best course of action.

Chapter 3:
Aromatherapy

Aromatherapy is a form of complementary and alternative medicine that makes use of the therapeutic effects of essential oils through their aroma. It's founded on the idea that specific aromas can profoundly affect our mental and physical well-being.

Essential oils are extremely potent plant extracts that can be distilled from a wide variety of plant components, including but not limited to the petals, leaves, stems, and roots. They can be obtained using methods such as steam distillation or cold-press extraction, and they retain the plant's inherent essence and smell.

There are several applications for essential oils in aromatherapy.

Most people use inhalation, wherein they take in the odor of essential oils either directly or after they have been diffused into the air. Diffusers, steam inhalation, or even just a few drops of oil on a tissue or cotton ball will do the trick.

Essential oils can be administered topically by massaging them into the skin or diluting them with a carrier oil like almond oil or coconut oil for a topical application. Some essential oils might irritate the skin, so it's vital to dilute them and do a patch test before using them on a larger area.

When taking a bath, it can be very soothing to add a few drops of essential oils to the water.

Relaxation, stress relief, better sleep, elevated mood, and other physical and mental sensations are some of the common uses of aromatherapy. It is widely held that various essential oils possess unique therapeutic benefits. For instance:

- ✓ Lavender is commonly used to aid with relaxation and sleep because of its sedative effects.
- ✓ Peppermint is a common remedy for a variety of ailments, including a lack of focus or concentration, a headache, or stomach pain.
- ✓ Commonly used to treat respiratory problems and clear the sinuses, eucalyptus has a reputation for having a stimulating and revitalizing aroma.
- ✓ The antibacterial qualities of tea tree oil have made it a popular topical treatment for skin ailments and a natural disinfectant.

Aromatherapy can be helpful as an adjunct treatment for some medical issues, but it should not be considered a replacement for conventional medicine. Always seek the advice of your doctor before beginning aromatherapy or using any essential oils, especially if you have any preexisting conditions.

Chapter 4:
Other Types Of Plant And Herbal Therapy

Plant and herbal treatment, often known as herbal medicine or herbalism, refers to the practice of treating medical conditions with plants and plant extracts. Here's a case in point for using herbs and plants medicinally:

Treatment of Insomnia with Valerian Root

1. Insomnia is a sleep disorder characterized by difficulty falling asleep or staying asleep. Valerian (Valeriana officinalis) is an herb commonly used in herbal therapy to promote relaxation and improve sleep quality. Here's how it can be utilized:
2. Identification and preparation: The herbalist identifies valerian as a potential remedy for insomnia based on its known sedative properties. They ensure they have access to high-quality valerian root, which is commonly available in the form of dried roots or capsules.
3. Consultation and assessment: The herbalist conducts a consultation with the individual suffering from insomnia to assess their specific symptoms, medical history, and any potential contraindications. They consider the person's overall health and other medications they might be taking.
4. Customized treatment plan: Based on the assessment, the herbalist creates a personalized treatment plan. In this case, they may recommend a valerian root preparation to be taken orally as a tea or in capsule form.
5. Administration: The individual follows the herbalist's instructions and takes the valerian root preparation as recommended. Typically, it involves consuming the tea or capsule a certain time before bedtime.
6. Monitoring and adjustment: The herbalist closely monitors the individual's progress and adjusts the treatment plan as needed. They may suggest changes in dosage or recommend additional herbal remedies to complement the valerian root, depending on the individual's response and any changes in symptoms.
7. Follow-up: Regular follow-up appointments are scheduled to evaluate the treatment's effectiveness and address any concerns or new symptoms that may have arisen.

Chapter 5:
Therapeutic Uses Of Herbal Ointments

Use of ointments for skin care and healing

Treatment of the main skin problems

Because of their capacity to act as a barrier, transport drugs or healing agents, and help skin retain moisture, ointments are frequently employed in skin care and healing. They are commonly used to heal a wide range of skin injuries and conditions. Here are some ways ointments can help with these problems:

- When treating burns, ointments containing aloe vera or silver sulfadiazine are used. They provide a soothing effect, cut down on pain, and help with healing by warding off infection and encouraging new skin to grow.
- Antibiotic ointments like bacitracin and neomycin are frequently used to prevent infection in cuts and wounds. These ointments serve to preserve the wounded area and speed up the recovery process.
- Hydrocortisone ointments are commonly used to treat the itching, redness, and inflammation that accompany rashes caused by things like allergic reactions or eczema. They alleviate pain and speed skin recovery.
- Ointments containing emollient components like petrolatum or lanolin are great for hydrating and soothing skin that is dry or injured. They provide a barrier that keeps moisture in and encourages the skin's barrier to heal.
- Chronic skin disorders like psoriasis or eczema can have their symptoms treated with ointments containing coal tar or corticosteroids. They help calm swelling, ease itching, and restrain rapid cell turnover in the skin.
- Even while ointments can aid in skin care and healing, it is crucial to use them in accordance with the directions provided by medical specialists or on the product labels. If you have any questions or worries about your skin, it's best to go to a doctor who can provide you individualized recommendations.

Applying ointments to relieve inflammation and pain

It's important to remember a few things when using ointments for pain and inflammation. Please note that while I can offer broad guidance, you should always seek the opinion of a licensed medical practitioner for specific recommendations. Listed below are some suggestions:

- Find the right ointment for your needs; there are several options, such as ointments containing topical steroids, NSAIDs, or counterirritants. The degree and source of inflammation or pain should guide your decision. Ointments containing nonsteroidal anti-inflammatory drugs (NSAIDs) can alleviate inflammation, counterirritants can alleviate pain by creating a cooling or warming feeling, and topical steroids can alleviate inflammation and itching.

- Just do as it says: Please refer to the enclosed directions and apply the ointment as directed. Take into account the suggested administration, the frequency of use, and any cautions or contraindications.
- It's important to wash and dry the affected region before applying the ointment. Rinse the area with water and a light soap, then dry it gently with a clean cloth.
- Use a tiny amount and spread it evenly over the affected area to create a thin layer of the ointment. Use clean hands or an appropriate applicator to rub it in gently. Avoid using too much, as doing so might not enhance efficacy and might create undesirable side effects.
- Be sure to wash your hands well after applying the ointment to get rid of any lingering residue. If you are using an ointment that contains substances that could be hazardous if consumed or that could irritate other regions of your body, this is an especially important precaution to take.
- Maintain coherence: Always apply at the suggested intervals. Different ointments have different recommended application frequencies and durations of usage. The efficacy of the ointment improves with consistent use.
- Keep an eye out for any unwanted effects: Notice how your body reacts to the ointment. Stop using and see a doctor if your symptoms of redness, rash, itching, or swelling get worse or appear for no reason.
- Keep in mind that ointments are intended solely for topical application. It is crucial to seek the advice of a medical practitioner and consider all available treatment options when dealing with chronic pain or other systemic problems.

Chapter 6:
Use of Ointments And Their Storage

How to store homemade ointments

To prevent contamination, use only clean, sterilized containers while keeping the ointments. They need to be washed in hot, soapy water, rinsed well, and then dried thoroughly.

1. Choose airtight containers to stop air, moisture, and pathogens from getting in. Ointments should be stored in glass or plastic containers with secure closures. Some of the active chemicals in ointments might be damaged by exposure to light, so it's best to keep them in a dark spot or use dark containers.
2. Ointment names, manufacturing dates, and ingredient lists should be prominently displayed on all packaging. In this way, you may monitor the formulations and their expiration dates.
3. Ointments should be kept in a cool, dry place, out of direct sunlight and away from any sources of heat. The ointment will lose its effectiveness if subjected to extreme temperatures, while direct sunshine and high humidity will cause it to dissolve. It's best to keep your food in a cool place, such a pantry, where you can use a cupboard or drawer.
4. Contamination can easily avoided by administering the ointment with clean hands or a sterilized spoon or spatula. Also, before sealing a container, check sure the aperture is free of debris.
5. Natural ointments have a shorter shelf life than mass-produced alternatives because of their dependence on perishable ingredients. When estimating how long your ointment will last, it's best to use the ingredient with the shortest expiration date as a benchmark. Homemade ointments are best used within six months to a year of preparation.
6. Keep an eye out for deterioration: check the ointments on a regular basis for any signs of deterioration, such as a change in color, texture, or smell. If you see anything out of the ordinary, you should stop using the cream immediately.

Application and correct use for each remedy create the correct recipe and with the right doses

1. Tea Made From Digestive-Friendly Herbs:

One cup of boiling water, one teaspoon each of dried peppermint leaves, chamomile flowers, and fennel seeds, and stir. Ten minutes of steep time and it's ready to be strained.

Drink the herbal tea if you have indigestion, bloating, or stomach pain. Relax and enjoy a gentle sip. Do not exceed two or three cups daily.

2. Lemon and Honey Cough Drops:

To prepare, combine half a lemon's juice with 2 tablespoons of honey. Add some grated ginger for flavor and health benefits, if desired.

If you have a cough or a sore throat, take 1–2 tablespoons of the syrup three or four times a day. Children younger than one year old should not consume honey.

3. Inhaling Eucalyptus Steam for a Stuffy Nose:

The recipe calls for boiling water to be infused with a few drops of eucalyptus oil or a handful of dried eucalyptus leaves.

To use, place your face (carefully, to avoid burns) over the pot and inhale the steam. Wrap a cloth around your head to keep the steam in. Nasal congestion may subside after using this method. Keep your breathing sessions to no more than ten minutes.

4. Applying Turmeric Paste to a Wound:

Prepare a thick paste by combining 1 teaspoon of turmeric powder with adequate water or coconut oil.

Use the paste on scrapes, insect bites, and other small wounds. A bandage should be applied and left on for a few hours. The antibacterial properties of turmeric may also make it useful for treating wounds.

Conclusion

In conclusion, aromatherapy is a popular method that has the potential to enhance one's state of mind and alleviate some physical discomforts. There is some evidence for its usefulness, but further study is needed to determine its precise mechanisms of action and their applicability to a wide range of health issues. Before adopting aromatherapy into your healthcare practice, it is best to speak with a trained medical expert.

BOOK 9: "HERBAL INGREDIENTS FOR COOKING AND THEIR HEALING PROPERTIES"

Chapter 1: Introduction To Cooking Herbs

Importance of fresh herbs in cooking and health

Fresh herbs improve the flavor of a dish by giving it more nuance, complexity, and brightness. Because of their individual aromas and flavors, herbs can greatly improve the quality of a dish.

Herbs have medicinal benefit because they contain many healthful nutrients like vitamins, minerals, and antioxidants. They are rich in phytochemicals, which may have beneficial effects on health. Fresh herbs can be a great source of these nutrients when added to your meals.

Sodium reduction: using fresh herbs in cooking instead of salt can help cut down on sodium intake. Herbs like basil, rosemary, and thyme have robust flavors that can stand in for some of the salt. People who have health issues that require them to limit their sodium intake may appreciate this.

Mint, ginger, and fennel are just a few of the herbs that have long been used for their ability to aid digestion. They are useful in relieving digestive issues such as indigestion, gas, and bloating. These herbs, whether eaten as part of a meal or savored as a herbal tea, have been shown to improve digestion.

Some herbs, such as garlic and oregano, have antibacterial capabilities due to their natural composition. Compounds in them aid in the battle against pathogenic bacteria, viruses, and fungi. Using these herbs in your cuisine may help maintain a healthy microbiome.

Fresh herbs not only improve a dish's flavor, but they also make it look more appetizing. A dish's aesthetic appeal and flavor can be improved by topping it with a sprinkle of freshly chopped herbs. They're pretty enough to use as garnishes, elevating a dish's visual appeal.

Calming herbs like lavender and chamomile have been shown to have beneficial effects in alleviating tension and facilitating relaxation. Herbal drinks and cooking with these herbs might help you unwind and feel at peace.

In order to preserve their flavor and freshness, fresh herbs require careful handling and storage before and after use. The freshest and best-quality herbs are those that have been harvested from one's own garden or purchased from reliable vendors.

Chapter 2:
How To Grow And Store Herbs At Home

Choosing the Right Location:

If you want your herbs to flourish, you should plant them in a spot that gets plenty of sunlight. Herbs thrive under bright sunlight for at least six hours a day.

Make sure the soil drains well there so your roots don't get sucked under. Add organic matter or build raised beds if your soil is too dense to work with.

Selecting Herbs:

Pick herbs that will thrive in your garden and in your dish. Basil, parsley, mint, rosemary, thyme, and chives are just some examples of easy-to-grow herbs that are widely used.

Think on the size and growth pattern of the herbs. Herbs with a tendency to spread aggressively, such as mint and oregano, may be better off growing in pots.

Planting and Caring for Herbs:

Get some herb seeds or start some herb plants from seed. Each herb has unique needs for planting distance, soil depth, and watering, so be sure to read the package directions before getting started.

Herbs need continuous watering; let the soil dry out a little in between soakings. Root rot is caused by overwatering, so be careful.

To prevent soil drying out, weed growth, and temperature swings, mulch should be used around the herbs.

Harvesting Herbs:

Herbs will grow bushier if you pick them on a frequent basis. Start at the top of the plant and pinch or cut off the outermost leaves or stalks.

It is preferable to remove entire stems rather than individual leaves when working with leafy herbs like basil and parsley.

Morning is the best time to gather herbs because that's when their volatile oils are at their peak. You should wash them gently in cold water and dry them off if necessary.

Storing Herbs:

Air Drying: Tie small bunches of herbs together and hang them upside down in a dry, well-ventilated area away from direct sunlight.

Common aromatic herbs and their healing properties, description of the healing properties of each herb

Antioxidant Herbs:

Rosemary: Rosemary contains antioxidants that help neutralize free radicals in the body, which can reduce oxidative stress and support overall health.

Thyme: Thyme is rich in antioxidants that protect cells from damage caused by free radicals, promoting healthy aging and supporting the immune system.

Oregano: Oregano is known for its high antioxidant content, which helps combat oxidative stress and supports the immune system.

Anti-inflammatory Herbs:

Basil: Compounds in basil with anti-inflammatory effects can aid in lowering systemic inflammation and bolstering cardiovascular health.

Inflammatory illnesses, such as arthritis and gastrointestinal issues, may benefit from sage's anti-inflammatory effects.

Turmeric is not an aromatic herb, but its active ingredient, curcumin, has potent anti-inflammatory effects. It's good for your joints and can help reduce inflammation.

Digestive Herbs:

Peppermint has a calming impact on the gastrointestinal tract. It's useful for soothing tummy pain, gas, and indigestion.

The digestive help of ginger has been appreciated for generations. It helps with digestion and can relieve nausea and bloating.

Fennel: The carminative characteristics of fennel seeds make them useful for treating gastrointestinal cramping, excess gas, and flatulence.

Calming and Relaxing Herbs:

Lavender has been shown to alleviate stress, ease muscle tension, and promote restful sleep.

Chamomile: Chamomile has been used for centuries for its sedative properties. It's been shown to aid with stress, insomnia, and tummy aches.

The moderate calming qualities of lemon balm make it an excellent stress reliever and sleep aid.

Immune-Boosting Herbs:

Echinacea: Echinacea is thought to strengthen the immune system, making it easier for the body to fend off illnesses like the common cold and the flu.

Allicin, the main ingredient in garlic, has antibacterial and antiviral activities and is responsible for the plant's immune-boosting characteristics.

The Chinese have long relied on the immune-boosting and infection-preventing properties of the plant astragalus.

Chapter 3: Characteristics Of The Most Used Aromatic Herbs In The Kitchen (Basil, Parsley, Rosemary, Thyme, Etc.)

Here are some characteristics of the most used aromatic herbs:

- Basil: Basil has a sweet and slightly peppery flavor with a hint of clove. It is commonly used in Italian cuisine, particularly in pasta sauces, pesto, and salads. Basil leaves are delicate and should be added at the end of cooking to preserve their flavor.
- Rosemary: Rosemary has a strong, pine-like flavor with a hint of citrus. It pairs well with roasted meats, potatoes, and bread. The leaves are woody and should be minced or crushed before using.
- Thyme: Thyme has a subtle, earthy flavor with a slightly minty and lemony undertone. It is commonly used in Mediterranean and French cuisines, particularly in stews, soups, marinades, and roasted meats. Thyme leaves are small and can be used whole or chopped.
- Oregano: Oregano has a pungent, slightly bitter flavor with a hint of spiciness. It is a staple herb in Italian, Greek, and Mexican cuisines, used in tomato-based sauces, pizza, grilled meats, and salads. Oregano leaves can be used fresh or dried.
- Parsley: Parsley has a fresh, vibrant flavor with a hint of bitterness. It is widely used as a garnish and to enhance the flavor of various dishes, including soups, salads, sauces, and marinades. Both the flat-leaf (Italian) and curly varieties are used in cooking.
- Sage: Sage has a strong, slightly bitter flavor with a hint of eucalyptus. It is commonly used in Italian and Mediterranean cuisines, particularly in stuffing, roasted meats, and sausages. Sage leaves are hearty and should be used sparingly.
- Mint: Mint has a refreshing, cool flavor with a hint of sweetness. It is commonly used in both savory and sweet dishes, including salads, drinks, sauces, and desserts. Mint leaves are delicate and should be added at the end of cooking to retain their flavor.
- Coriander (Cilantro): The flavor is fresh and lemony with a touch of earthiness. It is commonly used in salsas, curries, and salads in Mexican, Indian, and Southeast Asian cuisines. The cilantro plant is utilized for its leaves and stems, while the coriander seed is ground and used as a spice.

Basil

Basil is an important medical herb due to its antibacterial, anti-inflammatory, and antioxidant qualities. It's healthy for the heart, helps with respiratory issues, and enhances digestion.

Rosemary:

Healing properties: Rosemary has antioxidant, anti-inflammatory, and antimicrobial properties. It may help improve memory and concentration, relieve muscle pain, support digestion, and promote hair growth.

Thyme:

Thyme is a potent medicinal herb with antibacterial, anti-inflammatory, and antiseptic qualities in addition to its high antioxidant content. It's beneficial for the digestive system, helps calm coughs, and promotes healthy lungs.

Sage:

Healing properties: Sage has antioxidant and antimicrobial properties. It can help improve memory and cognitive function, soothe sore throat and mouth, and support digestive health.

Oregano:

Healing properties: Oregano is a potent antimicrobial herb with antioxidant and anti-inflammatory properties. It can support immune health, aid digestion, and help fight against infections.

Mint (Peppermint, Spearmint):

Healing properties: Mint has antioxidant, anti-inflammatory, and antimicrobial properties. It can help soothe digestive issues, relieve headaches, alleviate respiratory congestion, and promote relaxation.

Lavender:

Healing properties: Lavender has calming and soothing properties. It can help reduce anxiety and stress, promote sleep, relieve headaches, and soothe skin irritations.

Cilantro (Coriander):

Healing properties: Cilantro has antioxidant, anti-inflammatory, and antimicrobial properties. It may help detoxify the body, support digestion, and promote healthy cholesterol levels.

Dill:

Dill's medicinal benefits include its ability to fight infection, protect cells from damage, and reduce swelling and pain. It can help with digestion, ease nausea, ease menstrual cramps, and induce slumber..

Lemongrass:

Healing properties: Lemongrass has antioxidant, anti-inflammatory, and antimicrobial properties. It can support digestion, relieve anxiety and stress, promote healthy skin, and alleviate respiratory conditions.

Conclusion

Herbal ingredients have been used in cooking for centuries not only for their flavors but also for their potential healing properties. While it's important to note that the scientific evidence supporting the healing properties of these ingredients may vary, they are generally considered to provide various health benefits.

BOOK 10: INTRODUCTION TO HERBAL TEAS, TEAS AND HEALING INFUSIONS

Chapter 1: Explore The Therapeutic Benefits Of Herbal Teas

For generations, people have turned to herbal teas as a safe and effective way to improve their health. Leaves, petals, seeds, and roots are just some of the plant elements that can be infused in hot water to create these delicious beverages. They have a wide variety of therapeutic uses and are very delightful to eat. In this article, we will discuss the health benefits of some popular herbal teas.

The calming and soothing effects of chamomile tea are well-known. It is commonly used to help people unwind, lessen the effects of stress and anxiety, and get a better night's sleep. In addition to its other benefits, chamomile tea is great for digestion and settling the stomach.

Peppermint tea is energizing and calming at the same time. It has been used for centuries as a remedy for indigestion, gas, and nausea. It has been suggested that drinking peppermint tea can aid with both headaches and mental clarity.

The digestive advantages of ginger tea are well known. It has anti-inflammatory and digestive benefits and helps alleviate nausea. Those suffering from cold symptoms may also benefit from drinking ginger tea, which is well-known for its warming effects.

Tea made from lavender flowers is said to reduce stress and promote relaxation. It has the potential to ease tension, ease anxiety, and enhance sleep. Many people drink lavender tea before bedtime because it helps them relax and get a good night's sleep.

The Echinacea plant is used to make a tea with immune-enhancing effects known as "Echinacea Tea." It has the potential to improve immune function and lessen the duration and intensity of cold and flu symptoms.

The antioxidants and anti-inflammatory effects of Rooibos tea are well-known. Its sweet and nutty flavor makes it a popular treat. Caffeine-sensitive individuals may want to switch to Rooibos tea instead of black or green tea due to its lack of this stimulant.

Tea made from lemon balm is said to relieve stress and anxiety and has a pleasant citrus flavor. It could ease stress, lift your spirits, and put you at ease. Many people drink lemon balm tea to improve their mood and concentration.

Hibiscus tea, brewed from the flower's petals, is known for its sour, fruity taste. It has a lot of antioxidants, so it could aid with weight loss, heart health, and lowering blood pressure.

Detoxifying nettle tea is prepared by steeping dried nettle leaves in hot water. It has anti-inflammatory, anti-thrombotic, and blood-cleansing properties. The use of nettle tea is also associated with improved hair and skin health.

Dandelion Tea: A natural diuretic, dandelion tea can be brewed from the plant's roots or leaves. It has the potential to improve detoxification, aid digestion, and protect liver function.

Herbal teas may be helpful for some conditions, but they shouldn't be used in place of conventional medicine. Always check with your doctor before adding a herbal tea to your daily regimen, especially if you have any preexisting conditions or are taking any drugs.

Chapter 2:
Preparation And Maceration Of Herbal Teas For Maximum Potency

Herbal Teas Recipes

It's a beverage generally produced using the Camellia sasanqua plant leaves, in some cases enhanced with chamomile, ginger, or cinnamon.

The beverage is called red tea in English-talking nations since it is regularly presented in a unique way of red food shading. Like green tea, it contains cell reinforcements that are thought to assist with decreasing the danger of malignant growth and coronary illness. It is likewise used to make red tea weight reduction.

Red tea is a homegrown tea produced using the Camellia sasanqua plant, now and then enhanced with chamomile, ginger, or cinnamon. It has been used in Chinese medication for quite a long time to treat various illnesses.

The beverage is called red tea in English-talking nations since it is regularly presented with a unique sound of red food shading. Like green tea, it contains cell reinforcements that are thought to assist with lessening the danger of malignant growth and coronary illness. It is additionally used to make red tea weight reduction.

The utilization of spices in food varieties and drinks goes back millennia. Tea has been utilized in societies throughout the planet for its therapeutic worth since antiquated occasions when it was joined into the everyday diet of the Chinese ruler Shen Nung, who found that it could lighten migraines, and upset stomachs, advance standard defecations, and forestall fevers. It has additionally been utilized for quite a long time in Europe as a solution for hacks and colds. The act of making tea from spices ultimately spread to the Western world.

Respiratory Support Tea

Ingredients:

- ¼ tsp. marshmallow root.
- 1/3 tsp. mullein.
- ¼ tsp. rose hips.
- ¼ tsp. lemon balm.
- ¼ tsp. OSHA root.
- ¼ tsp. coltsfoot leaves.

Instructions:

1. Put some water on to boil.
2. Add marshmallow roots to Osha.
3. Put a lid on it and simmer it for 10 minutes.
4. Mix the remaining ingredients thoroughly.
5. Re-cover and steep for another 10 minutes.
6. Honey can be added to taste.
7. Place tea servings through a strainer.
8. Dole it out and savor it.

Cold Care Tea

Ingredients:

- ¼ tsp. sage leaves.
- ¼ tsp. calendula flower.
- ¼ tsp. elderflower.
- ¼ tsp. hibiscus flower.

Instructions:

1. Boil the water in a pot.
2. Add all the ingredients to the serving cup and mix well.
3. Pour boiling water into the serving cup with the mixture.
4. Cover the cup and steep it for 8 minutes.
5. You can mix in honey as per your taste.
6. Serve and enjoy it.

Cayenne Tea

Ingredients:

- 1/8 tsp. cayenne powder.
- 1 tsp. honey.
- 2 tsp. lemon juice.

Instructions:

1. Boil the water in a pot.
2. Add all the ingredients to the serving cup and mix well.
3. Pour boiling water into a serving cup with lemon mixture.
4. Cover the cup and steep it for 8 minutes.
5. Serve and enjoy it.

Calming Marshmallow Rose Tea

Ingredients:

- 1 tsp. marshmallow root.
- 1 tsp. rosebuds.
- 1 tsp. cassia cinnamon chips.
- 1 tsp. Tulsi leaves (holy basil).

Instructions:

1. Boil the water in a pot.
2. Add all the ingredients to the serving cup and mix well.
3. Pour boiling water into the serving cup with the mixture.
4. Cover the cup and steep it for 8 minutes.
5. You can mix in honey as per your taste.
6. Strain the tea.
7. Serve and enjoy it.

Lavender Tea

Ingredients:

- 2 c water.
- 5 tbsp. lemon balm.
- 2 tbsp. lavender flower, dried.
- 1 tbsp. honey.

Instructions:

1. Boil the water in a pot.
2. Add all the ingredients to the serving cup and mix well.
3. Pour boiling water into a serving cup with lemon balm mixture.
4. Cover the cup and steep it for 8 minutes.
5. You can mix in honey as per your taste.
6. Strain the tea.
7. Serve and enjoy it.

Easy Masala Tea

Ingredients:

- Cinnamon, one teaspoon's worth.
- Ginger, 1 teaspoon.
- Cardamom, 1 teaspoon.
- ½ clove.
- One teaspoon of black tea.
- 1/4 teaspoon of black pepper.
- two cups of water.
- 1 ½ c milk.

Instructions:

1. First, crush cinnamon, peppercorn, cardamom, and cloves in a mortar system.
2. Add water to a pan and bring it to a boil.
3. Add the crushed spices and ginger.
4. Reduce the flame to low and cover the pan.
5. Let it simmer for 20 minutes.
6. Stir in milk and tea leaves.
7. Cover the pan again and cook it for 7 minutes.
8. Remove the pan from the flame and let it steep for six more minutes.
9. You can add honey or sugar as per your taste.
10. Strain the tea in serving cups.
11. Serve and enjoy it.

Herbal Tea

Ingredients:

- 1/3 tsp. elderberries.
- 1/3 tsp. rose hips.
- 1/3 tsp. Echinacea.
- 1/3 tsp. chamomile.
- 1/3 tsp. astragals.

Instructions:

1. Boil the water in a pot.
2. Add all the ingredients to the serving cup and mix well.
3. Pour boiling water into the serving cup with the mixture.
4. Cover the cup and steep it for 8 minutes.
5. You can mix in honey as per your taste.
6. Serve and enjoy it.

Chapter 3: Herbal Teas For Common Ailments (Recipes And Ailments)

Teas

Poppy Seeds Tea

Ingredients

- Poppy seeds – 1.5 Tsp
- Cloves – 3 No's
- 1 teaspoon of cardamom powder
- 2 cups of water
- 2 teaspoons of honey

Preparation

1. To a pot of boiling water, add all the ingredients.
2. Give it ten minutes to steep.
3. Put the herbs in a sieve and drain them out.
4. To taste, add honey.
5. Five, eat up!

General Benefits

This tea helps to have a deep and peaceful sleep. Increase appetite and increase productivity. This tea helps to proper blood flow in nerves.

Earl Grey Black Tea

Ingredients

- Black tea - 1 Cup
- Bergamot Essential Oil - 20-22 drops

Preparation

1. Put the tea in a canning jar.
2. Put in some Bergamot oil, please.
3. Put the top back on and give it a good shake.
4. Permit a day of rest.
5. Brew your tea by boiling one teaspoon per cup of water for three to five minutes.
6. Prepare and savor.

General Benefits

Black tea's ability to dilate blood vessels and improve blood flow to the heart lowers the probability of cardiovascular problems including heart attacks and strokes.

Cranberry Nettles Tea

Ingredients:

- Unsweetened Cranberry juice - 6-8 oz
- Dried nettle leaf - 1 Cup
- 3Dried spearmint leaf - 3 tsp.
- Dried green leaf stevia - 2 tsp.

Preparation:

1. The nettles, spearmint, and stevia should be combined in a 2-quart mason jar with a tight-fitting lid.
2. Toss the herbs into a quart of freshly boiled water.
3. Give it at least half an hour to an hour to steep.
4. Put the herbs in a sieve and drain them out.

5. Fill the rest of the way with water and add 6-8 ounces of unsweetened cranberry juice.
6. Enjoy while chilled.

General Benefits

Sores and other mouth illnesses can be avoided by drinking this tea. Cancer patients, particularly those with stomach or breast cancer, can benefit from its use.

Russian Star Anise Tea

Ingredients

- Orange juice - 1 cup
- Lemon juice - ½ cup
- Star anise - 3 No's
- Cinnamon stick - a small piece
- Loose Tea or Black Tea - 1/2 cup or 4 teabags
- Hot water - 4 cups
- Honey – 2 Tsp

Preparation

1. Boil the water and add the ingredients to a tea strainer.
2. Let it steep for at least 10 minutes.
3. Strain the tea into the teacup and add the cinnamon stick and lemon slice for garnish.
4. Add honey as desired.
5. Serve and enjoy

General Benefits

Russia has its own unique way of serving tea, just as the British and other Asian nations. They stock their samovars with robust spices, dark black tea, and citrus juices.

Hibiscus Raspberry Green Tea

Ingredients

- Green tea - 6 Tsp
- Chamomile - 6 Tsp
- Dried Hibiscus Flower - 1/2 Cup
- Dried raspberries - 1-2 oz
- Honey - 3 Tsp

Preparation

1. Combine everything in a mason jar and keep it out of the light.
2. To prepare iced tea, use four to six tablespoons per quart of water. (One Tablespoon for Steaming Tea)
3. Set timer for 3 minutes and steep.
4. Put the herbs in a sieve and drain them out.
5. Honey can be added to taste.
6. Enjoy while chilled.

General Benefits

This tea has been shown to reduce both blood pressure and total blood fat. In addition, it helps you lose weight and improves your liver health.

Coconut Spritzer Tea

Ingredients

- Coconut Chai Tea - 1 Cup
- Mineral water - 1 Cup
- Honey - 3 -4 Tsp

Preparation

1. Add your chilled, brewed tea to a large jar.
2. Add in the mineral water and Honey to taste.
3. Serve Cold and enjoy.

General Benefits

This tea helps in lowering the bad cholesterol in the body and protects you from cardiovascular diseases.

Rose Black Tea

Ingredients

- Rose petals - 2 Tsp
- Black tea - 1 Cup
- Honey – 3 Tsp

Preparation

1. Place the rose petals and black tea in a glass jar.
2. Allow to steep 5-8 minutes.
3. Strain the Petals through a strainer.
4. Add honey as desired.
5. Serve and enjoy.

General Benefits

This tea helps in fighting inflammation, remove toxins. It boosts digestion and strengthens the immune system.

Almond Tea

Ingredients

- Black Tea Powder – 3 Tsp
- Milk – 2 Cups
- Lemon Juice – 2 Tsp
- Almond powder – 4 Tsp
- Water – 3 Cups
- Honey – 3 Tsp

Preparation

1. Boil the milk in a pan and add Almond powder and boil for 5 mins.
2. Add black tea powder in teapot and steep for 5-10 mins.
3. Pour the Almond milk into the teapot.
4. Strain the tea and add honey.
5. Serve and enjoy.

General benefits

This tea prevents you from anti-aging, detoxify, chronic disease, and rheumatism.

Lemonade Ice Tea

Ingredients

- Black or Green tea - 1 teabag
- Lemonade r- 2/3 cup
- Honey - 2 to 3 Tbs

Preparation

1. Make the black or green tea as usual and let cool.
2. Pour the tea in a mason jar and add lemonade and sugar or honey.
3. Add ice, put the lid on the jar, and shake the tea until it is blended well.

General Benefits

It cures Migraine headaches and helps in detoxification of the body. Also, it aids in lung cleansing.

Cold Care Tea

Ingredients

- Calendula flowers - 1 Tsp
- Sage leaves - 2

- Hibiscus flowers - 1Tsp
- Elderflowers - 1 Tsp
- Honey - 3 Tsp

Preparation

1. Boil the water and add the herbs.
2. Allow to steep 8-10 minutes.
3. Strain herbs and discard them.
4. Add honey as desired.
5. Serve and Enjoy.

General Benefits

If you are severely affected by nasty cold and cough then try this tea.

Dual Purpose Tea

Ingredients

- 1. Dried Chamomile Flowers – 2 Tsp
- 2. Water – 1 Cup
- 3. Honey – 3 Tsp

Preparation

1. Put the dried chamomile in a cup of boiling water.
2. give it at least 15 minutes to steep.
3. The spice needs to be strained.
4. To taste, add honey.
5. Prepare and savor.

General Benefits

This tea calms you from sickness, and stomach upset. And furthermore it diminishes the feminine cramps.

Menstrual Cramps Tea

Ingredients

- Licorice root powder – 1 Tsp
- Ginger Powder – 1 Tsp
- Pepper powder – 1 Tsp
- Water – 2 cups
- Coconut Milk – 1 cup
- Honey – 2 Tsp

Preparation

1. Add licorice powder and different fixings in the bubbling water.
2. Boil it for 10 mins.
3. Strain the spices through a strainer.
4. Add coconut milk.
5. Add honey as desired.
6. Serve and enjoy.

General Benefits

Licorice has mitigating properties, so it might assist with peopling who are nervous.

Basil Leaves Tea

Ingredients

- Basil Leaves – 5 No's
- Water – 1 cup

Preparation

1. Add basil leaves in the teapot.
2. Let it steep for 5-10 mins.
3. Strain the leaves through a strainer.
4. Add Honey as desired.
5. Serve and enjoy.

General Benefits

Basil Leaves go about as an adaptogen. An adaptogen is a characteristic substance that assists your body with adjusting pressure and advances mental equilibrium.

Guava Tea

Ingredients

- Guava Leaves – 6 No's
- Water – 2 cup
- Fenugreek– ½ Tsp
- Honey – 3 Tsp

Preparation

1. Add 2 cups of water and make it boil.
2. Add Guava Leaves and Fenugreek in the bubbling water.
3. Let it steep for 10 mins.
4. Strain the leaves through a strainer.
5. Add Honey as desired.
6. Serve and enjoy.

General Benefits

Guava is powerful in forestalling and treating enlarged gums and toothache. It assists with bringing down cholesterol and keeps the heart and vascular tissues sound. It cleans the intestinal system and diminishes stomach torment and diarrhea.

Earl Gray Black Tea

Ingredients

- 1. Black tea - 1 Cup
- 2. Bergamot Essential Oil - 20-22 drops

Preparation

1. Pour the tea into a glass jar.
2. Add the Bergamot fundamental oil.
3. Close the top and shake vigorously.
4. Allow resting for a day.
5. Steep one teaspoon of tea in water and bubble for 3-5 minutes.
6. Serve and enjoy.

General Benefits

Black tea will lessen the danger of coronary failures and strokes, as it can assist with expanding the supply routes, which lifts blood course to the heart.

Digestive system

Lung Blend Tea

Ingredients

- Echinacea– 1 part
- Elecampane – 1 part
- Ginger – 1 part
- Pleurisy roots – 1 part
- White Oak Bark – 1 part
- Cinnamon Bark – 1 part
- Orange strip – 1 part
- Fennel Seeds – 1 part
- Stevia – 1 pinch

Preparation

1. Blend every one of the fixings in an artisan jar.
2. Store the holder in a dim spot to keep away from direct sunlight. To Brew
3. Place all spices in a tea pack and cover with bubbling water.
4. Let steep something like 5-10 minutes.
5. Remove Tea sack and add Stevia or honey anything that to taste.
6. Serve and enjoy.

General Benefits

This tea is really great for breathing.

Soothing Tea

Ingredients

- Mint – 1 Part
- Hyssop – 1 Part
- Oregano – 1 Part
- Parsley – 1 Part
- Lemon Balm - 1 Part
- Honey – 3 Tsp

Preparation

1. Blend every one of the fixings in an impenetrable container.
2. Store the compartment in a dull spot to keep away from direct sunlight. To Brew
3. Place all spices in a tea pack and cover with bubbling water.
4. Let steep no less than 10-15 minutes.
5. Remove Tea pack and add honey.
6. Serve and enjoy.

General Benefits

Drinking this tea will help loosens up the stomach muscles.

Sun Brewed Black Tea

Ingredients

- Black tea - 2 Teabags
- Sliced organic product or berries - 1/2 Cup
- Spring water - 1 Gallon
- Honey – 3 Tsp

Preparation

1. Mix all fixings in the glass container, cover with a tight lid.
2. Allow the tea to sit in the sun for up to five hours.
3. Pour tea over glasses of ice and improve as desired.
4. Serve and enjoy

General Benefits

This tea expands focus and memory. This tea assists with lessening terrible cholesterol and raises great cholesterol.

Jack Frost Tea

Ingredients

- Dried Peppermint leaves - 1/4 Cup
- Dried Spearmint leaves - 1/4 Cup
- Honey - 3 Tsp

Preparation

1. Blend all fixings in a bowl.
2. Store in a water/air proof container.
3. Add 1 Tsp of spice blend in a medium saucepan.
4. Pour 1 cups of high temp water over herbs.
5. Bring to a speedy bubble and lower heat.
6. Allow stewing 10 minutes.
7. Strain spices and dispose of them.
8. Add Honey if you want.

General Benefits

This tea is a typical home solution for fart. This tea likewise eases agony and distress from gas and bloating.

Digestive Stimulator Tea

Ingredients:

- 1 parts spearmint leaves
- 1/8-part dried licorice root
- 3 cloves
- sprinkle of fennel seeds.

Preparation:

1. Mix the spearmint and licorice root together.
2. Store in a glass jar.
3. Use 1 tablespoon per cup when brewing tea.

General Benefits

This tea assists with lessening terrible cholesterol and raises great cholesterol

Peppermint Tea

Ingredients

- Dried Peppermint leaves - 1 Tsp
- Honey - 1 Tsp
- Water - 1 Cup

Preparation

1. Put one serving of peppermint in your tea sifter for some tea you want.
2. Steep leaves in steaming hot water from 5-10 minutes, as indicated by your ideal strength.
3. You can drink it unsweetened or add sugar, or honey as desired.
4. Serve and enjoy.

General Benefits

As a piece of the mint family, peppermint has been utilized for ages to relieve indigestion and respiratory problems.

Turmeric Tea

Ingredients

- Turmeric – 2 Tsp
- Cinnamon Powder – 1 Tsp
- Clove– 3 No's
- Nutmeg– A pinch
- Black Pepper – ½ Tsp

- Water – 2 Cups
- Honey – 3 Tsp

Preparation

1. Add 2 cups of water and make it boil.
2. Add cleaved every one of the fixings in the bubbling water aside from honey.
3. Let it steep for 10-15 mins.
4. Strain the spices through a strainer.
5. Add Honey as desired.
6. Serve and enjoy.

General Benefits

This Tea has a strong alleviating cure and has many mending properties. Upholds assimilation, insusceptible, and liver capacity. It has mitigating and anticancer properties. It is utilized in customary prescriptions as a therapy for some stomach related conditions.

Chapter 5:
Herbal Teas For Specific Ailments

Enhance herbal teas with additions.

Citrus Zest: Add a twist of citrus by grating the zest of lemon, lime, or orange into your tea. This can add a refreshing and tangy flavor to your herbal blend.

Honey or Agave Syrup: If you prefer your tea on the sweeter side, consider adding a drizzle of honey or agave syrup. These natural sweeteners can complement the herbal flavors and provide a touch of sweetness.

Fresh Herbs: Experiment with adding fresh herbs like mint, basil, or lavender to your tea. These herbs can infuse their unique flavors and aromas into the brew, creating a delightful blend.

Spices: Certain spices can enhance the warmth and complexity of herbal teas. Try adding a cinnamon stick, a few cloves, or a pinch of ginger to your tea for a cozy and aromatic twist.

Fruit Slices: Thinly sliced fruits, such as apples, berries, or peaches, can add a subtle fruity essence to your herbal tea. Infuse the tea with the fruit slices while brewing for a delicate infusion of flavor.

Coconut Milk: For a creamy and tropical twist, consider adding a splash of coconut milk to your herbal tea. It adds richness and a hint of coconut flavor, particularly delicious in teas with tropical or floral notes.

Vanilla Extract: A drop or two of vanilla extract can add a sweet and comforting flavor to your herbal tea. It pairs well with teas featuring chamomile, rooibos, or hibiscus.

Chai Spices: Create a spiced herbal tea by adding chai spices such as cardamom, cinnamon, cloves, and black pepper. This combination can provide a warming and aromatic experience.

Remember to adjust the quantities of these additions according to your taste preferences and the specific herbal tea you're enhancing. Enjoy exploring and finding the combinations that delight your senses!

Explore additional ingredients to enhance the healing properties of herbal teas

Addition of turmeric to herbal teas is beneficial because of turmeric's anti-inflammatory effects. It may also help with digestion and improve immunity.

Ginger: This potent herb has been used for centuries due to its ability to combat nausea, inflammation, and oxidative stress. Indigestion, nausea, and other gastrointestinal complaints may find especial relief.

The addition of cinnamon to herbal teas not only improves the taste, but also may have positive effects on health. In addition to perhaps aiding in blood sugar regulation and digestive health, cinnamon possesses antibacterial and anti-inflammatory qualities.

Citrusy and delicious, lemon is a great addition to herbal teas and helps them retain their medicinal qualities. Lemons' high levels of vitamin C and antioxidants make them useful for cleansing the body and boosting immunity.

Honey is a healthy alternative to refined sugars and can be used to sweeten herbal drinks. It has antimicrobial qualities and may ease a cough or sore throat. However, due to the risk of botulism, honey shouldn't be given to infants younger than one year old.

Peppermint is a well-liked herb for its sedative and stomach-settling properties. Peppermint leaves, either fresh or dried, can be used to herbal teas to ease gastrointestinal distress.

Echinacea is a popular herbal remedy for boosting the immune system and warding off illness. Echinacea's immune-boosting benefits are amplified when brewed with herbal teas.

Antioxidant-rich elderberry has long been used to help the body fight off infections and feel better throughout cold and flu season. Herbal teas can have even more of an immune-boosting effect if dried elderberries or elderberry syrup are added to the mix.

Chamomile is a mild herb with sedative qualities. It can help you unwind, calm your nerves, and have a good night's sleep. You may make a relaxing and pleasant tea by combining chamomile with other herbal teas.

Rosehips: These nutrient- and anti-oxidant-packed little guys are the rose plant's fruit. Dried rosehips are a great way to augment the nutrient content and health benefits of herbal drinks.

Chapter 6:
Herbal Infusions For Health And Well-Being

Benefits of Infusions

Infusions allow for the rapid and direct administration of fluids, nutrients, or drugs into the bloodstream. Bypassing the digestive system's slower absorption process compared to oral drugs, this approach provides a speedy commencement of effect.

Infusions allow for exact control over the amount of fluids or drugs given. The proper amount of medication may then be given to each patient because doctors can adjust the dosage based on their particular needs.

The effects of infusions are frequently experienced more quickly than those of other routes of administration since the chemicals are injected straight into the bloodstream. In times of crisis or when quick aid or action is urgently needed, this can be invaluable.

Increased Bioavailability Intravenous infusions have a higher bioavailability than other modes of administration because more of the delivered medication reaches its target. This is due to the fact that the drug enters the bloodstream unimpeded and is not subject to breakdown in the digestive system.

IV infusions are frequently used for the management of fluids and electrolytes in cases of severe sickness, electrolyte imbalance, or dehydration. Medical professionals are able to quickly rectify electrolyte imbalances and restore fluid balance with these products.

Some therapies need to be given over a lengthy period of time, or given repeatedly. A consistent therapeutic impact can be maintained with the use of infusions because of their slow and steady distribution throughout time.

For nutritional support, vitamins, minerals, and amino acids can be infused directly into the bloodstream by an infusion. When patients have problems digesting and absorbing meals, this technique is frequently used.

Bypassing the digestive system, infusions reduce the risk of adverse effects on the gastrointestinal tract that may be experienced when taking oral drugs. Those who have digestive issues including nausea, vomiting, or malabsorption can benefit greatly from this.

IV infusions allow for therapeutic versatility by allowing for the administration of a wide variety of drugs. Depending on the patient's condition, they can be used for a wide range of medical procedures, including the delivery of medication, transfusion of blood, chemotherapy, pain control, and immunotherapy.

Infusion

An infusion is prepared by mixing the herbs with water or oil and waiting for the chemical compounds to mix with the solvent. This process is known as steeping. Infusion is used to make herbal remedies. The advantage of infusion is that it is easy to prepare and has the strong medicinal quality of the herb.

A very small number of herbs can be used for infusion because they are made up of many herbs, which results in a very mild flavor. Herbal tea or herbal soup is made through the process of infusions.

Depending on the herb type, one can brew an infusion by placing herbs in a jug with clean water and placing it by sunlight for several hours, usually six to ten hours. When the water has reached full flavor, it can be drunk at once or have a second step.

Infusions can be used to address all symptoms of illness and can also be used at any time when needed. It is an excellent way of treating mild problems and preventing disease symptoms and serious disorders by just drinking herbal tea three times a day. Herbal teas are made by infusing herbs in boiling water for a few minutes and removing the herb from the mixture before drinking it.

Many materials used are leaves, flowers, berries, and seeds either in whole or when they are dried and pounded or ground. The liquid is boiled, and the herbs are added and allowed to steep for some time, usually 15-30 minutes. The herbs can be removed, or the liquid is strained and drunk either immediately or later.

Here is a list of herbs Infusions can be made with:

Sore Throat Infusion

Preparation:

- To prepare, bring two cups of water to a boil and stir in one teaspoon of fresh ginger.
- The steeping time is 10 minutes, so turn off the heat now.
- As needed, use 1–2 teaspoons of the mixture to ease the pain of a sore throat.

People who regularly take this infusion have fewer cases of the sore throat every year because they have strong bacterial resistance.

Infusion of Sage

Preparation:

- Put one ounce of sage leaves in a pot with two cups of water and bring it to a boil.
- The steeping time is 10 minutes, so turn off the heat now.
- For chest congestion, take 2 to 4 teaspoons of the combination three to four times daily.

People who regularly take this infusion have fewer cases of the sore throat every year because they have strong bacterial resistance.

Infusion of Fennel

Preparation:

- Put one teaspoon of fennel leaves in a pot with two cups of water and bring it to a boil.

- The steeping time is 10 minutes, so turn off the heat now.
- Cold, cough, and respiratory issues can be treated with 1–2 teaspoons of the mixture, as needed.

People who regularly take this infusion have fewer cases of constipation every year because they have strong bacterial resistance.

Infusion of Valerian

Preparation:

- Put two cups of water in a pot and bring it to a boil. Then, add one teaspoon of fresh parsley blossoms.
- The steeping time is 10 minutes, so turn off the heat now.
- If you suffer from insomnia, anxiety, or nervousness, try taking 1/2 teaspoon of valerian root with 2 to 4 teaspoons of chamomile tea.

People who regularly take this infusion have fewer cases of insomnia every year because they have strong bacterial resistance.

Infusion of Yellow Dock Tea

Preparation:

- Bring two cups of water to a boil and add one teaspoon of fresh dandelion.
- The steeping time is 10 minutes, so turn off the heat now.
- For conditions involving the liver, the skin, or the urinary tract, take 1–2 tablespoons three times daily.

People who regularly take this infusion have fewer liver disorders and skin problems every year because of strong bacterial resistance.

Infusion of Dandelion Tea

Preparation:

- Put two cups of water in a kettle and bring it to a boil. Then, add one teaspoon of fresh dandelion leaves.
- The steeping time is 10 minutes, so turn off the heat now.
- For conditions involving the liver, the skin, or the urinary tract, take 1–2 tablespoons three times daily.

People who regularly take this infusion have fewer liver disorders and skin problems every year because of strong bacterial resistance.

Baths

The skin is the body's biggest organ, with a complex structure and a wide range of characteristics and hues. The skin is a crucial component in the body's immune system, as it provides a physical barrier from the outside. There are also some special layers of the skin that contain various chemicals to protect us from diseases, worms, and microbes.

Bath treatment with herbs can be a great way to deal with the chills and make you feel very relaxed after a hard day's work. Using herbal baths can help you achieve healthy skin and helps maintain overall body health.

Herbs that can be used for baths are either made into decoctions, capsules, or tinctures.

Hot baths are essential because they can help dissolve the herbs and increase their effectiveness, thus improving the quality of the bath. It is important to avoid extreme hot baths because they raise body temperature and can cause hyperthermia.

The decoction can be used for baths as they are delicious and have skin-nourishing properties.

The most popular herbs for baths are mint and lemon balm. Mint extracts are used not only for baths but also for aromatherapy. Lemon balm can be used to relieve stress and improve blood circulation.

Here is a list of herbal baths that can help you achieve healthy skin:

Lavender Bath

Preparation:

- Add 1 to 2 cups of dried lavender flower to your bathtub.
- Boil a pot of water and add 1/2 cup of Epsom salt.
- Pour the mixture into the bathtub, and then get into the tub after you've added water.
- Soak for 5 to 10 minutes.
- Use with caution because the Epsom salt may irritate those who are sensitive to it.

Sage Bath

Preparation:

- Place 1/4 cup of dried sage in your bathtub and add hot water.
- Steep for 5 to 10 minutes before getting into the tub.
- For extra effect, you can leave the herbs in the tub after your bath.
- It is recommended not to use this herbal treatment if you are pregnant or breastfeeding because sage has properties that can make you feel like you're on an intense trip.

Rose Petal Bath

Preparation:

- Place 8 to 10 organic rose petals into your bathtub.

- Vitamin C in rose petals brightens and softens skin.
- Steep the rose petals in hot water for 3 to 5 minutes before getting into the tub.
- Rose glyceride is a substance in rose petals that can soothe irritations and inflammation caused by eczema and acne.

Ginger Bath

Ginger is an essential element to improving your skin's health.

The best ginger is fresh ginger and can be added to your bath either as a decoction or powder.

If you make the decoction, be sure to use two parts water for one part ginger root.

Preparation:

- For each bather, add 1/2 cup Epsom salt and 1 cup fresh ginger root.
- Use 3 to 4 cups of hot water for each person taking a bath.
- Steep in a pot for 5-10 minutes.
- When ready to take a bath, use 1/2 cup of the mixture with the Epsom salt and add it to your bathwater.
- Soak for 5-10 minutes before rinsing.

Precautions: do not use this herbal treatment if you have high blood pressure because ginger can increase blood pressure levels. Also, do not take this herbal bath if you are pregnant.

Conclusions

Herbal teas, teas, and healing infusions have been used for centuries in various cultures around the world for their potential health benefits. While the scientific evidence regarding their specific healing properties may vary, many of these beverages have been associated with positive health effects.

BOOK 11: NATURAL HERBAL ANTIBIOTICS

The use of natural remedies as an alternative to traditional antibiotics has gained popularity in recent years. Herbal antibiotics, sometimes called botanical antibiotics or herbal antimicrobials, are a type of natural antibiotic that is produced from plants and has antimicrobial properties that can be used to treat bacterial, viral, fungal, and parasitic illnesses.

Ayurveda, TCM, and Native American healing traditions are just a few examples of traditional medical systems that have relied on herbs and plants for hundreds of years. Many of these plants have shown strong antibacterial action, making them viable substitutes for or additions to conventional antibiotics.

Herbal antibiotics, as opposed to synthetic ones, are typically safer and less harmful. Both as a preventative tactic to boost immunity and a treatment for certain infections, they have multiple uses. Herbal medicines have their uses, but they may not be adequate for treating illnesses that could become fatal. It is essential to get medical attention from a qualified practitioner in such circumstances.

Examples of Natural Herbal Antibiotics:

Allium sativum (garlic): Garlic's antibacterial and immune-boosting characteristics have made it a popular therapeutic herb for millennia. The component allicin it contains is highly effective against bacteria, viruses, and fungi.

The immune-boosting effects of the herb echinacea (Echinacea purpurea) have made it a favorite among herbalists. Historically, it has been used to treat a wide variety of respiratory diseases caused by bacteria and viruses.

Goldenseal (Hydrastis canadensis): The chemical berberine found in goldenseal has been shown to have antibacterial effects against a wide variety of microorganisms. Historically, people have utilized it to heal their stomach and lungs.

Origanum vulgare (Olive) Oil: The active ingredients in oregano oil, carvacrol and thymol, are potent antimicrobials. It is typically prescribed for the treatment of gastrointestinal problems, respiratory infections, and fungal infections.

Ginger (Zingiber officinale) is a popular spice for its medicinal uses, including its ability to reduce inflammation and kill bacteria. The immune system is strengthened, and the signs of respiratory infections and stomach upset are lessened.

Curcumin, found in turmeric (Curcuma longa), is an active chemical with antibacterial and anti-inflammatory activities. In traditional medicine, it is used to combat infections and boost general well-being.

If you have a prior medical condition, use any medications, are pregnant, or nursing, herbal antibiotics should be used with caution and only under the guidance of a healthcare professional.

It's vital to remember that natural herbal antibiotics are not meant to replace conventional therapy, but rather to augment it. It is crucial to have a medical diagnosis, treatment, and advice when dealing with serious or persistent infections.

Chapter 1:
Introduction To Natural Herbal Antibiotics

Benefits of using herbs as natural antibiotics

Reducing the prevalence of bacteria that are resistant to antibiotics, which has been exacerbated by the careless and excessive use of synthetic antibiotics. Because of the complex mixture of compounds found in most herbal antibiotics, antibiotic resistance in bacteria is less likely to develop in response to their use.

Many herbs have antimicrobial properties that are broad in scope, making them effective against a wide variety of pathogens. They can be effective against many different kinds of infections thanks to this adaptability.

Synthetic antibiotics, while effective, can cause unwanted side effects like diarrhea and allergic reactions in some people. When used properly, herbal antibiotics rarely cause adverse reactions. Though some people may not react negatively to herbs, others may still be sensitive to them.

Some herbs not only have antimicrobial properties, but they also support the immune system, allowing the body to fight infections better. They have the ability to strengthen the immune system and improve general well-being.

The antimicrobial properties of many herbs used as antibiotics are only part of their overall health benefits. Garlic, for instance, is good for your heart, and ginger can help reduce inflammation. The use of herbs as antibiotics has many potential benefits.

In many cases, herbal antibiotics can be obtained with less difficulty and expense than conventional antibiotics. The reliance on pharmaceutical products can be reduced due to the widespread availability of medicinal herbs, some of which can even be grown at home.

Herbs have been shown to be effective as natural antibiotics; however, they should not be relied upon for treating life-threatening infections. Synthetic antibiotics and medical attention from trained professionals may be required in such situations. In addition, if you have any preexisting medical issues or are on any other medications, it is essential to speak with a healthcare expert or herbalist to verify correct usage, dosage, and safety.

Safety and efficacy of herbal antibiotics

Although there is limited scientific study on the antibacterial effects of specific herbs, the bulk of studies are exploratory in nature and have only been performed in test tubes or animal models. Herbal antibiotics have not been well studied for their efficacy or safety in humans.

Herbal antibiotics may only be effective against certain strains of bacteria or other diseases, and their activity spectrum may be quite limited. If you want to know if a herbal antibiotic will work against your infection, you need to know what kind of microbe is causing it.

Different plant species, cultivation methods, extraction techniques, and preparation processes can all affect the strength and quality of herbal antibiotics. Their efficiency and security may be compromised due to this variation.

The risk of adverse effects and drug interactions is present with herbal antibiotics, just as it is with conventional antibiotics. When used in excessive doses or for lengthy periods of time, certain herbs can have harmful effects or induce allergic reactions in some people. If you have any preexisting medical concerns or are already taking any pharmaceuticals, it is essential to speak with a healthcare practitioner prior to using herbal antibiotics.

Herbal remedies, in contrast to conventional pharmaceutical antibiotics, are not required to adhere to the same stringent standards. Herbal antibiotics on the market may have inconsistent dosing and composition due to varying quality control.

When treating serious or life-threatening diseases, conventional antibiotics should be used instead of herbal medications. However, under the supervision of a healthcare practitioner, they may play a role as supplementary or supportive therapies.

Chapter 2:
Common Antibiotic Herbs

Description of herbs with antibiotic properties

Antimicrobial and antibacterial properties of each herb

Garlic (Allium sativum): Garlic is a popular herb with potent antibiotic properties. It contains a compound called allicin, which exhibits antimicrobial activity against various bacteria, viruses, and fungi. Garlic is known to be effective against common pathogens like E. coli, Staphylococcus aureus, and Candida albicans. It also has immune-boosting properties.

Oregano (Origanum vulgare): Oregano is a culinary herb that possesses strong antimicrobial properties. It contains compounds such as carvacrol and thymol, which have been found to exhibit antibacterial and antifungal activity. Oregano oil is particularly potent and is used in natural remedies to combat infections caused by bacteria like Salmonella and Pseudomonas aeruginosa.

Thyme (Thymus vulgaris): Thyme is an aromatic herb known for its antibacterial properties. It contains thymol, carvacrol, and other compounds that possess antimicrobial activity. Thyme has been used traditionally to treat respiratory infections, skin infections, and digestive issues. It is effective against bacteria like Staphylococcus aureus and Escherichia coli.

Sage (Salvia officinalis): Sage is a herb with antimicrobial and antioxidant properties. It contains volatile oils, including thujone and cineole, which possess antibacterial and antifungal properties. Sage is often used as a natural remedy for throat infections, dental infections, and respiratory ailments. It has shown effectiveness against bacteria like Streptococcus pyogenes and Staphylococcus aureus.

Echinacea (Echinacea spp.): Echinacea is an herb commonly used to boost the immune system. It contains compounds like alkamides, caffeic acid derivatives, and polysaccharides that have immune-stimulating and antimicrobial effects. Echinacea is often used to prevent and treat respiratory infections, including those caused by viruses and bacteria.

Goldenseal (Hydrastis canadensis): Goldenseal is a herb native to North America that contains an active compound called berberine. Berberine has been shown to possess broad-spectrum antimicrobial activity against bacteria, fungi, and protozoa. Goldenseal is commonly used to support the immune system and treat infections of the respiratory and digestive tracts.

Chapter 3:
Preparation And Use Of Herbal Antibiotics (recipes - ailments etc.) (infusions, decoctions, tinctures, oils, etc.)

Herbal Teas

Herbal teas differ widely from general teas because they do not come from the same plant. They are the combinations of flowers, herbs, and dried fruits, which are brewed like tea. Herbal teas contain no caffeine, often lower blood pressure, have delicious flavors, and improve digestion. They also often contain no calories and no sugar.

Raspberry Tea

- Serving Size: 1
- Brewing Time: 10 minutes

Ingredients:

- 1 c. water
- ¼ c. dried raspberry leaves
- ¼ c. dried lemongrass
- ½ c. dried chamomile flowers
- ½ c. dried orange peel

Directions:

1. Mix all the dried herbs listed above.
2. Boil water.
3. Add 1 tsp of tea mixture to a cup.
4. Pour hot water over it. Cover and steep for 5-10 minutes. The longer the time, the more tannin is extracted.
5. Consume hot, cold, or iced.

Hibiscus-Ginger Tea

- Serving Size: 4 cups
- Brewing Time: 15 minutes

Ingredients:

- 4 c. water
- 1 tbsp. hibiscus leaves
- 1 tbsp. grated fresh ginger
- 3-5 mint leaves

Directions:

1. Boil water in a pot.
2. Take hibiscus and ginger and blend in another pot.
3. Pour hot water over the tea mixture, cover, and steep for 10-12 minutes.
4. The color of the tea will turn ruby red, then add mint leaves for fresh flavor.
5. Serve hot or cold.

Mint Tea

- Serving Size: 2
- Brewing Time: 8 minutes

Ingredients:

- 2 c. water
- 15-20 fresh mint leaves
- 2 lemon slices
- 1 tsp. honey (optional)

Directions:

1. In a teapot, boil the water.
2. Remove from heat and add mint leaves. 5 minutes covered in the pot Increase the time for a strong flavor of mint.

3. Pour in a cup or glass.
4. Add honey and garnish with a lemon slice.
5. Enjoy hot or iced.

Sweet and Spicy Herb Tea

- Serving Size: 1
- Brewing Time: 10 minutes

Ingredients:

- 1 c. water
- ½ tbsp. cloves
- 1 tbsp. dried stevia
- ¼ c. cinnamon stick
- ¼ c. dried orange zest
- ¼ c. dried chamomile flowers
- ½ c. dried lemon verbena

Directions:

1. Make the blend and use 1 tsp. Tea mixture.
2. Boil water and pour over tea.
3. Cover the pot for 5 minutes or longer.
4. Strain into a cup and serve hot. Alternatively, pour over ice in the glass and serve cold.
5. Enjoy the sweet and spicy taste.

Basil Tea

- Serving Size: 1
- Brewing Time: 5 minutes

Ingredients:

- 1 c. water
- 1 tsp. basil leaves
- ¼ tsp. dried ginger
- ½ tsp. cinnamon powder
- 1 tsp honey (optional)

Directions:

1. Boil the water and add the basil leaves, ginger, and cinnamon.
2. Steep it for 5 minutes.
3. Strain and add honey to improve the taste.
4. Pour in a cup and serve hot.

Decoctions

Decoctions are another form of herbal remedy. This is the extraction of medicinal qualities from herbs by steeping them in water until the water gets its color, smell, and taste traits. Decoctions are made through which plant material or herbal substance can release its active ingredients during boiling. In this way, various natural chemical components present inside the herb can be easily released by just mixing it with warm water. Decoctions are widely used sources of herbal medicine in herbalism. When roots or barks of plants contain medicinal benefits, it is hard to obtain extracts from these hard parts of plants, such as willow bark. Decoctions are used for extracting tannins, which are harsh and bitter and also help indigestion.

Decoctions have been used for millennia in herbal medicine to treat a variety of ailments. The process is also very useful for treating several health disorders, including blood purification, salves for skin problems such as acne and dermatitis, tonics for dryness, irritations such as eczema or psoriasis.

Often they are known to be useful for treating musculoskeletal problems such as rheumatism, arthritis, cramps, etc.

Making Herb-Infused Decoctions

Herbs can be used not only to make herbal decoctions but also to prepare infusions. This is the preparation process of herbs by boiling the leaves with water, usually for a longer time than what is needed to make decoctions. In this way, the active ingredients would be more effective because they concentrate inside the water and are not simple in the herbs themselves. Decoctions are made by boiling herbs in water until the water gets its color, smell, and taste traits. In this way, various natural chemical components present inside the plant can be easily released by mixing them with warm water. Decoctions are widely used sources of herbal medicine in herbalism. However, they can also be made from bark or roots or barks that do not contain as many medicinal benefits as extracts from leaves, flowers, seeds, etc.

Here is a list of Decoctions for you to try out;

Basil Decoction

Method:

- Boil 2 – 3 tbsp of Basil leaves in a cup of water.
- Steep for 10-15 minutes with a lid.
- To make the decoction more concentrated, add more Basil leaves.
- Take your hot decoction and strain it using a strainer or cheesecloth into an empty cup.
- Thoroughly clean up the filter if used before storing it for later use.
- Drink this hot herbal tea twice daily for best results.
- Other components for your decoction include mint, rosemary, and lavender.
- Also, note that Rosemary can be used instead of Basil for a more robust decoction.

German Chamomile Decoction

Method:

- Boil 1 – 2 tbsp of Chamomile flowers in a cup of water.
- Steep for 10-15 minutes with a lid.
- Take your Hot Chamomile decoction and strain it using a strainer or cheesecloth into an empty cup.
- Thoroughly clean up the filter if used before storing it for later use.
- Drink this hot herbal tea twice daily for best results.
- Other ingredients you may want to include in your decoction are mint leaves, rosemary, or lavender.
- Also, note that Rosemary can be used instead of Chamomile for a more robust decoction.

Chicory Decoction

Method:

- Boil 1 – 2 tbsp of Chicory roots in a cup of water.
- Steep for 5-10 minutes with a lid.
- Take your hot decoction and strain it using a strainer or cheesecloth into an empty cup.
- Thoroughly clean up the filter if used before storing it for later use.
- Drink this hot herbal tea twice daily for best results.
- Other ingredients you may want to include in your decoction are mint leaves, rosemary, or lavender.

- Chicory can be used instead of Chamomile for a more robust decoction.

Ginger Decoction

Method:

- Boil 1 – 2 tbsp of Ginger in a cup of water.
- Steep for 10-15 minutes with a lid.
- Take your hot decoction and strain it using a strainer or cheesecloth into an empty cup.
- Thoroughly clean up the filter if used before storing it for later use.
- Drink this hot herbal tea twice daily for best results.
- Other ingredients you may want to include in your decoction are mint leaves, rosemary, or lavender.

Ginkgo berry Decoction

Method:

- Boil 1 – 2 tbsp of Ginkgo in a cup of water.
- Steep for 10-15 minutes with a lid.
- Take your hot decoction and strain it using a strainer or cheesecloth into an empty cup.
- Thoroughly clean up the filter if used before storing it for later use.
- Drink this hot herbal tea twice daily for best results.
- Other ingredients you may want to include in your decoction are mint leaves, rosemary, or lavender.

Ginseng Decoction

Method:

- Boil 1 – 2 tbsp of Ginseng in a cup of water.
- Cover with a lid and steep for 10-15 minutes.
- Take your hot decoction and strain it using a strainer or cheesecloth into an empty cup.
- Thoroughly clean up the filter if used before storing it for later use.
- Drink this hot herbal tea twice daily for best results.
- Other ingredients you may want to include in your decoction are mint leaves, rosemary, or lavender.

Horsetail Decoction

Method:

- Boil 1 – 2 tbsp of Horsetail in a cup of water.
- Cover with a lid and steep for 10-15 minutes.

- Take your hot decoction and strain it using a strainer or cheesecloth into an empty cup.
- Thoroughly clean up the filter if used before storing it for later use.
- Drink this hot herbal tea twice daily for best results.
- Other ingredients you may want to include in your decoction are mint leaves, rosemary, or lavender.

Irish Moss Decoction

Method:

Boil 1 – 2 tbsp of Irish moss in a cup of water.

Cover with a lid and steep for 10-15 minutes.

Take your hot decoction and strain it using a strainer or cheesecloth into an empty cup.

Thoroughly clean up the filter if used before storing it for later use.

Drink this hot herbal tea twice daily for best results.

Other ingredients you may want to include in your decoction are mint leaves, rosemary, or lavender.

Popsicles

Popsicles can be made from various sources, such as fruit juice, herbs, fruits, and vegetables. Popsicles are mainly made from fresh ingredients to provide health benefits with no preservatives or artificial flavorings.

Popsicles can be made by using fresh herbs as an ingredient in the mixture of the frozen solid state of water. Herb-infused popsicle recipes can be found online. Herb-infused popsicles usually have different flavors like mint or orange. Some other popular flavors include pineapple and strawberry, which is a combination of both lemon and orange.

The use of herbs on popsicles can provide some great benefits. Herbs have properties such as antioxidant, anti-inflammatory, antibacterial, antiviral, and analgesic effects. A mixture of herbs can provide a unique taste to your popsicles.

Ginger and mint popsicles are among the most common herb popsicles sold in grocery stores because of their refreshing taste and health benefits. Ginger is known to have properties with anti-inflammatory effects and improve digestive problems. Mint has antioxidant properties which help protect the cells from damage by free radicals. Mint also has antibacterial and anti-inflammatory properties.

Making Herb-Infused Popsicles

Herbs can be used not only to flavor our foods but also can be used in herbal medicine. Herbal medicine is a form of complementary treatment that employs herbs in combination with other drugs. In most cases, it is a form of alternative medicine that relies on the healing power of plants rather than modern medication or surgery. In this kind of therapy, modern medicine and herbs are combined to help patients improve their health and regain their wholeness from illness. Herbal medicine is also used to give the body a boost of energy and rejuvenation.

The medicinal herbs can be infused in popsicles. Preserves and herbs are used because they combine well with popsicle ingredients.

Popsicle molds can be purchased or are homemade from old molds that you can buy at craft stores. Popsicle sticks, parchment paper, and sticks can also be purchased at craft stores. Colorful popsicles may be made by adding food coloring.

Ginger Mint Popsicles

- 1 cup of coconut water or any fruit juice of your choice (if you are on a low-calorie diet, you can replace it with water)
- 2-inch ginger root, peeled, sliced into 1/4 pieces
- 4 to 6 fresh mint leaves

Process: Add freshly sliced ginger and mint leaves to the blender. Pour in the fruit juice or coconut water. Blend until smooth. Pour into popsicle molds and freeze overnight.

Cucumber and Herb Popsicles

- Juice or coconut water, 1 cup
- Two peeled and quartered cucumbers
- 2-3 sprigs of fresh mint

Process: Place the jars in the blender. Add in mint leaves and make sure that they are completely blended. Pour in fruit juice or coconut water. Blend until smooth. Pour into popsicle molds and freeze overnight.

Fruit and Herb Popsicles

- 1 cup of fruit juice or coconut water
- 2-inch piece of fresh ginger, peeled, sliced into 1/4 pieces
- 5 to 6 fresh mint leaves

Process: Place the jars in the blender. Add in mint leaves and ginger. Make sure that all the pieces are completely blended. Pour in fruit juice or coconut water. Blend until smooth. Pour into popsicle molds and freeze overnight.

Herbal Popsicles

- 1 cup of fruit juice or coconut water
- 5 to 7 fresh mint leaves

Process: Place the jars in the blender. Add mint leaves and make sure that they are completely blended. Pour in fruit juice or coconut water. Blend until smooth. Pour into popsicle molds and freeze overnight.

Cucumber and Mint Popsicles

- 1 cup of fruit juice or coconut water
- 1–a 2-inch piece of fresh ginger, peeled

- 5 to 7 mint leaves

Process: Place the jars in the blender. Add ginger and mint. Make sure that they are completely blended. Pour in fruit juice or coconut water. Blend until smooth. Pour into popsicle molds and freeze overnight.

Breast milk

Infants can also use herbal medicine if their mums have been using herbs. Breast milk contains many herbs, which are essential for the well-being of infants. Infants can be given herbal teas or capsules to help clear symptoms of colds and flu and reduce allergic reactions.

A mother and her child can both benefit from the positive effects of natural herbs. They both can avoid using pharmaceutical drugs and chemicals to treat conditions that are often caused by stress, diet, pollutants, or aging.

Another significant benefit is to insert potent herbal antibacterial medicine inside an infant to make them more immune to side effects of getting sick from antibacterial is to introduce them from the mother's breast milk. It will boost the natural immunization responses in both mother and her infant. Common herbs commonly used in the skin and associated with breast milk are alel5, oil of citronella, essential oils including lemon, lavender, and other herbs.

The advantages of using herbal infant teas made by mothers are that they are just made using natural extracts from plants.

In terms of safety, herbal infant teas are safe for both mother and the baby as long as they are made using natural and non-toxic ingredients.

Herbal infant teas can interact with other herbs or medications used by the mother. Therefore, mothers must take herbs without interactions with other medicines while breastfeeding simultaneously.

Here is a list of breast milk herbal that can be beneficial to infants:

Lemon Balm

Lemon balm has been found to help infants with colic, fussiness, and other digestive problems. Lemon balm has also been known to soothe infant fussiness and relieve cramps. Studies have shown that lemon balm can help stimulate breast milk secretion and increase nutrients in the milk of nursing mothers who take them.

Method:

- Mix 2–3 drops of lemon balm essential oil or 1/4 teaspoon of finely powdered lemon balm powder into 4 ounces of breastmilk.
- Heat the breast milk in the microwave or on the stove, whichever is most convenient.
- Baby food, please.
- Do it again every two hours as needed throughout the day.

- If the mother is breastfeeding a premature infant, she should not use this herbal remedy.

Chamomile

Chamomile is one of the most common herbs used in treating children who are suffering from colic, fever, and teething. Chamomile is also known to help reduce swelling, soothe irritable newborns, and soothe fevers. Chamomile can also be used for making herbal infant teas or tinctures.

Method:

- Add 1/4 teaspoon of finely ground Chamomile or 2 to 3 drops of Chamomile essential oil to 4 ounces of breastmilk.
- Warm the breast milk either by the microwave or on the stove.
- Serve your baby.
- Repeat every two hours during the day and as needed for relief.
- Do not use this herbal treatment if the mother is breastfeeding a preterm infant.

Calendula

Calendula is also known as marigold. Calendula can be used to make herbal teas for infants or be added to a bath in a little bit of water. Calendula has strong anti-inflammatory properties.

Method:

- Add 1/4 teaspoon of finely ground calendula or 2 to 3 drops of calendula essential oil to 4 ounces of breastmilk.
- Warm the breast milk either by the microwave or on the stove.
- Serve your baby.
- Repeat every two hours during the day and as needed for relief.
- Do not use this herbal treatment if the mother is breastfeeding a preterm infant.

Washcloths

Washcloths are used to gently clean the baby's face, lips, eyes, and genitals. They can be used in the bath area as well. They can be used on a critically ill patient who cannot survive an active bath. In this comfortable way, medicine can easily be applied to the skin, and thus it can be transferred to a deeper area of the body through diffusion. Washcloths can be warm by using hot infusions of medicine when specific heating impacts are needed, or they can be cold when benefits of cold are needed. It all depends upon personal choice as well as symptoms of illnesses. For acute injuries, for example, brushing and combat sports fights, cold washcloths with specific benefits of ice and anti-inflammatory medicine can be a smart choice to limit swelling and bruising and impede bleeding from fresh wounds. Cold also has anesthetic properties, which make it a natural painkiller.

When used warm, washcloths can stimulate blood flow due to vasodilatory effects as well as a soothing response of the body can also be obtained. Herbal washcloths can be applied to the area of an injury.

Here are different ways to make herbal washcloths to be used for different conditions:

Eyewash

Preparation:

- The eye spray bottle only needs a few drops of water added to it.
- Put peppermint oil into the remaining space in the bottle.
- To clean your eyes, use these eye drops.

This is very good for people who suffer from dry eyes, as they can treat them with one quick and simple treatment. Refrigerate in an airtight container after each use to ensure potency.

The eyewash can also be used for other purposes, such as treating conjunctivitis, blepharitis, and other eye issues.

Tongue wash

Preparation:

- Fill the tongue spray bottle with water.
- Fill the rest of the bottle with Thyme essential oil.
- Use this tongue spray to clean the area around the mouth, and in its presence, you would feel a soothing sensation on your tongue.

This is a very good treatment if your mouth is filled with bad breath and a cleansing of the inside of your mouth. After usage, keep in an airtight container for two weeks.

Tongue wash can be used on other body parts such as the inner thigh area, groin area, armpit, and any other areas that may need a light cleaning and soothing.

Armpit wash

Preparation:

- Add a few drops of water to the armpit spray bottle.
- Add Lavender essential oil to the bottle.
- Use this armpit spray to clean your armpits, and you will feel a soothing sensation on your skin.

This is very good for people who work in the construction field, as it will help remove odors from the body and develop an antibacterial treatment for skin infections. In an airtight container, it lasts two weeks.

The armpit wash can also be used on other body areas such as the groin area, inner thigh area, and back of the neck to get a good cleaning.

Inner thigh wash

Preparation:

- Fill the inner thigh spray container with water.
- Add Lavender essential oil to the bottle.
- Use this inner thigh spray to clean the area around your groin, and it will make you feel a soothing sensation.

This is very good for people who play sports, as it will help remove sweat and bacteria that may cause infections. It can create an antibacterial treatment for skin infections. After usage, keep in an airtight container for two weeks.

The inner thigh wash can be used on other areas such as the armpit, groin, inner wrist, and any other not-to-be-replaced areas.

Inner wrist wash

Preparation:

- Fill the inside wrist spray bottle with water.
- Add Lavender essential oil to the bottle.
- Use this inner wrist spray to clean the area around your hand, making you feel a soothing sensation.

This is very good for people who work in the construction field, as it will help remove odors from the body and develop an antibacterial treatment for skin infections. After usage, keep in an airtight container for two weeks.

The inner wrist wash can also be used on other body areas, such as the groin area, armpit, inner thigh area, or any other not-to-be-replaced areas.

Tinctures

Tinctures are drops of herbs in liquid form, which is usually alcohol or vinegar. These drops are directly inserted into the mouth with a dropper. Tinctures are more potent than teas, especially when extracting aromatic oils and resins from the plant and barks. Tinctures can come in liquid, tablet, caplet, capsule form as well as in liquid form.

Tinctures are very popular among people because they do not require big preparation time and provide noticeable effects within minutes after application.

Tinctures can be used to treat many symptoms of different diseases, such as indigestion, stomach aches, sugar disorders, or headaches.

Vinegar can be used to make tinctures; vinegar is an essential part of herbal medicine, and it is usually used in the process of making tinctures.

Tinctures are important at home, especially for first aid, because they contain the most potent herbs in just a few drops. Tinctures are easy to travel with because they are liquid and do not take up too much space.

Find a list of herbs below that can be used to create different tinctures for various purposes.

Indigestion Tincture

Preparation:

- Add one tablespoon of dried mint leaves to one-half cup of water in a pot.
- Bring it to a boil, turn off the stove, and let it steep and cool down for about 10 minutes.
- Line the alembic with cheesecloth, and then add mint mixture through it into your bottle of choice.
- Now, screw the cap on firmly and store it in a cool and dark place for at least 2 weeks.
- Take 2 spoonfuls of tincture into the mouth, swish it around to spread it evenly on your teeth, gums, and other parts of your mouth.
- After that, you can take more tinctures as required depending on how well you feel after the first application.
- You can also add Tincture to your food or juices.
- Unlock Bactericidal Properties

Cough and Cold Tincture

Preparation:

- Mix one tablespoon of Chamomile with one cup of water in a pot.
- Boil the mixture for about five minutes and then cover it until cooled for at least ten minutes.

- Use 2-3 drops of tincture as needed for cough or cold.

Unlock Anti-inflammatory Properties

Painkiller Tincture

Preparation:

- Mix one tablespoon of Chamomile with two cups of water in a pot.
- Boil the mixture for about five minutes and then cover it until cooled for at least ten minutes.
- Use 2-3 drops of tincture as needed for headaches, cramps, or other types of pain.

Chapter 4: Correct Use Of Herbal Antibiotics For Different Conditions (Describe Them)

In place of synthetic antibiotics, herbal antibiotics are a safe and effective solution for many medical issues. It's worth noting that while herbal antibiotics may be helpful in some cases, this doesn't mean they'll work in all. A medical expert should be consulted prior to the use of any natural antibiotics. For various ailments, the following natural antibiotics come highly recommended:

Allium sativum (garlic): Garlic has broad-spectrum antibacterial activities and is a powerful natural antibiotic. Colds, sinusitis, and bronchitis are just some of the respiratory illnesses that it can treat. It has been found that garlic can help with gastrointestinal infections such food poisoning and parasites.

Commonly used to boost the immune system, echinacea (Echinacea spp.), may be useful in warding off and treating upper respiratory tract illnesses like the common cold and flu. In addition, it can be used in combination with other treatments for UTIs.

Sinus infections, bronchitis, and traveler's diarrhea are just some of the respiratory and gastrointestinal ailments that goldenseal (Hydrastis canadensis) is used to treat. Topical use for skin infections and wounds is also possible.

Another herb with antibacterial qualities is Oregon grape (Mahonia aquifolium), which is useful for treating bacterial and fungal diseases. It is effective against infections of the urinary tract, the digestive tract, and the skin.

Olive leaf (Olea europaea) extract has been shown to be effective against bacteria, viruses, and fungi. Infections of the respiratory system, the sinuses, and the herpes simplex virus can all benefit from its use.

Andrographis paniculata, more often known as andrographis, is used to treat a variety of respiratory tract illnesses in traditional medicine. It's immunomodulatory and effective against malaria.

Oil of oregano (Origanum vulgare) includes chemicals with potent antibacterial activity, including carvacrol and thymol. It is effective against bacterial, fungal, and viral infections of the respiratory, digestive, and skin systems.

Although it does not work like an antibiotic, cranberry (Vaccinium macrocarpon) is useful for warding off and treating UTIs. It has chemicals that stop bacteria from sticking to the lining of the urinary tract, which helps avoid infections.

Keep in mind that there is some debate over the efficacy of herbal antibiotics, and that everyone's body reacts differently to them. Factors including dosage, quality of the herbal medicine, and interactions or contraindications with preexisting prescriptions or medical conditions should be taken into account. If you want to make sure you're using herbs safely and effectively, it's best to talk to a doctor or an experienced herbalist.

Chapter 5:
Herbal Antibiotics For Specific Infections And Ailments
(Recipes And Ailments)

For respiratory infections (cold, sinusitis, cough, etc.)

for urinary tract infections, skin and digestive tract infections etc.

Remedies for Common Ailments

Allergies

Mucus production, eye irritation, and a runny nose are common symptoms of allergies. Changing your diet during allergy season can also be helpful in addition to using the therapies provided. Avoiding mucus-inducing foods like milk and other dairy products may speed up the healing process.

Asthma is frequently made worse by allergies. If your asthma persists despite using these therapies, you should consult a medical professional or herbalist.

Consult a medical professional if your symptoms worsen while using medication for allergies or asthma. Consult your doctor before trying any home treatments for severe allergies. Do not substitute a herbal cure with any prescribed medications, especially steroids or inhalers.

Nettle, elderflower, and echinacea are some of the plants used to treat allergies. Nettle, chamomile, and echinacea are some of the herbs used to treat asthma.

General Asthma Remedies

Take 400-600 cc of nettle infusion daily, but for no longer than three months. Make an infusion using 20 g of dried or 30 g of fresh herbs. Warm a teapot and put them in it. Put some boiling water in a pot. After letting it steep for 10 minutes, pour some into a cup, taking care to use less than the recommended amount. Sugar or honey can be added if preferred. The extra infusion can be kept in the refrigerator for up to 24 hours.

Nettle and elderflower infusion is the second all-purpose cure.

This infusion calls for 300 ml of water to 1 tsp of dried or 2 tsp of fresh of each plant. One dose is all that is needed. Prepare the infusion by pouring boiling water over the strained herbs. Steep the mixture for 5-10 minutes with the lid on before discarding the herbs and filter. Sugar or honey can be added if preferred.Take 400-600 cc of nettle infusion daily, but for no longer than three months. Make an infusion using 20 g of dried or 30 g of fresh herbs. Warm a teapot and put them in it. Put some boiling water in a pot. After letting it steep for 10 minutes, pour some into a cup, taking care to use less than the recommended amount. Sugar or honey can be added if preferred. The extra infusion can be kept in the refrigerator for up to 24 hours.

Nettle and elderflower infusion is the second all-purpose cure.

This infusion calls for 300 ml of water to 1 tsp of dried or 2 tsp of fresh of each plant. One dose is all that is needed. Prepare the infusion by pouring boiling water over the strained herbs.

Steep the mixture for 5-10 minutes with the lid on before discarding the herbs and filter. Sugar or honey can be added if preferred.

Hay Fever

Prepare 300–450 ml of elderflower infusion daily. To reduce allergy symptoms, consume the infusion daily for a few months leading up to allergy season. Make an infusion using 20 g of dried or 30 g of fresh herbs. Warm a teapot and put them in it. Put some boiling water in a pot. Ten minutes of infusion time is required before dosage. If you need to, you can sweeten it with honey or another sweetener. The extra infusion can be kept in the refrigerator for up to 24 hours.

Wheezing

Infuse some thyme and nettle leaves together. The infusion calls for 15 g of each plant per pot. Throw them into a teapot of hot water. Boil 710 ml (about 2 cups) of water and add it to the pan. Infuse for 10 minutes. Take sips of it all day long. If more sweetness is desired, feel free to add honey.

The second remedy is a German chamomile infusion. To prepare the infusion, use 2 heaping tsp of chamomile to 150 ml of water. One single dosage is contained herein. Put the herbs in a sieve and pour boiling water over them to make an infusion, much like you would with tea. Put a lid on it and let it steep for ten minutes. Before discarding the herbs and strainer, take a deep breath of the steam. Take the infusion, and if you must, sweeten it with honey or something else.

Asthma for Infections

Several variations of this treatment are available. Echinacea is available in both pill and tincture form. Put around 500 milligrams of echinacea powder into a capsule shell. Just three times a day, take one capsule.

The same quantity of powder can also be used to flavor food or drink. Half a teaspoon of 1:5 tinctures should be taken with water twice daily.

Ear, Nose, and Throat

Chest infection/bronchitis

Mucus can be effectively treated with eucalyptus leaves. In addition to relieving various respiratory issues, it has antiseptic properties. The root elecampane has been found to be effective for treating a wide variety of chest conditions.

Do not take elecampane if you are pregnant or nursing. Children and newborns are also not recommended to be given eucalyptus.

Thyme infusion is the first treatment option. You can have as much as 750 ml per day, but three servings of 100 ml each is a decent starting point. Make an infusion using 20 g of dried or 30 g of fresh herbs. Warm a teapot and put them in it. Put some boiling water in a pot. Let it steep for 10 minutes before pouring it into a cup, but don't drink more than one cup. If you'd like, you can add sugar to the infusion.

A decoction of elecampane is useful for treating coughs and bronchitis. For severe coughs and bronchitis, try mixing in 5 grams of eucalyptus leaf and 5 grams of licorice powder. Consume daily doses of around 300 ml of the decoction. Make a decoction by combining 20 grams of elecampane root with 750 milliliters of water in a saucepan (or 15 grams of elecampane with 5 grams of eucalyptus for acute coughs). To prepare, bring to boiling, then simmer for 20-30 minutes. We need to get it down to a mere 500 mL of liquid. Remove the herbs and strain the mixture through a fine mesh sieve. Any remaining decoction can be stored for up to 48 hours in the fridge.

Do not take this medication if you are expecting a child.

You can make a soothing chest rub by combining 2 tablespoons of olive oil with 5 drops each of thyme and eucalyptus essential oils. Apply to your upper body as often as twice a day. Don't use it if you're expecting, and never put it in your mouth.

Fever

You can make an infusion of yarrow and elderberry; Pregnancy contraindicates the use of this treatment. Half a teaspoon of yarrow and half a teaspoon of elderberry per 100 ml of water will provide the infusion. One single dosage is contained herein. Put the herbs in a sieve and pour boiling water over them to make an infusion, much like you would with tea. Put a lid on it and let the herbs steep for 10 minutes before you remove them and the strainer. Honey or another sweetener can be used if necessary. Every day, you're allowed to drink up to 600 cc of water.

If you don't have access to a doctor, try baking a full onion at 400 degrees for 40 minutes as a home treatment. Combine equal parts onion juice and honey. The treatment can be taken every hour in increments of one or two teaspoons, but no more than eight times daily.

A chilly bath can help bring down a fever without the use of herbs.

A combination of yarrow, boneset, and cayenne can be used to treat a high fever.

The boneset herb is new to this publication. For this treatment, you'll need to make advantage of the plant's aerial components. If you are expecting a child, you should not use this treatment. 1 teaspoon of dried boneset, 1 teaspoon of dried yarrow, and a pinch of cayenne pepper should be added to 150 milliliters of water to make the infusion. One single dosage is contained herein. Put the herbs in a sieve and pour boiling water over them to make an infusion, much like you would with tea. Put a lid on it and let the herbs steep for five minutes before you strain them out. If you want more taste, feel free to add honey, ginger, or cinnamon.

The maximum daily dose of the infusion is 600 ml.

Congestion and sinusitis

Inhaling the steam from infusions or essential oils is a proven method for relieving congestion.

Inhaling the steam from an infusion is the first line of defense. The infusion can be made using 15 g of dry herbs and 750 ml of water. Prepare the infusion by pouring boiling water over the strained herbs. Steep the mixture for 5-10 minutes with the lid on before discarding the herbs and filter. Then, take a 10-minute steam bath.

German chamomile can be used instead by following the same procedures. In place of the herbs, you can use 5–10 drops of eucalyptus or chamomile essential oil and continue with the rest of the steps outlined above.

Sore Throat and Laryngitis

A sore throat can be alleviated by any of these treatments, and laryngitis, too. Gargling with warm water and salt might also help with laryngitis symptoms.

Gargling with 20 cc of lemon juice can help alleviate a sore throat. You can weaken it with water and honey if it's too potent. Another option is to gargle with a mixture of 5 teaspoons of lemon juice and a pinch of cayenne pepper powder.

Making a sage infusion is another option. If you are expecting a child, do not use this medicine. One teaspoon of dried herb or two teaspoons of fresh herb per 250 ml of water is all that's needed to make the infusion. One single dosage is contained herein. Put the herbs in a sieve and pour boiling water over them to make an infusion, much like you would with tea. Put a lid on it and let the herbs steep for 10 minutes before you remove them and the strainer. Gargle and drink the infusion once it has cooled enough that it won't burn your throat. Add 5 cc of vinegar and honey to boost its efficacy.

Garlic, ginger, and lemon juice are another option. A garlic clove needs to be crushed to extract the juice. Hold off for ten minutes. The crushed garlic and fresh ginger should be combined with 1 lemon's juice and 150 ml of warm water. Consume as much as 450 ml daily. You can also use this cure to treat a cold.

Echinacea root decoction gargled as a treatment is another option. Twenty grams of dried root and seven hundred and fifty milliliters of water will make a decoction.

To prepare, bring to boiling, then simmer for 20-30 minutes. We need to get it down to a mere 500 mL of liquid. After straining the mixture, save the liquid and toss the roots. Any remaining decoction can be stored for up to 48 hours in the fridge. Use a daily gargling routine of 3.5 tbsp.

Chapter 6:
Using Herbal Antibiotics, Drug Interactions And Precautions To Take

Herbal antibiotics are non-chemical treatments said to be effective against germs. Although they have their uses, they should be used with caution because they might cause drug interactions and other problems. Here are a few things to keep in mind about herbal antibiotics, potential drug interactions, and safety measures:

Always seek the advice of a skilled healthcare expert, such as a naturopathic physician or integrative medicine practitioner, before starting treatment with any herbal antibiotics. They will be able to provide you advice tailored to your own health situation, current medications, and possible drug interactions.

It is essential to do research and select trustworthy sources when making decisions about the use of herbal antibiotics. You should research the medicines' efficacy, safety, and any interactions by consulting scientific studies, reviews, and reputable resources.

Keep in mind that several medications, including prescription drugs, over-the-counter treatments, and even other herbal supplements, may interact negatively with herbal antibiotics. They might alter the way these drugs are metabolized, absorbed, or even how well they work. St. John's Wort, garlic, ginkgo biloba, and echinacea are just a few of the common plants that are known to interact. Never take a herbal antibiotic without first discussing it with your healthcare physician.

Antibiotic resistance should be taken into account because it is becoming an increasingly serious problem around the world. Herbal antibiotics may seem like a healthy choice, but they can actually promote antibiotic resistance if they are misused. Avoid using natural antibiotics for longer than required and stick to the stated dosages and times.

Herbal medicines, like conventional antibiotics, may cause adverse effects including allergies. These may change with the type of herb utilized. Typical adverse reactions consist of stomach pain, itching, and hives. If you have any negative reactions, you should stop using it and see a doctor.

Women who are pregnant or nursing should avoid using natural antibiotics unless absolutely necessary. It's possible that the mother or the baby could be harmed by using certain herbs while pregnant or breastfeeding. Herbal therapies should never be used during these times without first consulting a medical practitioner.

Standardization Herbal product quality control and standardization varies greatly. Try to find brands that produce items in accordance with good manufacturing practices (GMP) and have them independently tested. This can help guarantee that the herbal antibiotics you use are effective and safe.

Always consult with your doctor before using any herbal antibiotics to treat a serious infection or condition. It is important to collaborate with a healthcare expert to determine the most appropriate and effective treatment strategy, however they may play a role as supplementary or supporting therapies.

Conclusions:

Overview of Natural Herbal Antibiotics, exploring the most common herbs with antibiotic properties, methods of preparation and usage, as well as tips for applying herbal antibiotics for specific infections and ailments.

BOOK 12:
THE ESSENTIAL OILS

Introduction

Many people wish to use natural remedies in place of the chemical-ridden over-the-counter medications. Though it can be difficult to find useful information on essential oils, this guide hopes to add a little help when it comes to using them for ailments such as headaches. You will learn what types of oils are used for headaches and how many drops you should apply for each ailment.

Native American essential oils have been consumed throughout history, and native peoples have used these plants since before Columbus arrived in America. Native Americans have been known to use these oils for various reasons, from pain relief to energy. Many methods are used to produce essential oils, including distilling, extracting and cold pressing.

The plant matter is usually either dried or partially dried to make it easier to digest or absorb into your body. Everyone's body interacts differently with these oils, so the amount you consume will depend on your body chemistry.

Chapter 1:
Essential Oils As Natural Remedies, Description

The Impact of Essential Oils on the Body

Essential oils from plants have been used for centuries by Native American herbalists. Pure essential oils are used by some Native American herbalists, while others take a more holistic approach and create their own formulae by combining different herbs with other natural components like plants, flowers, roots, stones, and water. Herbal and natural ingredient combinations might vary, with the idea being that each contributes something unique to the blend's therapeutic effects. These combinations are growing in popularity since they not only aid in healing the body but also fuel it with antioxidants, leading to increased energy and general well-being.

Among Native American herbalists, "fresh feet" is a popular mix. This mixture's history is shrouded in mystery, although it has been employed by Native American herbalists and healers for centuries. Colds, the flu, sore throats, infections, and other attacks produced by germs or toxins in the body are all treatable with a pair of clean feet. Nasal congestion caused by infections can be alleviated by inhaling the vapor into the upper respiratory system. Coughing due to asthma and other lung problems can also be alleviated, as can bronchitis brought on by temporomandibular joint dysfunction. It also soothes sunburns, rashes, and burns caused by insects.

Put some eucalyptus oil, some pine oil, and some peppermint oil into a small basin and use that to prepare clean feet. Sinus congestion can be alleviated by placing a cloth over the head and around the neck and inhaling the fumes of this mixture. The effectiveness of inhalation treatments can be further increased by adding a few drops of this mixture to an aroma diffuser.

Advantages of Essential Oils and Aromatherapy

Since ancient times, Native American herbalists have relied on plant oils for medicinal purposes. While some Native American herbalists employ only pure essential oils, others adopt a more holistic approach, creating their own formulae by mixing together a wide variety of herbs with other natural components like plants, flowers, roots, stones, and water. Different combinations of herbs and natural components can be used to boost the therapeutic effects of the whole. Such concoctions are becoming increasingly popular in the twenty-first century due to their ability to restore health and energy by feeding the body with antioxidants.

The term "fresh feet" refers to a mixture utilized by numerous Native American herbalists. No one knows for sure where this mixture came from, but Native American herbalists and healers have relied on it for centuries. Colds, the flu, sore throats, infections, and other attacks caused by germs or poisons can all be remedied by soaking one's feet in a bucket of cool water. Inhaling the vapor into the upper respiratory system can help clear congested sinuses caused by illnesses. Asthma-related cough and bronchitis are two more respiratory disorders that this treatment can ease. It's great for soothing bug bites, burns, rashes, and sunburns, too.

Essential oils like eucalyptus, pine, and peppermint, mixed in equal parts, can be used to prepare clean feet. To alleviate sinus pressure, drape a cloth over your head and around your neck and inhale the fumes from this mixture. You can also increase the efficacy of inhalation treatments by adding a few drops of this blend to an aroma diffuser.

Safety and precautions when using essential oils

1. Because of their potency, essential oils should never be applied directly to the skin without first being diluted. Essential oils are highly concentrated and should be diluted before being applied externally. Standard adult dilution is 2-3 drops of essential oil per teaspoon (5 ml) of carrier oil. When applying to children or people with sensitive skin, a lower dilution ratio is suggested.
2. A skin test should be done before applying an essential oil topically. Apply a little amount of the diluted oil to a test area of skin (such as the inner forearm) and wait 24 hours to see if any adverse reactions develop, such as redness, itching, or swelling.
3. Essential oils should be kept away from the eyes, ears, and other mucous membranes. In the event of accidental contact, the afflicted area should be flushed with a carrier oil or water and, if necessary, medical help should be sought.
4. It is not advised to use essential oils while pregnant or nursing because of the potential danger they provide to the developing fetus or infant. Essential oils are not recommended during pregnancy or when nursing.
5. Be careful when handling essential oils if you know you have an allergy to any of the plants or scents they come from. You might consult a dermatologist or an allergist, or you could do a patch test.
6. Essential oils should be stored in a cool, dark place away from direct sunlight. Keep them away from kids and pets in case of accidental intake. Because of their potency, essential oils should never be applied to the skin, and users should always thoroughly wash their hands after handling them.
7. Be sure to only purchase from reputable brands that provide information about the origin, safety, and purity of their essential oils if these factors are important to you. Look for oils labeled as "100% pure" or "therapeutic grade." Oils that have been diluted or are of poor quality could be harmful to your health.
8. It's possible that certain essential oils could have an adverse reaction with a preexisting condition or medication. Essential oils can have a broad variety of impacts; if you have any preexisting health conditions or use any

medications, you should talk to your doctor before using them.

9. Essential oils should be used sparingly and in accordance with the recommended dosage. Essential oils are potent, but remember that more isn't necessarily better because there are potential risks associated with using too much of them.
10. Using an aromatherapy diffuser? Get lots of air circulation going in there. Long or repeated exposure to the fumes of highly concentrated essential oils can irritate the respiratory systems of some persons.

Chapter 2: Most Popular Essential Oils

Popular essential oils

Lavender oil is well-known for its calming and soothing properties, making it one of the most popular essential oils. Its relaxing, floral aroma is often used to assist individuals de-stress, wind down, and fall asleep. Lavender oil's effectiveness in relieving headaches and boosting mental health goes beyond its conventional applications.

Tea tree oil, sometimes called melaleuca oil, is a powerful essential oil with a fresh, medicinal aroma. Its antimicrobial properties have made it highly sought after for centuries. When applied topically, tea tree oil can help with a wide variety of skin issues, including acne, wounds, and infections. Its antiseptic qualities also make it a good addition to all-natural cleaning products.

The oil of the peppermint plant has a strong, refreshingly minty aroma. Its rejuvenating and invigorating effects make it a popular choice. Peppermint oil's soothing properties extend beyond its use as a headache remedy and cognitive enhancer. It also aids in digestion and removes odors from the mouth.

The eucalyptus leaf oil smells similar to camphor but is much stronger and more refreshing. Its useful effects on the respiratory system mean it is frequently used in products like chest rubs and inhalers. Eucalyptus oil's anticongestive, expectorant, and sedative properties make it a useful treatment for respiratory illnesses including the common cold.

Lemon oil, made from the rinds of lemons, has a zesty, uplifting aroma. It's well-known for restoring energy and lifting spirits. Lemon oil has been shown to improve mood, concentration, and nerves. It is also commonly used to clean the air because of its lovely scent.

Because of its comforting, woodsy scent, frankincense has been used for religious and spiritual purposes for centuries. It's believed to have relaxing and calming effects on the body and mind. The anti-inflammatory, meditative, and focus-increasing properties of frankincense oil extend beyond its cosmetic uses.

Essential oils have a wide range of applications, but they require careful handling to prevent adverse reactions. Essential oils are highly concentrated, thus it is recommended to dilute them before using them topically and to conduct a patch test to ensure there will be no negative reactions. If you have any health concerns, are pregnant, or planning to become pregnant, it is best to talk to a qualified aromatherapist or doctor.

Therapeutic properties and uses of each oil

Effective combinations of oils for specific purposes

Lavender Oil:

Therapeutic benefits include sedative and relaxing effects.

Its many applications range from facilitating sleep and relaxation to calming nerves and relieving tension and pain.

Peppermint Oil:

Properties used in treatment: cooling, stimulating, and restorative.

Benefits include alleviation of headaches and migraines, enhanced focus and mental acuity, relief from digestive distress, and relief from muscle aches and pains.

Eucalyptus Oil:

Antiseptic, expectorant, and decongestant are some of the therapeutic properties.

Benefits include easing symptoms of a cold or cough, protecting against bug bites, increasing concentration, and fostering overall well-being.

Tea Tree Oil:

Antimicrobial, antifungal, and antiseptic therapeutic properties.

Acne, skin infections, itching, irritation, healing of cuts and wounds, prevention of fungal infections (such as athlete's foot), and usage as a natural household cleaner are all possible benefits.

Chamomile Oil:

Properties used for therapy include being calming, relaxing, and anti-inflammatory.

Benefits include easing anxiety and tension, easing skin diseases like eczema and dermatitis, and alleviating stomach aches and cramps.

Lemon Oil:

Possesses recuperative qualities, including stimulating and purifying effects.

Benefits include an uplifted disposition and sharpened focus, a strengthened immune system, improved digestion, and the ability to be included into all-natural household cleaners.

Effective combinations of oils for specific purposes:

- Relaxation: Lavender, Chamomile, and Bergamot.
- Respiratory Support: Eucalyptus, Peppermint, and Tea Tree.
- Pain Relief: Peppermint, Lavender, and Marjoram.
- Focus and Concentration: Rosemary, Peppermint, and Lemon.
- Skin Care: Tea Tree, Lavender, and Frankincense.

Essential oils are extremely potent, so please exercise caution when using them. They should be diluted before usage, and a patch test should be done to check for sensitivities or reactions. You should also talk to an aromatherapist or doctor if you have any preexisting diseases or serious health issues before utilizing essential oils.

Chapter 3:
Using Essential Oils

How to Use Essential Oils

1. Air Freshener Spray

There are so many options for house fragrances now that it might be overwhelming. The market offers a wide variety of products to eliminate unpleasant odors from a space, including sprays, oils, plug-ins, and incense. The problem is that many of these items include chemicals and pollutants that are detrimental to human health. Essential oils are very concentrated, so only a few drops can fill your room with a pleasant aroma. All you need is an empty spray bottle, some water, your preferred essential oil, and a splash of pure alcohol like vodka to make your own air freshener spray. Sprays containing essential oils like lavender, lemon, lime, rosemary, clary sage, clove, and orange are very popular.

2. Bath Salts

You have probably heard of the soothing effects of a A soak in a tub filled with lavender or peppermint essential oils. After a long day, soaking in one of these baths is the perfect way to unwind and restore your body and mind. A bacterial infection can also be treated with one of these baths. Since oil and water do not mix, using essential oils in a bath probably won't do you much good. Actually, it might cause very serious skin irritation or even burns. It may not effectively combine with water, but you can reduce the risk of discomfort by first mixing it with a carrier oil. The best way to ensure that the essential oil you use in your bath diffuses evenly and completely throughout the water is to combine it with some bath salts.

Infuse your preferred bath salts with 10–20 drops of oil, such as lavender or rosemary, before using them. Dead sea salt, Epsom salt, and regular sea salt are the three most popular choices for combining oils with bath salts.

3. Candles

Scented candles are sometimes burned for aromatherapy purposes, such as enhancing mood and relieving stress, or to get rid of unpleasant scents in the room. It's simple and cheap to make your own candles. These fragrant candles can also serve as thoughtful presents for friends and family. Pick the right essential oil for your needs based on your intended outcome. For more information on how to put various oils to use, read the preceding chapter.

You can experiment with other proportions, but the standard recommendation is one ounce of oil per one pound of wax. It's worth noting that since burning candles exposes the oils directly to heat, the oils may be destroyed, leaving you with little or no aroma. You might try using candles to spread pleasant aromas about the house, despite the fact that this is not the best method for doing so.

4. Gel Sprays

Essential oils can provide a natural and cost-effective hair maintenance technique for dreadlocks. Essential oils like tea tree oil, lavender oil, rosemary oil, and peppermint oil are combined with a base like Aloe Vera gel to create the most popular modern mixtures for gel sprays. When it comes to treating or alleviating the following conditions, organic Aloe Vera is by far superior to its synthetic cousin.

- Burns
- Fungus
- Scalp itchiness
- Eczema
- As a hand sanitizer

Besides Aloe Vera, other bases used for making a DIY gel spray include: rich creams, lotions and heavy butters.

5. Humidifier

Aromatherapy is the practice of employing essential oils in a diffuser to treat mental and physical illness, improve air quality, and achieve emotional harmony. The essential oil's potency is preserved since most diffusers use cold air to disperse the oil's particles. However, humidifiers use warm air, which might degrade the oil's particle structure and render it ineffective. Humidifiers run nonstop, so your body never gets a chance to take in the oil mist. Essential oils with a high citral content, for example, have been shown to degrade plastics and could eventually ruin your humidifier. Because of these factors, essential oil humidifiers are not always the best choice.

6. Massage Oils

An individual's sense of well-being and capacity to deal with life are both improved by the extraordinary harmony provided by aromatherapy massage. Essential oils and carrier oils can be used to create a wide variety of massage oils. There must be a million different ways to make aromatherapy massage oils. If smell is a major factor in your purchasing decision, it is recommended that you test out various essential oil and carrier oil scents before committing to one. It's best to take it slow while blending oils and sniff the finished product as you go. It will be easier to reproduce the results if you write down the amounts or ratios you used. Sweet almond oil, cold-pressed coconut oil, grapeseed oil, jojoba oil, and olive oil are some of the most common carrier oils used in aromatherapy massage oils.

Easy DIY Diffuser Blends You Can Make Yourself

Diffusing a single oil is fine, but are there any others that would be preferable? Using a diffuser to spread a variety of oil scents! Some well-liked combinations for a diffuser are as follows:

Rejuvenating Freshness

Enter the summer with a smell that stimulates your entire brain. Your heart will be filled with love and tranquility after drinking this. Mix 3 drops of lavender oil, 2 drops of lemon oil, 2 drops of grapefruit oil, and 2 drops of spearmint oil in a diffuser.

Dissolve the Stench

Sports uniforms, pets, and the garbage can all contribute to the unpleasant smells in the home. Two drops each of lemon and tea tree oils, together with identical amounts of lime and cilantro oils, can work wonders throughout the house.

Is It Allergy Season Again? No Problem

Both summer and winter allergy seasons can be extremely unpleasant. Allergies can be reduced or avoided altogether with the help of the right combination of essential oils. Diffuse a combination of lemon oil, lavender oil, and peppermint oil (three drops each) to alleviate allergy symptoms.

Eliminate the Bugs

Pests such as cockroaches, mosquitoes, ants, and houseflies can be a tremendous pain at home. Typical bug hiding areas include the aforementioned shadows, crevices, trash cans, and sink bases. One drop each of lemongrass oil, basil oil, thyme oil, and eucalyptus oil makes a great diffuser blend for this.

Essential Oil Blending: A Guide

Essential oil blending can be a very peaceful experience if you know what you're doing, or it might give you a headache if you don't. Here, you'll get the lowdown on mixing and matching various essential oils with ease.

Essential Oils: Where to Keep Them

Essential oils should be kept in a cool, dry, dark place because they can become hazardous if exposed to moisture. However, keep in mind that you shouldn't take the advice to the letter. There is a higher concentration of bacteria in this region since the illumination is different from the main room. Instead, essential oils should be stored in a dark, cold place that is shielded from light.

How to Select Essential Oils

Hundreds of different essential oils exist today. Pick those that appeal to you most or that can help you overcome a health issue. You should always have some on hand for regular use, and some reserved for times when you're feeling under the weather. Essential oils are sold in many different retail settings, including health food stores, aromatherapy shops, and even internet pharmacies.

Check the aroma first; a powerful mixture can be exactly what you need. Inquire as to whether or not it contains any synthetic substances, such as petroleum, which may be absorbed by the skin and lead to irritation or other issues before making a purchase.

How to Mix Essential Oils

You should know a few things before you start mixing essential oils. To begin, you need know that pure essential oils should never be applied directly to the skin or used inside. Always dilute with a carrier oil or blend.

Jojoba, olive, peanut, sesame, and avocado oils are all examples of carrier oils. It is usually dependent on the chemical composition and percentages of each ingredient within the blend as to whether or not essential oils can be blended directly with others without dilution.

However, some essential oils cannot be absorbed by the skin unless they are combined with a carrier oil. For instance, when applied undiluted to the skin, lavender can be irritating because it is a skin sensitizer.

Because of this, you should first combine a dilution of 1 part oil to 5 parts carrier oil. A pestle and mortar, or even an empty eggshell, will do the trick, but be warned that it will take more work. You can also use an electric mixer to combine oils. Before blending, swirl the oils into the water base to fully incorporate.

The potency of essential oils can vary widely. Less than 2 percent of the phenols that give an essential oil its unique character can be found in modern essential oil brands. Because of this, some experts advise watering down essential oils before blending them. If you've never mixed your own concoctions before, it's smart to ease into the process by using a small dilution and gradually increasing it.

How to Apply Essential Oils

Only under medical supervision may diluted mixes be applied gently to the skin or consumed orally. Read and adhere to the bottle's directions carefully.

Not all essential oils can handle high temperatures. Applying peppermint oil to the chest and neck might help relieve a cold, but doing so in direct sunlight can cause irritation. Even in the heat of summer, a freshly mixed blend will keep well if kept in a cool, dark spot until usage.

How, therefore, do essential oils bring about all of these advantages?

How Essential Oils Work to Promote Health

Essential oils primarily exert their effects by stimulating the limbic system of the brain via olfactory receptors in the nose. Because of the limbic system's central role in controlling our emotions, being exposed to certain scents can trigger a range of physiological responses. The olfactory receptors in the body are directly affected by the actions of essential oils, which can either stimulate them or inhibit them.

So, how can we choose the right oil?

Essential oils are most commonly associated with their health benefits due to their aroma. Because almost all of us have developed a strong sense of smell for foods and spices, most of us can tell within seconds if an oil has a particular aroma. This is because our bodies react differently to various aromas, which in turn can cause a wide range of health problems. Many people, for instance, experience a surge of adrenaline when they smell cinnamon, which means that it can enhance their focus and concentration. This causes our adrenal glands to secrete hormones that boost blood pressure and heart rate. Because of the potential for this to raise blood pressure, anxious people should exercise caution when taking cinnamon to treat hypertension or sleeplessness.

Chapter 4:
Essential Oils For Specific Needs

Essential oils for stress and anxiety relief (recipes and explanations)

Essential oils have been used for centuries to promote relaxation, reduce stress, and alleviate anxiety. Here are a few recipes and explanations for essential oils commonly used for stress and anxiety relief:

Lavender Relaxation Blend:

- Essential oil of lavender, three drops
- Add 2 drops of chamomile oil.
- Essential oil of bergamot, 2 drops

Lavender is renowned for its calming properties and can help reduce nervous tension. Chamomile has a soothing effect on the mind and body, while bergamot has mood-lifting qualities.

Citrus Uplifting Blend:

- Essential oil of sweet orange, 3 drops
- Essential oil of lemon, 2 drops
- Two drops of pure grapefruit oil

Citrus oils are known for their uplifting and energizing effects. They can help boost mood, reduce stress, and create a sense of well-being.

Calming Woodsy Blend:

- Essential oil of cedar, 3 drops
- Two drops of pure vetiver oil
- Two drops of pure frankincense oil

Cedarwood has a grounding effect, promoting a sense of stability and calmness. Vetiver is deeply relaxing and helps quiet an overactive mind. Frankincense has been used for centuries to induce feelings of peace and tranquility.

Floral Serenity Blend:

- Essential oil of ylang-ylang, three drops
- Essential oil of geranium, 2 drops
- Two drops of pure clary sage oil

Ylang-ylang is known for its soothing and sedative properties, helping to ease anxiety. Geranium promotes emotional balance and relaxation, while clary sage can help relieve nervous tension and stress.

When using essential oils for stress and anxiety relief, you can try the following methods:

Diffusion: Add the recommended number of drops to a water-filled diffuser and enjoy the aroma throughout the room.

Just place a few drops on some tissue or a cotton ball and breathe it in.

Spend 15 to 20 minutes soaking in a warm bath with 5 to 10 drops of the mixture.

Dilute the mixture with a carrier oil and use it for a relaxing massage (such coconut or jojoba oil).

Essential oils can have varying effects on various people. It is recommended to perform a patch test and see a medical professional if you have any known allergies or sensitivities before using essential oils for the treatment of stress and anxiety.

Essential oils for natural cleaning and disinfection

Tea tree oil is a powerful natural disinfectant due to its potent antibacterial characteristics. It's effective against microbes like bacteria, viruses, and fungi. Put some in a spray bottle of water and use it to disinfect the kitchen counter, the bathroom sink, and other surfaces that bacteria like to hang out on.

Oil from lemons has a pleasant citrus aroma and is used for its antibacterial and grease-cutting abilities. It's useful for cleaning a wide variety of surfaces free of grease, filth, and stains. Make an all-purpose cleaner by adding a few drops of lemon oil to a solution of water and vinegar.

Antibacterial and antiviral capabilities are just two of the many benefits of eucalyptus oil, which also has a pleasant scent. It has dual use as a disinfectant and an insect repellant. To make a cleaning spray, combine a few drops of eucalyptus oil with a gallon of water in a spray container.

Oil of lavender has an uplifting aroma and some minor antibacterial benefits. It may not be as effective as other oils for disinfecting, but it can give your house a nice scent while you clean. A few drops can be added to your own homemade detergent or fabric softener.

Peppermint oil provides an energizing and refreshing aroma and is antibacterial. It can be combined with other ingredients to make an all-purpose cleaner, or used alone as a natural carpet deodorizer. Its aroma has also been shown to discourage insects.

Oil from the thyme plant contains potent antibacterial qualities that aid in the destruction of microorganisms. It kills bacteria and fungi like no other. You may make a powerful disinfectant spray by combining a few drops with water and vinegar.

Always test a tiny inconspicuous area as a patch before using essential oils undiluted for cleaning or disinfecting sensitive surfaces. Essential oils should be kept in a cool, dark place, out of the reach of heat and light.

Essential Oils for Pain and Inflammation Relief

Essential oils have been used as a natural treatment for various ailments, ranging from headaches to muscle aches, for millennia. Essential oils have their uses, but they shouldn't replace your doctor or traditional treatment. If your pain is persistent or severe, you should see a doctor. However, the following essential oils have been shown to reduce swelling and pain:

The menthol in peppermint oil gives it analgesic and cooling properties. When used topically, it helps soothe sore muscles and joints by reducing inflammation and pain. When massaged into the skin after being diluted with a carrier oil (such as coconut or almond oil), peppermint oil can provide a cooling and refreshing effect.

In addition to its calming and relaxing benefits, lavender oil has been demonstrated to reduce pain. This could help alleviate symptoms of fatigue, muscle tension, and headaches. Applying diluted lavender oil to the temples, neck, or wherever pain is felt will help.

Eucalyptus oil is an efficient pain treatment due to its anti-inflammatory and analgesic properties. The pain of arthritis and sore muscles are two of the most common reasons for using it. Eucalyptus oil, diluted with a carrier oil, can be massaged into the skin.

Due to its anti-inflammatory and analgesic properties, rosemary oil is effective in relieving the pain associated with arthritic conditions and muscle strains. It is suggested that diluted rosemary oil be used topically.

Chamomile oil's anti-inflammatory properties could make it useful for treating pain and swelling. Particularly effective in soothing sore muscles and joints by lowering inflammation. Dilute chamomile oil with a carrier oil before using it on your skin.

Always perform a skin test before using an essential oil for the first time on your skin to be sure there are no adverse reactions. Those who are expecting a child, breastfeeding a child, or who have preexisting health conditions should see a medical professional before using essential oils.

Chapter 5:
Tools For Working With Essential Oils

Essential tools and materials

Oils of a purely aromatic nature: Get your oils from trusted vendors to ensure the best quality. Make sure they aren't watered down with anything else.

Amber or cobalt blue glass bottles or containers are perfect for storing essential oils. These canisters shield the oils from light, extending their shelf life.

Essential oils should be diluted with a carrier oil before being applied topically. Oils like sweet almond, coconut, jojoba, and grapeseed are all examples of carrier oils.

Pipettes and droppers are useful for precisely dosing out essential oils. Some essential oils might cause plastic to react, thus using a glass pipette or dropper is recommended.

Diffusers and inhalers are used to spread essential oils into the air, releasing their pleasant aroma. While diffusers may be found in many homes and offices, inhalers are more compact and can be carried in a pocket or handbag.

Spray bottles: Spray bottles are great for making homemade cleaning solutions with essential oils, as well as for generating room sprays and linen sprays. If you want the greatest results, use spray bottles made of glass or PET plastic.

Use labels and marker markers to clearly identify the contents of each bottle and blend. Label everything with a permanent marker or an oil-resistant label.

To prevent oil contamination, use separate mixing bowls and stirrers (preferably made of glass or stainless steel) when preparing your own mixes or recipes.

Case or box for storing essential oils to keep them safe and secure. To avoid the annoying clinking of bottles, search for a solution that includes dividers or separate slots.

In order to learn about various oils, their qualities, safety rules, and suggested dilution ratios, it is helpful to have a credible book, internet resource, or essential oil reference guide on hand.

When working with higher volumes of essential oils, it is important to take precautions by using safety equipment such as gloves, safety goggles, and a face mask.

How to store and organize essential oils and supplies.

Select a cool, dark, and dry environment to store essential oils to protect them from deterioration caused by heat, light, and moisture. Look for a box, a shelf, or a drawer that fits all these requirements.

Essential oils degrade when exposed to light, so store them in dark glass containers. Keep your oils out of direct sunlight by storing them in amber or cobalt blue glass containers. Essential oils can destroy some forms of plastic, so it's best to store them in glass or metal.

Make sure the bottles are properly labeled so that you can always tell which oils are which. Mark the oil with its name, botanical name, purchase date, and other information using waterproof labels or adhesive tape. The oil you need will be easy to find and mistakes will be minimized.

Classify oils as follows: Sort your essential oils into different bins, such as those for citrus, flowers, woods, etc. This categorization can aid in the speedy discovery of oils that meet specific needs.

Think about getting a box or container to store your oils and accessories in. This can help you maintain order in your collection. In order to keep bottles from rolling around inside the container and breaking, many of them incorporate slots or dividers.

Keep your carrier oils and other materials in different places: Separate from your essential oils should be your carrier oils, such as jojoba or sweet almond oil, and other equipment including droppers, pipettes, and blending tools. These items can be stored and quickly retrieved in a separate container or drawer.

Put commonly used items, such as empty bottles, droppers, and pipettes, in close proximity to your essential oils. This lessens the likelihood of losing or misplacing them and increases the likelihood that you will have easy access to them when you need them.

Keep an inventory: It can be good to keep track of your essential oils and other supplies. Write down the information of your purchase, such as the quantity and date. This way, you can keep tabs on your stock, reorder when necessary, and save money.

Obey all precautionary measures: Take all necessary precautions when keeping essential oils. Some oils are combustible, so keep them far from any flames or other sources of heat. Also, keep oils away from kids and pets to avoid any potential for spills or ingestion.

Chapter 6:
DIY Essential Oil Blends

Create your own blends of essential oils (recipes, descriptions, etc.)

Energizing Citrus Blend:

- Essential oil of grapefruit, 5 drops
- Add 3 drops of pure lemon oil
- Essential oil of peppermint, 2 drops

Description: This blend combines the refreshing and uplifting properties of citrus oils with the invigorating scent of peppermint. It helps to enhance focus, boost energy levels, and promote mental clarity.

Relaxing Lavender Chamomile Blend:

- Lavender oil, around 4 drops' worth
- Four drops of pure Roman chamomile oil
- Two drops of pure Bergamot oil

Description: This soothing blend combines the calming and sedative effects of lavender and chamomile with the uplifting and citrusy aroma of bergamot. It promotes relaxation, relieves stress and anxiety, and encourages restful sleep.

Purifying Tea Tree Blend:

- Essential oil of Tea Tree, 6 drops
- Add 3 drops of pure lemon oil
- Two drops of pure Eucalyptus oil

Description: This blend harnesses the cleansing and purifying properties of tea tree oil along with the refreshing scent of lemon and eucalyptus. It helps to purify the air, boost immunity, and support respiratory health.

Romantic Floral Blend:

- Rose essential oil, 4 drops
- Essential oil of Ylang Ylang, three drops
- Two drops of pure jasmine oil.

Description: This romantic blend combines the rich and floral aromas of rose, ylang-ylang, and jasmine. It creates a sensual and soothing ambiance, promotes feelings of love and intimacy, and uplifts the mood.

Focus and Clarity Blend:

- Add 4 drops of peppermint oil, if desired.
- Add 3 drops of rosemary oil.
- A few drops of pure lemon oil

Description: This blend combines the stimulating and invigorating properties of peppermint, rosemary, and lemon. It helps to enhance mental clarity, improve focus and concentration, and boost cognitive function.

Calming Serenity Blend:

- Lavender oil, around 4 drops' worth
- Add 3 drops of pure Frankincense oil.
- Essential oil of vetiver, 2 drops

Description: This blend combines the soothing and relaxing properties of lavender and frankincense with the grounding and earthy aroma of vetiver. It helps to promote deep relaxation, reduce stress and anxiety, and create a serene atmosphere.

Fresh Morning Blend:

- Essential oil of lemon, 5 drops
- Essential oil of peppermint, 3 drops
- Essential oil of rosemary, 2 drops

Description: This invigorating blend combines the energizing and uplifting scents of lemon, peppermint, and rosemary. It helps to awaken the senses, boost mood and motivation, and provide a refreshing start to the day.

Revitalizing Forest Blend:

- Pine oil, around 4 drops' worth
- Essential oil of cedar, 3 drops
- Two drops of pure Eucalyptus oil

Description: This blend captures the fresh and revitalizing essence of a forest. The combination of pine, cedarwood, and eucalyptus oils creates a grounding and rejuvenating aroma, promoting a sense of vitality and clarity.

Harmonizing Balance Blend:

- Essential oil of geranium, 4 drops
- Bergamot oil, three drops
- Two drops of pure Patchouli oil

Description: This blend combines the floral notes of geranium, the uplifting scent of bergamot, and the earthy aroma of patchouli. It helps to balance emotions, promote harmony, and create a peaceful and balanced atmosphere.

Uplifting Citrus Spice Blend:

- Add 4 drops of pure Sweet Orange oil to your bath.
- Add 3 drops of pure cinnamon oil.
- 2 drops of pure ginger oil

Description: This blend combines the bright and cheerful aroma of sweet orange with the warm and spicy scents of cinnamon and ginger. It creates a joyful and uplifting atmosphere, boosts mood, and adds a touch of cozy comfort.

Remember to dilute these essential oil blends appropriately before using them, either in a carrier oil or with a diffuser. The suggested dilution ratio is usually 2-3 drops of the blend per 10 ml of carrier oil.

Conclusions

In conclusion, while essential oils can provide pleasant aromas and potentially offer certain benefits, it is important to approach their use with caution. Consultation with professionals, proper dilution, and considering individual sensitivities are crucial steps to ensure safe and responsible use. Remember that essential oils should not replace conventional medical treatments and should be used as a complementary approach under appropriate guidance.

How to make tinctures, essential oils, infusions, and natural antibiotics is covered in the following chapter. Preparation instructions, recipes, and tips for combining herbs to achieve desired effects are all included.

BOOK 13: INTRODUCTION TO NATURAL MEDICINE FOR CHILDREN

When you have a child, you'll quickly learn how important it is to keep a supply of necessities on hand. As a parent, it's helpful to be prepared for any number of medical emergencies involving your child, such as a fall, a scratch while playing, a fever or discomfort, touching something extremely hot (like a pot or oven), getting a horrible sore, needing an immune system boost, and so on.

You probably have a box of medicines or a first aid bag with various helpful goods, but did you know that your own house can serve as a makeshift pharmacy? It's useful for treating both acute and chronic conditions. Some of these home treatments also have experimental study support. However, if the symptoms persist, it's best to get your child checked out by a doctor as soon as possible.

Supplements and Homemade Hand Sanitizer + Immune-Building Herbs for Kids

Do you know during the cold and flu season, it's necessary to keep your kid's immune system running high? You should also know it's equally necessary to have your children wash their hands constantly, most especially during this pandemic. Here are remarkable herbs and supplements that are potent immune-builders and a do-it-yourself recipe for hand sanitizer that your children can use.

Immune-Building Herbs and Supplements

- Elderberry
- Echinacea
- Golden Seal
- Vitamin C
- Vitamin D
- Oregano Oil
- Black Seed Oil
- Hand Sanitizer

Do you know how you can make an exceptional recipe for a powerful hand sanitizer? Instead of rubbing alcohol on your kid's hands (which is not as perfect), why not try making yours?

Recipe type: Homemade Hand Sanitizer

Ingredients:

- Strong Vodka, 3 ounces
- 5-10 drops of pure lavender essential oil 1 ounce of pure aloe vera gel
- 30 drops Oil extracted from tea trees
- Oil rich in vitamin E, equivalent to 1/4 teaspoon

Instructions:

1. Essential oils can be combined in a little glass jar. Then combine the alcohol with the mixture once more.

2. After that, pour in some aloe vera gel and give it a good shake.
3. Before using, give the mixture a gentle shake.

Kids with Sleep Issues and Sleep Apnea

Is that so? Sleep apnea can and does occur in children. Signs and symptoms may include:

Most evenings, they snore loudly.

They can halt in their breathing, snort, and gasp for air.

Sleeping with a large amount of perspiration

Pose their heads in odd ways while they sleep.

Sleep was broken up for the most part.

It might contribute to daytime fatigue and behavioral issues at school if it is not detected and treated promptly. Children who snore loudly are twice as likely to suffer academic difficulties, according to recent studies.

When children don't get enough sleep, they are more likely to exhibit hyperactivity, difficulty focusing, and ADD/ADHD symptoms the next day. There is some evidence linking childhood sleep apnea to impaired growth and cardiovascular health.

Some of the following symptoms may indicate that your child suffers from sleep apnea.

- Problems rousing oneself from sleep Morning and all day headache Sensitivity, irritability, hostility, and discomfort
- issues with behavior or social interactions at home or in school
- The child speaks with a nasal tone and opens their lips wide when they breathe.

Natural Remedies for Kids with Sleep Apnea

I. Using CPAP Mask

The first step is to take your child to a doctor for testing. Your child may require emergency tonsillectomy if they are experiencing breathing difficulties. The doctor can also prescribe a CPAP mask in a child's size (continuous positive airway pressure device).

II. You should try and learn the Didgeridoo

I get it; you don't have this lying around the house. If your child has sleep apnea, a strange Wind instrument called a Didgeridoo might assist with symptoms in the short term. You may not have heard of it either.

Recent research suggests that mild sleep apnea sufferers can benefit from 4 months of didgeridoo practice, leading to improved sleep and less daytime sleepiness. It's a valid question to wonder how exactly it operates. Playing the instrument can help you feel more in control of the situation by avoiding your child's upper airway from becoming constricted during inhalation. Hey! You should know that children and adults alike have used the extra effort of learning to play an instrument as a means of improving their breathing and lung capacity for many years.

Petroleum Jelly and Listerine for Sores (Bliss)

Do you aware that blisters hurt and can make your kid feel uncomfortable? Do you want a quick fix?

In addition to its many other uses, Listerine can help dry out any sores your kids may have.

Cotton balls dipped in antiseptic can be applied to your child's blisters twice or thrice daily until they dry up and the pain goes away. Additionally, a new study found that applying petroleum jelly to a blister provided temporary relief from discomfort. The good news is that Listerine has been used successfully for a long time to treat simple wounds (blisters). This tried-and-true treatment is ideal for soothing your child's blisters.

Lemon Balm for Cold Sores

Lemon balm's efficacy as a remedy has been well-documented for quite some time. Cold sores can be very painful, especially for younger children and young adults. Herpes simplex virus (HSV) enters a developing child's tissues, where it might remain latent until reawakening throughout adolescence.

Possible causes of a cold sore include:

- Lack of protection from the sun
- Chronic lung illness
- Psychological stress

It has an antiviral impact due to its high polyphenol content, and it also has a pleasant flavor and aroma. There was no recurrence of cold sores after treatment with lemon balm, according to a recent study. Try some lemon balm ointment; it's great for so many different things, including soothing kids' chapped lips, cuts, small burns, and scrapes.

Using Ginger for Motion Illness

Are you taking the kids on a trip? You'll need ginger, the most sought-after herb. Capsules or syrup made from ginger root! All of these remedies will help your child feel more stable or prevent motion sickness.

Ginger is one of those useful treatments to have on hand, whether in your purse, kitchen, or emergency medical pack at home. If you're going on a trip with kids, you should all take some ginger pills in case anyone becomes car sick. Rub some ginger oil on your child's feet if you wish to employ essential oils for rapid relief.

When compared to anti-nausea medication, one study indicated that ginger was more effective in treating motion sickness. It was also discovered that ginger was effective in preventing seasickness.

Using a Duct Tape for Warts

This may come as a surprise, but I can assure you it has miraculous results. Do you know that there is little evidence to support the claim that duct tape may remove warts? Although it isn't as effective as just freezing them to death, it achieves its purpose. Over 80% of patients' warts disappeared using duct tape in less than three months, according to a recent study.

How to use it to get rid of warts on your kids:

- The wart and the skin around it should be kept clean and tidy.
- Then, cut a piece of duct tape slightly larger than the wart and press it into the affected area.
- If the wart is still present after three days, remove the tape and wipe it with a sandpaper board or pumice stone.

Banana Peel for Warts (and so much more)

If you don't have any duct tape handy, you can try using a particularly ripe banana peel to remove that pesky wart.

To begin, simply rub the inner surface of the peel on the child's wart on a daily basis.

Additionally, bananas can aid in:

An insect bite or poison ivy rash can be treated by massaging the inside part of a banana peel over the affected area.

Knowing that banana peel also has anti-acne properties is helpful. Adolescents can benefit from anti-microbial and anti-inflammatory properties by massaging the inner portion of the peel over their faces.

Papaya for Smoother Skin

Do you know that young people, especially, tend to want smooth skin? Helpful in this regard is the practice of exfoliation; papaya can serve as an effective exfoliant for the skins of children and young adults. Papain, the active element in papaya, removes the dead skin cells that cause a dull, rough appearance on the skin. To calm, soften, and polish their skin, try this fruity facial on your children and young adults.

- Prepare ripe papaya by washing and peeling it.
- Two teaspoons should then be blended completely in a food processor.
- Mix in a dried teaspoon of oatmeal to make a paste.
- After washing your face, apply and let it sit for 10 to 15 minutes.
- The paste can be scrubbed away with a wet rag or rinsed off with warm water.

Surely you are aware Papaya is a miraculous fruit that can clear even minor acne problems in children and young adults. Blend the papaya until smooth, add the oatmeal, and apply the mixture to your face if you wish to give a blender a try. It's a gentle exfoliant that helps get rid of dead skin cells that can block pores and lead to acne breakouts.

Treatment for Minor Burns: Mustard, Egg White, and Lavender Oil

Does your kid or teen like helping you in the kitchen? If so, be ready to treat the minor burns that are likely to occur:

Lavender Essential Oil

Did you know that a few drops of lavender oil on a burn will quickly alleviate the pain? When applied to a burn quickly, lavender oil can prevent blistering.

The white part of Egg

If your kid gets a burn, instantly grab an egg, leave the yolk and egg, and put it on the kid's skin. Be assured The burn will go away, the skin will recover, and the pain will end. If you or your children suffer from mild burns, egg white is a fantastic home cure. Simply apply with a soothing, even motion, and the burn will feel better immediately and completely. Mustard and lavender oil are also effective.

Mustard

If your child gets burned, don't be afraid to spread some mustard on the sore spot. The mustard will ease the pain and scorching after the initial burn. There is no art that explains why this is so effective, but there are plenty of suggestions.

Remedy for Bites and Stings

Is that so? Adolescence isn't complete without a few wasp, bee, or insect stings, right? Knowing that certain children can have a strong reaction to bites and stings can be helpful. Some cases are so severe that they require medical intervention. Get the kid to the doctor ASAP if he or she develops a cold rash, itching, or difficulty breathing after being stung or bitten. Try these homeopathic remedies for reduced itching and pain from bites and stings.:

Poison Ivy Stings

Even if you don't believe it, onions can reduce the swelling and pain associated with poison ivy bites in children. This is all that is required of you:

- To begin, halve the onion and apply the halves directly onto the skin.
- Then, use soap and water to thoroughly clean the area.
- At last, apply a paste made of sterile water and sodium bicarbonate to the affected area.

Bee Stings

My mother used bee stings on me and my siblings when I was a kid; a mixture of dirt and baking soda diluted with water. She slapped the mud or soda onto the bee sting, and the pain and redness subsided within a few minutes. Using mud is controversial since it could contain contaminants (and is messy), therefore sodium bicarbonate is a safer bet (baking soda).

Wasp Stings

As a mother, you need to think and act immediately when your child is stung by a wasp. Vinegar or lemon juice can be applied undiluted to the skin with a cotton ball. It will immediately neutralize the toxin.

Pure Essential Oils and Herbs for Headaches

Is your family prone to frequent headaches? Alcohol, chocolate, cheese, and caffeinated drinks can all bring on a headache. Also, there are a lot of potential problems (tension, vascular, hormonal, migraine, tension, and cluster).

Understanding that children and adolescents may have trouble expressing the onset of their headaches is helpful. If you think your kid has a headache, try one of these common herbal or essential oil treatments. However, some headaches are so bad that a cup of tea or some essential oils won't cut it. A severe headache in a child warrants prompt medical attention.

Chapter 1-2-3-4-5-6-7: Natural Remedies For Common Childhood Pathologies (Recipes, Etc.)

Abscess

Cold and Cough:

Honey: For kids older than one, this sweetener can help ease their cough. Warm water or herbal tea with a teaspoon of honey added is a good remedy.

Congestion and coughing can be alleviated by inhaling steam from a bowl of hot water or a warm shower.

Sore Throat:

Encourage your youngster to gargle with a mixture of half a teaspoon of salt and warm water. Be sure they don't put the concoction in their mouths.

For a soothing remedy, try this: dissolve a teaspoon of honey and a few drops of lemon juice in a cup of hot water. Your child's sore throat will feel better after drinking this concoction.

Upset Stomach:

Ginger: Ginger has been shown to reduce nausea and stomach pain. Give your child a little bit of real ginger ale or ginger tea.

Peppermint may assist with stomach aches; try drinking peppermint tea or using diluted peppermint oil. Make sure the peppermint is safe and effective for kids.

Skin Irritations:

Colloidal oatmeal added to a bath can help soothe skin irritations including eczema and rashes that cause itching.

Applying pure aloe vera gel (either directly from the plant or from a reliable source) can help calm minor skin irritations.

Fever:

Keep your child well hydrated by giving him or her plenty of fluids to drink when he or she has a fever. It may help to drink fluids like water, herbal tea, or fruit juice watered down.

Applying a cool, moist cloth to your child's forehead or underarms can assist reduce his or her body temperature.

Fresh Yarrow Poultice

Makes 1 poultice.

- Chopped fresh yarrow leaves, one tablespoon

1. Cover the abscess with a clean, soft cloth after applying the chopped leaves. Ten to fifteen minutes is sufficient time for the poultice to work.
2. Perform this procedure twice or thrice daily until the abscess has completely healed.

Echinacea and Goldenseal Tincture

Makes about 2 cups.

- Two cups of plain 80-proof vodka Two ounces of finely chopped dried echinacea root Three ounces of dried goldenseal root

1. Mix the echinacea and goldenseal in a sterile pint jar. Fill the jar up with vodka

so that the herbs are completely submerged.

2. Put the lid on the jar and give it a good shake. Keep it in a dark, cool cabinet for 6-8 weeks, shaking it several times a week. If some of the vodka evaporates, just add more until the jar is full again.
3. Cheesecloth can be dampened and used to cover the opening of a funnel. The tincture should be transferred using the funnel to a clean pint jar. Wring the cheesecloth until no more liquid drains from the roots. Remove the tincture to dark glass bottles and discard the roots.
4. Take 10 drops orally twice or thrice day for 7-10 days to treat an abscess.

Acne

Calendula Toner

Makes about ½ cup.

- Ingredients: 2 tbsp. of calendula oil, 1/3 cup of witch hazel

1. Shake the ingredients gently in a dark glass bottle.
2. After washing your face or other affected areas, add 5 or 6 drops to a cotton cosmetic pad and gently pat in. Add more or less to suit your needs.
3. To keep acne at bay, do this treatment twice a day. If you want a chilled experience, keep the bottle in the fridge.

Agrimony-Chamomile Gel

Makes about ⅔ cup.

- Agrimony, dry, 2 tablespoons
- 2 tablespoons chamomile flowers, dried
- Aloe vera gel, 1/4 cup (1/2 cup) water

1. Put the agrimony and chamomile in a saucepan with the water. Over high heat, bring the ingredients to a boil before turning the heat down to a simmer. Reduce the ingredients by half in a saucepan, then set them aside to cool completely.
2. Cheesecloth can be dampened and used to cover the opening of a funnel. Use the funnel to transfer the contents to the bowl. Wring the cheesecloth with the herbs in it until no more liquid comes out.
3. Whisk in the aloe vera gel until fully incorporated. Put the gel in a clean container, such as a glass jar. Put the lid on the jar and put it in the fridge.
4. Apply a small application twice a day using a cotton cosmetic pad to the afflicted areas.

Allergies

Common allergens include cat dander, pollen, and dust, and they provoke aberrant immunological responses in some people. It can be challenging to avoid exposure to allergens due to their widespread presence in the environment, including in food and drink. Herbal medicines are much more gentle than conventional treatments, which typically involve suppressing your immune reaction to allergens.

Feverfew-Peppermint Tincture

Makes about 2 cups.

- Feverfew, dried, 2 ounces; peppermint, dried, 6 ounces

- 2 cups of plain vodka (80 proof)

1. Mix the feverfew and peppermint in a sterile pint container. Pour the vodka into the container until it is completely full.
2. Put the lid on the jar and give it a good shake. Keep it in a dark, cool cabinet for 6-8 weeks, shaking it several times a week.
3. Cheesecloth can be dampened and used to cover the opening of a funnel. The tincture should be transferred using the funnel to a clean pint jar. Extraction of liquid from herbs by wringing. Throw away the used herbs and pour the tincture into dark glass bottles.
4. When allergy symptoms appear, take 5 drops orally. Mix it with some water or juice if the flavor is too intense for you.

Garlic-Ginkgo Syrup

Makes about 2 cups.

This syrup will stay fresh for up to 6 months when refrigerated.

- Ingredients: 2 ounces of chopped fresh or freeze-dried garlic 2 ounces of crushed or chopped ginkgo biloba 2 cups of water
- 1 pound of native honey

1. Put the water, garlic, and ginkgo biloba in a saucepan. Reduce the liquid by half by bringing it to a simmer over low heat while partially covered.
2. Pour the contents of the saucepan into a glass measuring cup, then strain it back into the pan using cheesecloth dipped in water and squeezed until dry.
3. When the temperature hits 105°F to 110°F, remove the mixture from the heat and stir in the honey.
4. Refrigerate the syrup by placing it in a clean bottle or jar.
5. To relieve allergy symptoms, take 1 tablespoon three times a day by mouth.

Precautions Do not use if you are taking a monoamine oxidase inhibitor (MAOI) for depression. Ginkgo biloba enhances the effect of blood thinners, so talk to your doctor before use. Children under age 12 should take 1 teaspoon three times per day.

Asthma

Inflamed airways in the lungs and narrowed bronchial tubes are hallmarks of this persistent disease. Some persons with asthma also suffer from panic attacks whenever breathing becomes difficult because of how terrifying asthma episodes may be.

Ginkgo-Thyme Tea

Makes 1 cup.

- 1 cup of water, boiled
- Dried ginkgo biloba, one teaspoon
- Dried Thyme, 1 Teaspoon

1. A big cup should be filled with the boiling water. Tea should be steeped for 10 minutes after the dried herbs are added and the mug is covered.
2. Take it easy and enjoy the steam as you sip your tea. Perform as many as four times daily.

Peppermint-Rosemary Vapor Treatment

Makes 1 treatment.

Two drops of peppermint essential oil and four drops of rosemary essential oil can be used as a substitute for the fresh herbs in this remedy.

- Four cups of boiling water (not boiling)
- 1/2 cup of fresh peppermint leaves, crushed
- 1/2 cup of fresh rosemary, chopped

1. Place all the ingredients in a wide, shallow bowl and mix well. Make yourself at home in front of the bowl by setting it down on a table.
2. Cover your head and the bowl with a big towel. Take in the aroma of the herbs as they evaporate. If the fumes get too intense, you should step outside for a moment of fresh air. After the water has cooled, you can stop the treatment.
3. When asthma symptoms return, use as often as necessary. You can use this therapy as often as you wish because it is so mild.

Precautions If you suffer from epilepsy, you should not use rosemary. Seizures can be avoided by using oils such as jasmine, ylang-ylang, chamomile, and lavender; however, oils such as rosemary, fennel, sage, eucalyptus, hyssop, camphor, and spike lavender have been linked to epileptic episodes.

Athlete's Foot

The fungus responsible for this irritating and occasionally painful infection prefers humid, warm, dark environments. It's important to get it treated before it spreads under your toenails and becomes permanently disfiguring.

Fresh Garlic Poultice

Makes 1 treatment.

- 1 squeezed garlic clove
- 1 tsp. raw honey

1. Mix the garlic and honey in a separate bowl. Apply the mixture with a cotton cosmetic pad to the afflicted region.
2. Slip on a clean pair of socks and kick up your feet for 15 to 60 minutes while the poultice does its work. After you're done, go wash and dry your feet. Goldenseal Ointment should be used afterward. The treatment should be repeated once or twice a day (here). Carry on for 3 days after the signs of illness have subsided.

Precautions In certain people, eating garlic could trigger a skin rash.

Goldenseal Ointment

Makes about 1 cup

- One-and-a-half cups of extra-virgin olive oil, light
- Goldenseal root, dried and diced 2 ounces 1-ounce beeswax

1. Put the olive oil and goldenseal in a slow cooker and turn it on low. Set the slow cooker to its lowest setting, cover, and let the roots sit in the oil for 3 to 5 hours. Take the oil off the heat and let it cool down in the infusion.

2. In the bottom of a double boiler, heat a few inches of water to a simmer. Turn down to a low simmer.
3. Cover the top of the double boiler with cheesecloth. Once the cheesecloth has absorbed all of the infused oil, you can discard it. Throw away the used cheesecloth and herbs.
4. To the base of the double boiler, add the beeswax and the oil that has been infused. Slowly reheat on low heat. Beeswax should be taken off the heat as soon as it has melted fully. Rapidly transfer the liquid to sterilized, dry containers, and cool to room temperature before sealing.
5. Cotton cosmetic pads should be used to apply a quarter teaspoon to the afflicted areas. You can apply it as often as three times a day, with the last time being right before bed. Put on a clean pair of socks over the ointment to keep from falling.

Precautions Avoid use if you are expecting a child or nursing a baby. Avoid if you suffer from hypertension.

Backache

Passionflower–Blue Vervain Tea

Makes 1 cup

- 1 cup of water, boiled
- 1/2 a fresh passionflower leaf 1 tsp.
- 1 tsp. of blue vervain in its dry form

1. A big cup should be filled with the boiling water. Put the dry herbs in the mug, cover it, and let the tea soak for ten minutes.
2. Take it easy and savor each sip of tea. Do up to twice a day if desired.

Ginger-Peppermint Salve

Makes about 1 cup.

- One-and-a-half cups of extra-virgin olive oil, light
- Chopped dried gingerroot and peppermint leaves equal 1 ounce.
- Beeswax, 1 ounce

1. Olive oil, ginger, and peppermint can be combined in a slow cooker. Turn the slow cooker's heat setting to low, cover, and leave the herbs to steep in the oil for three to five hours. Take the oil off the heat and let it cool down in the infusion.
2. In the bottom of a double boiler, heat a few inches of water to a simmer. Turn down to a low simmer.
3. Cover the top of the double boiler with cheesecloth. Once the cheesecloth has absorbed all of the infused oil, you can discard it. Throw away the used cheesecloth and herbs.
4. To the base of the double boiler, add the beeswax and the oil that has been infused. Slowly reheat on low heat. Beeswax should be taken off the heat as soon as it has melted fully. Rapidly transfer the liquid to sterilized, dry containers, and cool to room temperature before sealing.
5. One teaspoon should be massaged into the afflicted region using your fingers or

a cotton cosmetic pad. Add more or less to suit your needs. You can give yourself this therapy up to four times daily.

Precautions If you have gallstones, gallbladder disease, or a bleeding issue, ginger should be avoided.

Bee Sting

Fresh Plantain Poultice

Makes 1 treatment.

- One Tablespoon of Fresh Plantain Leaves, Finely Chopped

1. Cover the area with a soft cloth after applying the chopped leaves to the wound. Ten to fifteen minutes is sufficient time for the poultice to work. Do as often as necessary until the pain has completely subsided.

Comfrey-Aloe Gel

Makes about ¼ cup

When kept in the refrigerator, it stays fresh for about 2 weeks.

- 2 tsp dried comfrey leaves 1/4 cup water
- Aloe vera gel, 2 teaspoons

1. Put the comfrey and water in a pan and heat it up. The mixture should be brought to a boil over high heat before the heat is turned down to low. Reduce the ingredients by half in a saucepan, then set them aside to cool completely.
2. Cheesecloth can be dampened and used to cover the opening of a funnel. Use the funnel to transfer the contents to the bowl. Wring the cheesecloth full of the comfrey liquid until no more comes out.
3. Whisk in the aloe vera gel until fully incorporated. Place the completed gel in a clean glass container. Refrigerate the jar after you've secured the lid.
4. Apply a tiny coating to the affected region with a cotton cosmetic pad as needed until the discomfort and swelling have subsided.

Bloating

Peppermint-Fennel Tea

Makes 1 cup.

- 1 cup of water, boiled
- 1/2 tsp. fresh mint leaves
- 1/4 teaspoon crushed fennel seeds

1. A big cup should be filled with the boiling water. Put in the fennel and peppermint, cover the mug, and let the tea sit for 10 minutes.
2. Unwind with some tea. This treatment is gentle enough to be used as often as necessary.

Dandelion Root Tincture

Makes about 2 cups.

- Ingredients: 2 cups of plain 80-proof vodka 8 ounces of coarsely chopped dandelion root

1. The dandelion root should be placed in a clean, dry pint jar. Pour in the vodka

until it reaches the top of the jar; this will ensure that the roots are completely submerged.

2. Close the lid and give the jar a good shake. Keep it in a dark, cool cabinet for 6-8 weeks, shaking it several times a week. If some of the vodka evaporates, just add more until the jar is full again.
3. Cheesecloth can be dampened and used to cover the opening of a funnel. Use the funnel to transfer the tincture to another clean pint jar. Wring the cheesecloth until no more liquid drains from the roots. Throw away the roots and pour the tincture into bottles made of black glass.
4. When gas is a problem, take 1 teaspoon orally once or twice day. If you find the flavor too overpowering, dilute it with some water or juice.

Bronchitis

Rosemary–Licorice Root Vapor Treatment

Makes 1 treatment.

- Amounting to 5 cups, water
- dried licorice root, diced (1/4 cup)
- 1/3 cup dried or 1 cup fresh rosemary leaves, chopped

1. The dried licorice root and water should be mixed together in a saucepan. Get it boiling, then turn the heat down low. Maintain a low boil for 10 minutes.
2. Add the rosemary leaves to the water and licorice root in a shallow basin.
3. Cover your head and the bowl with a big towel. Take in the aroma of the herbs as they evaporate. If the fumes get too intense, you should step outside for a moment of fresh air. After the water has cooled, you can stop the treatment.
4. As often as required. You can use this therapy as often as you wish because it is so mild.

Goldenseal-Hyssop Syrup

Makes about 2 cups

- Goldenseal root, dried, 1 ounce; hyssop, dry, 1 ounce; chop
- 4 cups of coffee
- Honey, 1 pound

1. Goldenseal and hyssop are combined with water in a saucepan. Reduce the liquid by half by bringing it to a simmer over low heat while partially covered.
2. Pour the mixture from the measuring cup back into the pot through a cheesecloth that has been soaked with water and wrung out until no more liquid comes out.
3. Stirring frequently, heat the mixture until it reaches 105 to 110 degrees Fahrenheit, then remove it from the stove.
4. Refrigerate the syrup by placing it in a clean bottle or jar.
5. To relieve symptoms, take 1 tablespoon three to five times daily.

Chickweed-Mullein Compress

Makes 1 treatment.

- Chopped chickweed equaling 2 tablespoons

- Fresh mullein leaf, cut to a fine powder (1 teaspoon)

1. Cover the burn with a cotton cloth and apply the freshly chopped plant stuff. Ten to fifteen minutes is sufficient time for the poultice to work. Do this as often as every 2 to 3 hours, or as needed, until the pain goes away.

Fresh Aloe Vera Gel

Makes 1 treatment.

- Aloe vera plant

1. Take an aloe vera leaf and snip off a one-inch portion from the very tip. The plant will benefit from having the rest of the leaf, so don't remove it.
2. Cut an opening in the leaf with a sharp knife. Scoop the gel from the center of the leaf and apply it to the burn and the area around it using your fingers or a cotton cosmetic pad. You should do this once or twice a day until the burn has healed.

Chest Congestion

Hyssop-Sage Infusion

Makes 1 quart.

- 4 cups of water, boiled
- Hyssop, dried, four teaspoons
- Sage, dried, four tablespoons

1. Boil some water and add the dried herbs to a teapot. Put a lid on the saucepan and let the infusion sit for 10 minutes.
2. Take it easy and enjoy a cup of the infusion while you breathe in its calming aroma. The leftovers are OK to reheat in the microwave or store in the refrigerator for later consumption.

Precautions Hyssop should not be taken by anyone who is epileptic or pregnant.

Angelica-Goldenseal Syrup

Makes about 2 cups.

- 1 ounce of chopped angelica
- 1 ounce of minced dried goldenseal root
- 2 glasses of water
- Honey, 1 pound

1. Put the water and herbs in a saucepan. Reduce the liquid by half by bringing it to a simmer over low heat while partially covered.
2. Fill a glass measuring cup with the contents of the saucepan, and then strain the liquid back into the pot by pouring it through a cheesecloth that has been soaked with water and wrung out thoroughly.
3. Stirring frequently, heat the mixture until it reaches 105 to 110 degrees Fahrenheit, then remove it from the stove.
4. Refrigerate the syrup by placing it in a clean bottle or jar.
5. To relieve symptoms, take 1 tablespoon three to four times daily. One teaspoon, twice or three times a day, is the recommended dosage for kids under the age of 12.

Precautions Avoid use if you are expecting a child or nursing a baby. Angelica shouldn't be taken alongside blood-thinning medication. If you have hypertension, you should not take goldenseal.

Chicken Pox

Comfrey-Licorice Bath

Makes 1 quart.

- Apple cider vinegar, organic, unfiltered, 4 cups
- Comfrey tincture, half a teaspoon
- 1/2 tsp tincture of licorice root

1. Put the tinctures and vinegar in a clean, dry container. Keep the lid tightly on and put it somewhere cool and dark until you need it.
2. Pour one cup of the mixture into a tub of lukewarm water and soak. Put in a minimum of 20 minutes of soak time. Calendula-Goldenseal Gel (found here) can be used as a follow-up if desired.

Precautions If you have hypertension, diabetes, kidney illness, or heart disease, you should not use licorice root.

Calendula-Goldenseal Gel

Makes about 2 cups.

- Calendula, 1 ounce dried
- One ounce of minced dried goldenseal root Two glasses of water
- Aloe vera gel, 1 1/2 cups

1. Put the water, calendula, and goldenseal in a saucepan. The mixture should be brought to a boil over high heat before the heat is turned down to low.
2. Reduce the volume of the mixture by half by simmering it, and then set it aside to cool.
3. Cheesecloth can be dampened and used to cover the opening of a funnel. Use the funnel to transfer the contents to the bowl. Wring the cheesecloth with the herbs in it until no more liquid comes out.
4. Whisk in the aloe vera gel until fully incorporated. Place the completed gel in a clean glass container. Refrigerate the jar after you've secured the lid.
5. Apply a thin application two or three times a day using a cotton cosmetic pad to all afflicted areas.

Precautions Avoid use if you are expecting a child or nursing a baby. Avoid if you suffer from hypertension.

BOOK 14: INTRODUCTION TO NATURAL MEDICINE FOR PETS

The term "natural medicine" is commonly used to describe the practice of using non-conventional methods to improve the health of one's pet. Herbal medicine, acupuncture, homeopathy, nutritional therapy, and other practices are all included under this umbrella. The goal of natural medicine for pets is to complement the body's own healing processes and provide perpetual good health.

Basics of Holistic Veterinary Care:

Natural medicine offers a holistic approach, meaning it considers not just the pet's physical health but also its mental and emotional state. Instead than merely masking symptoms, it seeks to address the root of the problem.

Customized Care: Each pet is given the attention and care that they deserve as an individual. When developing a treatment plan, the veterinarian takes into account the animal's breed, age, medical history, lifestyle, and current health status.

Maintaining health and avoiding illness are important tenets of natural medicine's emphasis on preventative care. It recommends being proactive by changing one's diet, exercising regularly, and adopting other healthy habits.

Natural Veterinary Care Routines:

Supplementing a pet's health in various ways is possible with the help of herbs and plant extracts. The calming effects of chamomile and the immune-enhancing properties of echinacea are only two examples. Teas, tinctures, and supplements are just some of the ways that herbal medicine can be taken in.

Acupuncture is a form of alternative medicine in which tiny needles are inserted into a patient's skin at strategic areas to increase blood flow and aid healing. It has positive effects on pain relief, blood flow, and general health.

Homeopathy uses natural chemicals as medicine, following the law of "like heals like." Symptoms in a healthy animal are utilized as a dose to trigger the body's natural healing processes.

Nutritional therapy: feeding your pet a diet tailored to its species is a cornerstone of holistic pet care. The goal of nutritional therapy is to provide your pet with a healthy, natural diet that is tailored to their individual needs. Raw food diets, home-cooked meals, and premium commercial pet foods all fit under this category.

Massage, hydrotherapy, and chiropractic care are just a few examples of the physical therapy procedures that can be used to help patients recover from injuries and surgeries more quickly and with less discomfort.

Stress Reduction: Natural medicine recognizes the impact of stress on pets' health and utilizes various techniques to promote relaxation and reduce anxiety. These may include aromatherapy, music therapy, and behavior modification techniques.

It is important to note that while natural medicine can be beneficial for pets, it should never replace conventional veterinary care. It is essential to work with a qualified veterinarian who is knowledgeable about natural medicine to ensure the best care for your pet's specific needs.

Chapter 1-2-3-4-5-6: Natural Remedies For Common Pet Diseases (Recipes, Etc.)

While natural remedies can provide some relief for common pet diseases, it's important to note that they are not substitutes for professional veterinary care. If your pet is unwell, it's always recommended to consult a veterinarian for an accurate diagnosis and appropriate treatment. However, here are some natural remedies that may help alleviate symptoms associated with common pet diseases:

Digestive Upset:

Probiotics: These can promote a healthy gut by restoring the balance of beneficial bacteria. Look for pet-specific probiotics.

Slippery elm: This herb can soothe the digestive tract and alleviate diarrhea. Give as directed by your vet or follow product instructions.

Skin Allergies:

Oatmeal baths: Soothing oatmeal baths can relieve itchiness and irritation. Use colloidal oatmeal specifically formulated for pets.

Coconut oil: Applying coconut oil topically may help moisturize and soothe irritated skin. Consult your vet for appropriate use.

Ear Infections:

Apple cider vinegar (ACV) rinse: Dilute ACV with water (1:1 ratio) and use it to gently clean your pet's ears. This can help maintain a healthy pH and prevent infection.

Calendula or mullein oil: These natural oils have antimicrobial properties and can be used sparingly after consulting with your vet.

Urinary Tract Infections (UTIs):

Cranberry supplements: Cranberry extracts or supplements may help prevent or manage UTIs by inhibiting bacterial growth. Consult your vet for proper dosage.

Arthritis and Joint Pain:

Omega-3 fatty acids: Fish oil supplements rich in omega-3 fatty acids can have anti-inflammatory properties and support joint health. Follow your vet's recommendations for dosage.

Gentle exercise and weight management: Regular, low-impact exercise and maintaining a healthy weight can help alleviate joint pain in pets.

Anxiety and Stress:

Lavender oil: Use pet-safe lavender oil to provide a calming effect. Consult your vet for appropriate usage, such as diffusing or using a diluted spray.

Adaptil or Feliway: These synthetic pheromone products can help reduce anxiety in dogs and cats, respectively. Follow the product instructions.

Remember, while these natural remedies can provide some relief, they may not be suitable for every pet or every situation. It's crucial to consult with your veterinarian before trying any natural remedies and to follow their guidance for the best care of your pet.

Conclusion

Animals can benefit from a wide variety of complementary and alternative treatments, many of which go under the umbrella term of "natural medicine." Even while there are many natural cures out there, you shouldn't count on them to take the place of veterinarian care. It is important to use natural medicine cautiously and only after consulting with a trained veterinarian as a supplementary therapy to conventional therapies.

Herbal supplements, essential oils, acupuncture, chiropractic care, and homeopathy are just some of the more popular alternative treatments for pets. Many different health conditions, including pain, inflammation, anxiety, digestive problems, and immune system support, can be helped by aiding the body's natural healing processes, which these therapies are designed to do.

Before giving any treatment to your pet, you should talk to a vet who is familiar with alternative medicine. They will be able to assess your pet's general health, provide an acceptable dosage, and advise you on any possible drug interactions.

In addition, you should know that not all natural therapies are secure or helpful for your cat. It's possible that some substances are hazardous to animals, and it's possible that the claims made for some treatments lack sufficient scientific evidence. When treating your pet with natural remedies, it's important to do your homework, talk to an expert, and proceed with caut

Dear reader, thank you so much for delving into 'The Herb Bible.' Your support means the world to me! I hope this book has sparked your interest in the fascinating world of herbs and natural wellness.

Your feedback is valuable, so I invite you to share your experience through a review. As a token of gratitude, you can download the 'Guide to Anti-Inflammatory Herbs' for free.

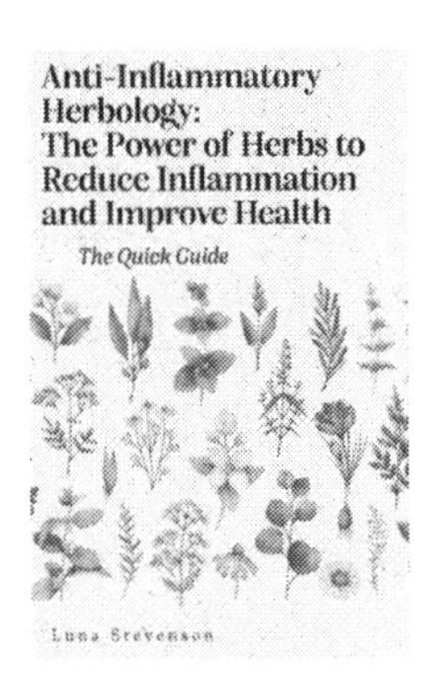

It's a special gift for you, a way to further explore the benefits of herbs. Thank you again for choosing this book and being a part of this incredible journey into the world of herbs!

BOOK 15: CULTIVATION OF MEDICINAL HERBS

Growing herbs for medical purposes has been done for ages all over the world. Plants with chemicals with therapeutic characteristics are known as medical herbs, medicinal plants, or herbal medicines. These plants have a long history of therapeutic use, and their uses range from curing specific conditions to bolstering general health and happiness.

There are many benefits to growing herbs for medical use. It enables better quality control and standardization of herbal treatments while easing the burden on wild plant populations. Farmer income isn't the only benefit that comes from growing medicinal herbs; doing so also helps to keep ancient herbal practices alive.

There are a number of factors to think about when planting medicinal plants. It is critical to pick the right plant species in consideration of their usefulness as medicine, their adaptability to the local ecosystem, and the needs of the market. Successful cultivation requires a thorough familiarity with the necessary growing parameters, including soil type, light levels, water availability, and temperature.

Field culture, greenhouse cultivation, and hydroponics are all viable options. Greenhouse gardening allows for year-round output and is more controlled than field cultivation, which includes growing medicinal plants directly in the ground. Hydroponics is a way of growing plants without the use of soil.

Once the herbs have been cultivated, the next procedures include harvesting and processing. The effectiveness and quality of the medicinal chemicals in a plant depend on its being harvested at the ideal time and using the right methods. Herbs are usually preserved for storage and distribution by drying, grinding, and packaging after harvesting.

Interest in natural and alternative medicine has contributed to the growth of the global market for medicinal plants. Herbal treatments are popular due to their perceived therapeutic value, low risk of adverse effects, and historical relevance. However, it should be noted that rules and quality requirements exist to safeguard consumer safety in the production and marketing of medical herbs.

Chapter 1:
Growing Medicinal Herbs At Home

It's possible to reap several benefits from growing your own medicinal plants at home. You may control the environment in which the herbs grow, so increasing their potency as medicine. Here are some guidelines to help you get going:

1. Selected Herbs: Choose the therapeutic plants that you will cultivate. Chamomile, lavender, peppermint, echinacea, lemon balm, and sage are just some of the popular choices. Find out what each herb needs in terms of sunlight, soil type, water, and temperature by doing some research.
2. Pick a method of cultivation: Depending on the environment and area, herbs can be grown either indoors or outdoors. Hydroponics and other containers are great for indoor growing, while a proper garden bed or a separate herb garden are necessities for outdoor cultivation.
3. In order to foster growth, you must: Make sure the herbs get enough of light. Herbs require at least four to six hours of sunlight per day. Indoor growers need invest in grow lights to simulate natural sunlight. Make some organic-rich soil or potting mix that drains nicely. Care for the plant properly by keeping it at the right temperature and humidity.
4. Herbs can be grown from either seeds or young plants purchased from a nursery. If planting seeds, be sure to use the exact depth and distance recommended on the seed packet. Carefully place the transplants in the soil or containers you've already prepared.
5. Fertilizing and watering: Herbs like it when you don't drown them. Root rot is caused by overwatering, so be careful. Water the soil only when it has dried out little. To nourish your plants, try using compost or organic fertilizers. For best results, fertilize your herbs according to their individual instructions.
6. Care and upkeep, or pruning: Herbs can be kept from getting leggy with regular pinching or trimming. It's important to prune away any leaves that are unhealthy or have died. In the event that pest management is required, organic measures should be used.
7. When the herbs have reached their maximum potency, harvest them. When to utilize what portion of the herb will determine how long it takes (leaves, flowers, roots, etc.). Learn how to properly harvest each herb by doing some homework. Leave enough of the plant's foliage so that it can continue growing.
8. The collected herbs' therapeutic virtues are best preserved if they are dried and stored properly. They should be hung upside down in small groups in a cool, dark place with good air circulation. After the herbs have dried, put them in airtight containers and keep them in a dark, cool place.

Chapter 2: Collection And Storage Of Medicinal Herbs

To maintain their quality, effectiveness, and shelf life, medicinal plants must be collected and stored properly. Some rules to follow when amassing and preserving therapeutic plants:

Collection:

- ✓ Accurately identify the plant: Be absolutely sure you know what kind of plant you're going to be collecting. When in doubt, look to reliable plant identification resources or consult with experts.
- ✓ Pick your moment wisely: Consider the plant's growth stage, the weather, and the section of the plant that will be used to determine when to harvest the herb (leaves, flowers, roots, etc.).
- ✓ Methods of harvesting: To prevent unnecessary plant damage, always use clean, sharp equipment like pruning shears or knives. Leave enough of the plant unharvested so that it can thrive in the future.
- ✓ Avoid pollutant exposure: Herbs should be gathered from locations that are not subject to heavy traffic or the use of pesticides or herbicides. Choose a spot that is far from factories, busy streets, and farms where chemicals may be used.

To wash and dry:

- ✓ Clean the herbs: get rid of any dirt, bugs, or damaged pieces.
- ✓ Wash the herbs gently in clean water to remove any dust or dirt that may have settled on their surface, if necessary. In general, it's best to avoid washing herbs, as doing so may cause them to lose their therapeutic characteristics or to spoil.
- ✓ Methods of drying: It's possible to dry herbs using either low heat or the air. Traditionally, herbs would be tied in small bundles and hung upside down in a dry, well-ventilated area, out of direct sunlight, to dry via air drying. Following the manufacturer's instructions, dehydrators can also be used to hasten the drying process.
- ✓ Keep an eye on the drying: Verify on a regular basis that the herbs are drying uniformly and showing no signs of mold or spoilage.

Storage:

- ✓ Herbs should be kept in clean, dark, and airtight jars or glass containers away from light and moisture. Keep your herbs in glass or ceramic containers, as plastic and metal can degrade their flavor over time.
- ✓ Clearly label each jar with the name of the herb inside and the harvest or use-by date. This allows you to monitor the herbs' potency and freshness.
- ✓ Conditions for storing: Store the containers in a place that is cold, dry, and dark. Herbs lose quality when exposed to elements including heat, sunshine, and moisture.

- ✓ Herbs with a long shelf life are hard to come by. Herbs can keep their medicinal properties for up to two years if properly dried and kept. Look for changes in aroma, color, and texture to determine if the herbs need to be thrown out.

Chapter 3: Practical Examples Of Crops

1. Peppermint (Mentha x piperita): Peppermint is known for its soothing properties and can be used to relieve headaches, indigestion, and congestion. It's relatively easy to grow and can be propagated from cuttings or purchased as seedlings.
2. Chamomile (Matricaria chamomilla): Chamomile is often used to promote relaxation and alleviate anxiety. The flowers can be dried and used to make a calming tea. Chamomile is typically grown from seeds and prefers well-drained soil and full sun.
3. Echinacea (Echinacea purpurea): Echinacea is believed to boost the immune system and can be used to help prevent or reduce the severity of colds and flu. It requires well-drained soil and plenty of sunlight to grow successfully.
4. Lavender (Lavandula angustifolia): Lavender is well-known for its calming and soothing properties. The flowers can be used to make sachets, oils, or teas. Lavender prefers well-drained soil and full sun.
5. Lemon balm (Melissa officinalis): Lemon balm has a calming effect and can be used to relieve stress and improve sleep quality. It's a hardy herb that grows well in a variety of conditions, but it prefers partial shade and moist soil.
6. Calendula (Calendula officinalis): Calendula is known for its healing properties and can be used topically to soothe skin irritations and promote wound healing. It's relatively easy to grow and prefers full sun.
7. Sage (Salvia officinalis): Sage has antimicrobial properties and can be used as a natural remedy for sore throat or to aid digestion. It's a hardy perennial herb that requires well-drained soil and full sun.
8. Aloe vera (Aloe vera): Aloe vera has soothing and healing properties and is commonly used to treat burns, sunburns, and skin irritations. It's best grown in containers indoors or in warm climates outdoors.
9. Rosemary (Rosmarinus officinalis): Rosemary is known for its aromatic scent and is believed to improve memory and concentration. It requires well-drained soil and full sun to grow successfully.
10. It is common practice to treat mild to moderate depression using St. John's wort (Hypericum perforatum). It thrives in sunny locations with well-drained soil..

Conclusions

This comprehensive resource describes in depth the various medicinal plants, their healing properties, and the various applications for which they might be used.

Beginning with a comprehensive overview of medicinal herbs and natural medicine, this book lays the groundwork for appreciating the value of these treatments for overall health.

The extensive research, straightforward writing, and applicable advice in "Herbal Remedies Natural Medicine Bible" set it apart. This book is a must-have for anyone interested in learning more about the benefits of herbal remedies and other forms of natural medicine for enhancing health and well-being.

Finally, medicinal plants with therapeutic characteristics cannot be reliably supplied without the production of medicinal herbs. It entails many steps, such as picking the right plant species, learning about their needs as they grow, using the right methods to cultivate them, and then collecting and processing them in the right way. Cultivating medical herbs can contribute to the economy, plant biodiversity, and the passing down of useful knowledge at a time when demand for herbal remedies is on the rise.

Conclusion

In sum, "Herbal Remedies: Natural Medicine Bible" is an all-encompassing resource for learning about and benefiting from herbal medicines. It advocates a holistic approach to healing that centers on the use of plant-based remedies for a wide range of health issues.

All sorts of herbs and their healing powers are discussed throughout the book. The author describes in depth the history, chemical make-up, and therapeutic potential of each herb. As an added bonus, the book includes instructions for making and carefully administering herbal treatments.

The resource succeeds largely because of its focus on tailoring care to each individual. It takes into account the fact that different people have varying responses to herbs. The book urges readers to evaluate their personal health situations and seek the advice of medical experts when necessary.

In addition, "Herbal Remedies: Natural Medicine Bible" advocates for a well-rounded approach to healthcare by praising both conventional and natural treatments. It emphasizes the possible synergies between the two techniques, urging readers to incorporate herbal treatments into their entire healthcare practices.

Herbal cures have the potential to improve health in a number of ways, but it's important to remember that they're not risk-free, either. The book stresses the significance of understanding one's dosage, possible adverse effects, and drug interactions. It also stresses the significance of exercising restraint and accountability when utilizing herbal treatments.

Made in the USA
Middletown, DE
04 December 2023